SEX IS FUN!

SEX IS FUN!

Creative Ideas for Exciting Sex

KIDDER KAPER

Illustrated by Josh Lynch

AVERY

a member of Penguin Group (USA) Inc.

New York

AVERY
Published by the Penguin Group
Penguin Group (USA) Inc., 375 Hudson Street, New York, New York 10014, USA • Penguin Group (Canada), 90 Eglinton Avenue East, Suite 700, Toronto, Ontario M4P 2Y3, Canada (a division of Pearson Penguin Canada Inc.) • Penguin Books Ltd, 80 Strand, London WC2R 0RL, England • Penguin Ireland, 25 St Stephen's Green, Dublin 2, Ireland (a division of Penguin Books Ltd) • Penguin Group (Australia), 250 Camberwell Road, Camberwell, Victoria 3124, Australia (a division of Pearson Australia Group Pty Ltd) • Penguin Books India Pvt Ltd, 11 Community Centre, Panchsheel Park, New Delhi–110 017, India • Penguin Group (NZ), 67 Apollo Drive, Rosedale, North Shore 0632, New Zealand (a division of Pearson New Zealand Ltd) • Penguin Books (South Africa) (Pty) Ltd, 24 Sturdee Avenue, Rosebank, Johannesburg 2196, South Africa

Penguin Books Ltd, Registered Offices: 80 Strand, London WC2R 0RL, England

Illustrations by Josh Lynch

Published simultaneously in Canada

ISBN 978-1-58333-392-1

147905709

To my wife, who has been my greatest supporter and critic.
Thanks for helping me keep it fun.

Contents

FOREWORD & FOREWARNED

This book is for all of you who are looking for creative ways to spice up your sex lives. If you are reading this, we assume that you believe that sex is fun. Therefore, we're not going to spend a chapter wasting your time or our ink trying to convince you of the importance of being creative in the bedroom. If you need convincing, we suggest you look elsewhere. We also won't be passing judgment on sexual acts between consenting adults. Frankly, we don't care who you are or what you are into. We don't care if you are straight, gay, bi, transsexual, female, male or have both sets of genitals. We are publishing this book for people who think that getting it on is a great way to spend their time. Therefore, we've designed the book for everyone who likes getting it on. If this means that we draw a chapter featuring women with women, men with men or, God forbid, a straight couple, just try to find a way to adapt the chapter to fit you and your partner(s).

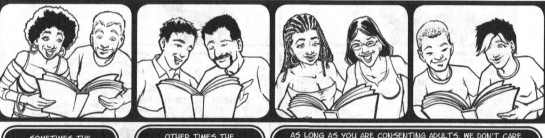

SOMETIMES THE SCENARIO WILL FEATURE A HETEROSEXUAL COUPLE.

OTHER TIMES THE SCENARIO MAY FEATURE A HOMOSEXUAL COUPLE.

AS LONG AS YOU ARE CONSENTING ADULTS, WE DON'T CARE WHO YOU ARE OR WHAT YOU ARE INTO, SO PLEASE DON'T GET TOO CONCERNED ABOUT THE SEXUAL PREFERENCE OR GENDER IDENTITY OF OUR CARTOONS.

Of course, we want you to be safe, so we've created a book of activities that can be practiced safely, sanely and consensually. This doesn't mean that there aren't some ideas in this book that may be beyond your comfort level or ability. You've got to decide for yourself what you are interested in trying and if you can do so safely. This isn't a book dedicated to safer sex practices, either. All of the characters in this book are sterilized, fluid-bonded cartoons in closed polyamorous relationships. They have all been tested and found to be free of all cartoon-related diseases, so if you see a drawing where one or two forgot to put on a condom,

just remember that if you are not sterilized and in fluid-bonded, polyamorous relationships, you will need to incorporate safer sex practices.

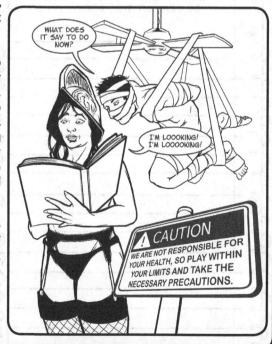

WHAT DOES IT SAY TO DO NOW?

I'M LOOOKING! I'M LOOOOKING!

⚠ CAUTION
WE ARE NOT RESPONSIBLE FOR YOUR HEALTH, SO PLAY WITHIN YOUR LIMITS AND TAKE THE NECESSARY PRECAUTIONS.

We want you to have fun with this book and don't want you to feel like we are just rehashing old ideas. Therefore, we have fully illustrated complete scenarios that leave little to the imagination. This doesn't mean that you can't use your own imagination to take the ideas further or that you have to follow our script to the letter. We encourage you to use these ideas as starting points and then mix and match to your own tastes. Not every scenario in this book is going to inspire all readers, but we do believe we've put together a very well-rounded book that will take you and your partner(s) into new and exciting territory.

This new territory may be exciting, but it can also be intimidating. Please keep this in mind when introducing new forms of sex play to your partner(s). Having a good conversation about what you want to try and reading this book together can help a timid partner feel more comfortable. Make sure to follow your common sense and foster good communication with your partner(s) about any sexual activities you choose to try. Don't forget to have fun, because sex is fun!

ABOUT THE INTERACTIVE PAGES

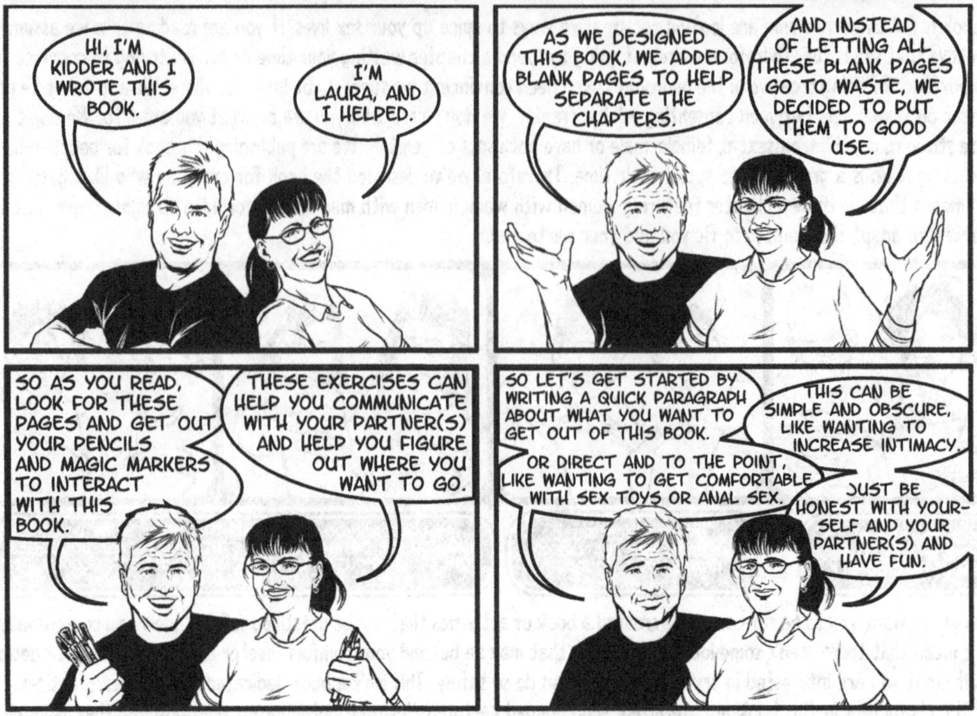

HI, I'M KIDDER AND I WROTE THIS BOOK.
I'M LAURA, AND I HELPED.
AS WE DESIGNED THIS BOOK, WE ADDED BLANK PAGES TO HELP SEPARATE THE CHAPTERS.
AND INSTEAD OF LETTING ALL THESE BLANK PAGES GO TO WASTE, WE DECIDED TO PUT THEM TO GOOD USE.
SO AS YOU READ, LOOK FOR THESE PAGES AND GET OUT YOUR PENCILS AND MAGIC MARKERS TO INTERACT WITH THIS BOOK.
THESE EXERCISES CAN HELP YOU COMMUNICATE WITH YOUR PARTNER(S) AND HELP YOU FIGURE OUT WHERE YOU WANT TO GO.
SO LET'S GET STARTED BY WRITING A QUICK PARAGRAPH ABOUT WHAT YOU WANT TO GET OUT OF THIS BOOK.
THIS CAN BE SIMPLE AND OBSCURE, LIKE WANTING TO INCREASE INTIMACY.
OR DIRECT AND TO THE POINT, LIKE WANTING TO GET COMFORTABLE WITH SEX TOYS OR ANAL SEX.
JUST BE HONEST WITH YOURSELF AND YOUR PARTNER(S) AND HAVE FUN.

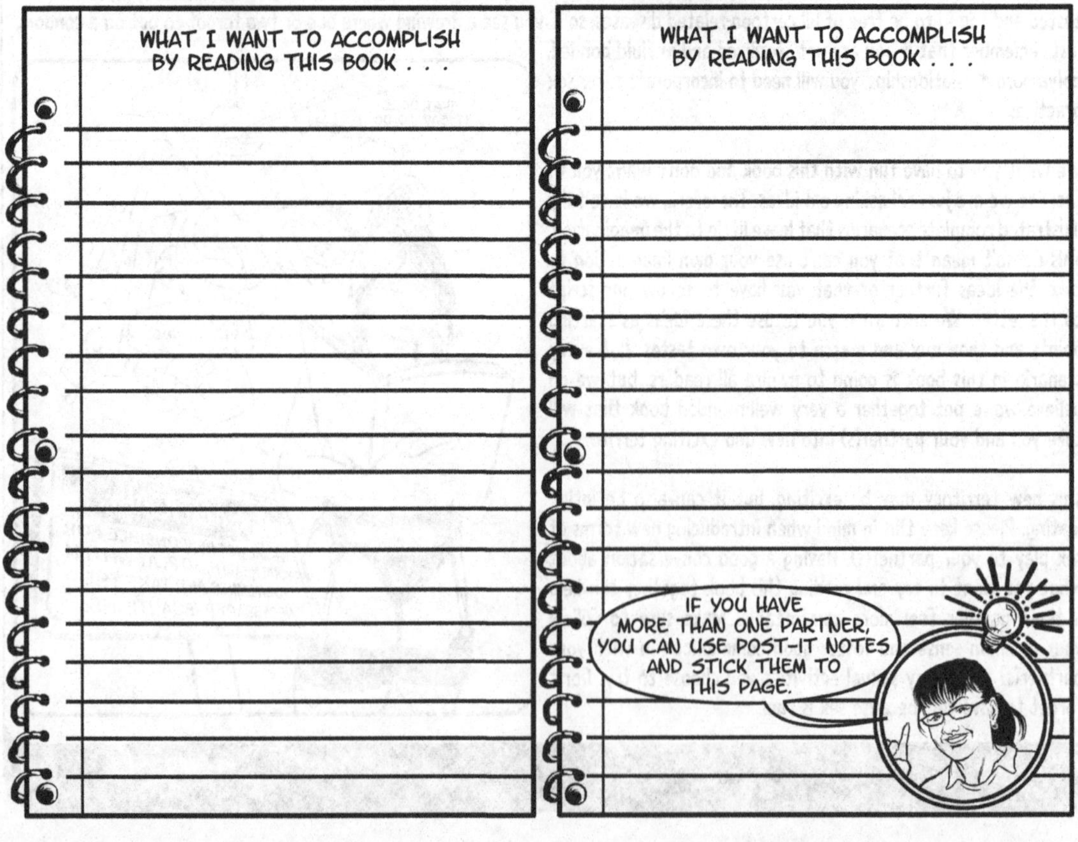

WHAT I WANT TO ACCOMPLISH BY READING THIS BOOK . . .
WHAT I WANT TO ACCOMPLISH BY READING THIS BOOK . . .
IF YOU HAVE MORE THAN ONE PARTNER, YOU CAN USE POST-IT NOTES AND STICK THEM TO THIS PAGE.

HOW TO ENJOY SEX SAFELY AND RESPONSIBLY

PLAY SAFELY AND HAVE FUN

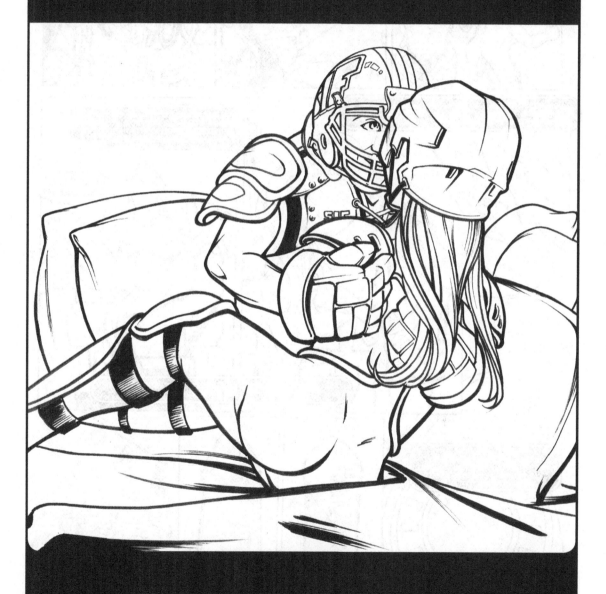

WE'LL SHOW YOU HOW . . .

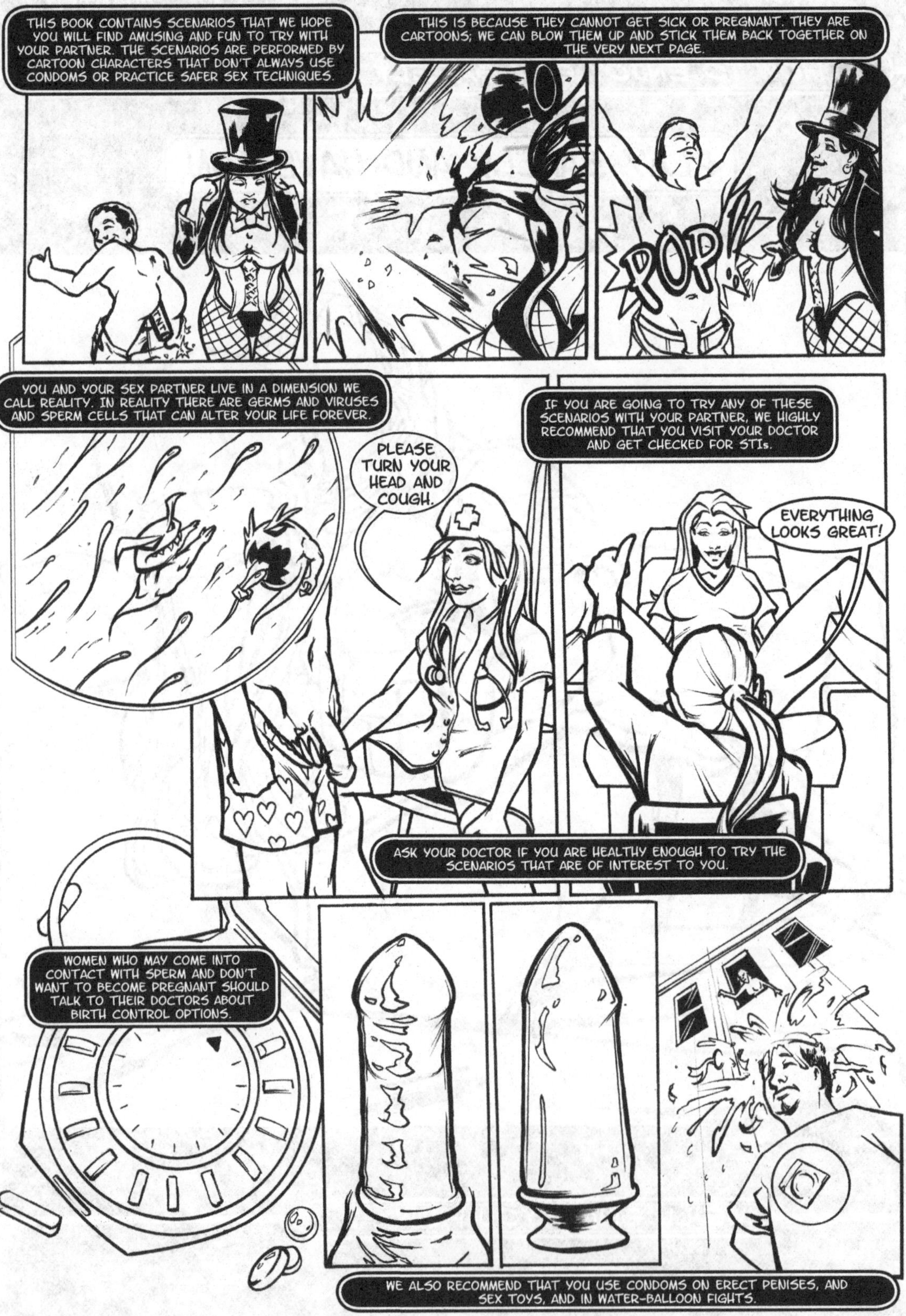
THIS BOOK CONTAINS SCENARIOS THAT WE HOPE YOU WILL FIND AMUSING AND FUN TO TRY WITH YOUR PARTNER. THE SCENARIOS ARE PERFORMED BY CARTOON CHARACTERS THAT DON'T ALWAYS USE CONDOMS OR PRACTICE SAFER SEX TECHNIQUES.
THIS IS BECAUSE THEY CANNOT GET SICK OR PREGNANT. THEY ARE CARTOONS; WE CAN BLOW THEM UP AND STICK THEM BACK TOGETHER ON THE VERY NEXT PAGE.
POP!!
YOU AND YOUR SEX PARTNER LIVE IN A DIMENSION WE CALL REALITY. IN REALITY THERE ARE GERMS AND VIRUSES AND SPERM CELLS THAT CAN ALTER YOUR LIFE FOREVER.
PLEASE TURN YOUR HEAD AND COUGH.
IF YOU ARE GOING TO TRY ANY OF THESE SCENARIOS WITH YOUR PARTNER, WE HIGHLY RECOMMEND THAT YOU VISIT YOUR DOCTOR AND GET CHECKED FOR STIs.
EVERYTHING LOOKS GREAT!
ASK YOUR DOCTOR IF YOU ARE HEALTHY ENOUGH TO TRY THE SCENARIOS THAT ARE OF INTEREST TO YOU.
WOMEN WHO MAY COME INTO CONTACT WITH SPERM AND DON'T WANT TO BECOME PREGNANT SHOULD TALK TO THEIR DOCTORS ABOUT BIRTH CONTROL OPTIONS.
WE ALSO RECOMMEND THAT YOU USE CONDOMS ON ERECT PENISES, AND SEX TOYS, AND IN WATER-BALLOON FIGHTS.

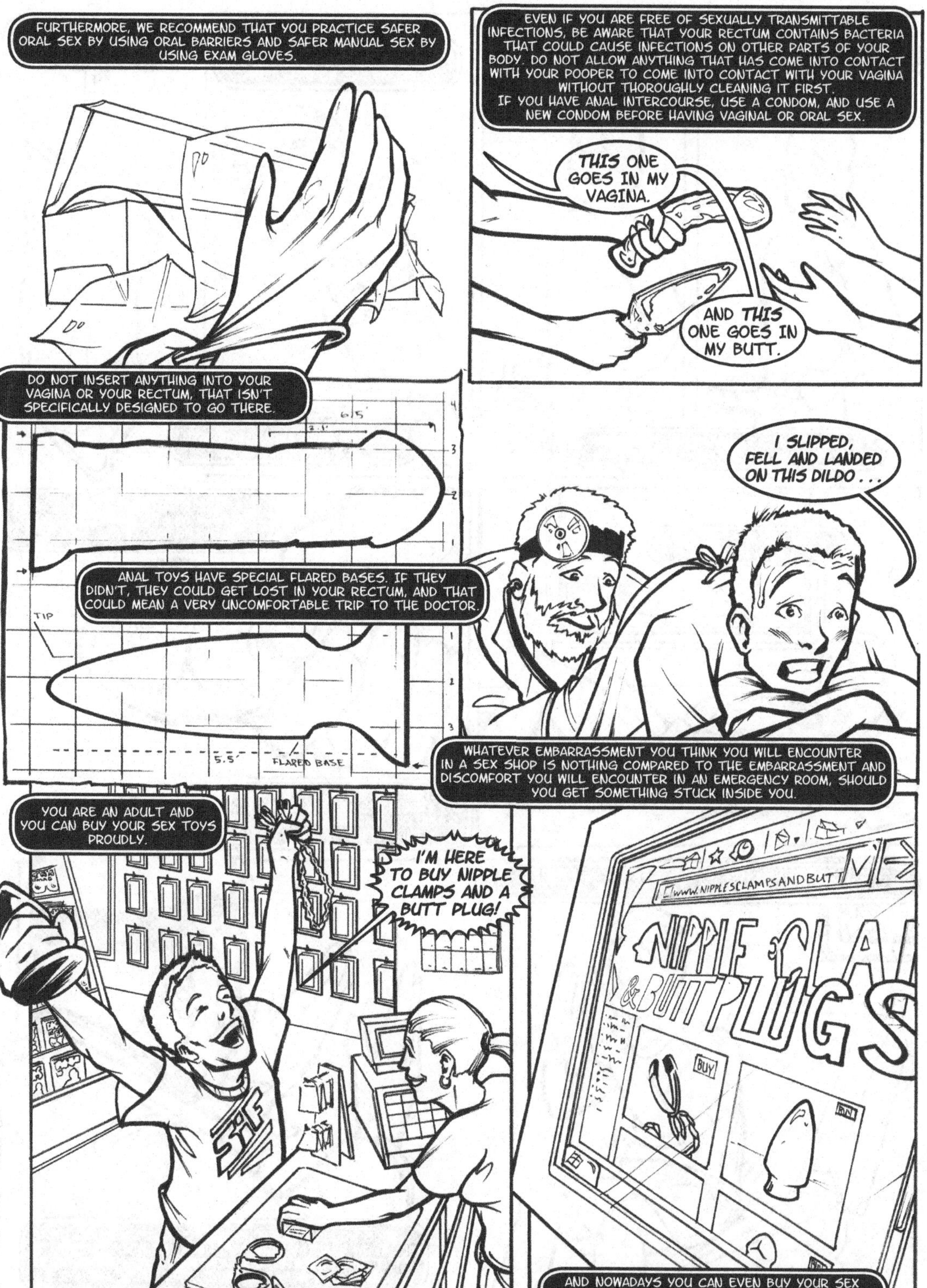
FURTHERMORE, WE RECOMMEND THAT YOU PRACTICE SAFER ORAL SEX BY USING ORAL BARRIERS AND SAFER MANUAL SEX BY USING EXAM GLOVES.
EVEN IF YOU ARE FREE OF SEXUALLY TRANSMITTABLE INFECTIONS, BE AWARE THAT YOUR RECTUM CONTAINS BACTERIA THAT COULD CAUSE INFECTIONS ON OTHER PARTS OF YOUR BODY. DO NOT ALLOW ANYTHING THAT HAS COME INTO CONTACT WITH YOUR POOPER TO COME INTO CONTACT WITH YOUR VAGINA WITHOUT THOROUGHLY CLEANING IT FIRST.
IF YOU HAVE ANAL INTERCOURSE, USE A CONDOM, AND USE A NEW CONDOM BEFORE HAVING VAGINAL OR ORAL SEX.
THIS ONE GOES IN MY VAGINA.
AND THIS ONE GOES IN MY BUTT.
DO NOT INSERT ANYTHING INTO YOUR VAGINA OR YOUR RECTUM, THAT ISN'T SPECIFICALLY DESIGNED TO GO THERE.
6.5
TIP
5.5
FLARED BASE
ANAL TOYS HAVE SPECIAL FLARED BASES. IF THEY DIDN'T, THEY COULD GET LOST IN YOUR RECTUM, AND THAT COULD MEAN A VERY UNCOMFORTABLE TRIP TO THE DOCTOR.
I SLIPPED, FELL AND LANDED ON THIS DILDO . . .
WHATEVER EMBARRASSMENT YOU THINK YOU WILL ENCOUNTER IN A SEX SHOP IS NOTHING COMPARED TO THE EMBARRASSMENT AND DISCOMFORT YOU WILL ENCOUNTER IN AN EMERGENCY ROOM, SHOULD YOU GET SOMETHING STUCK INSIDE YOU.
YOU ARE AN ADULT AND YOU CAN BUY YOUR SEX TOYS PROUDLY.
I'M HERE TO BUY NIPPLE CLAMPS AND A BUTT PLUG!
WWW.NIPPLESCLAMPSANDBUTT
& BUTT PLUGS
BUY
AND NOWADAYS YOU CAN EVEN BUY YOUR SEX TOYS ONLINE.

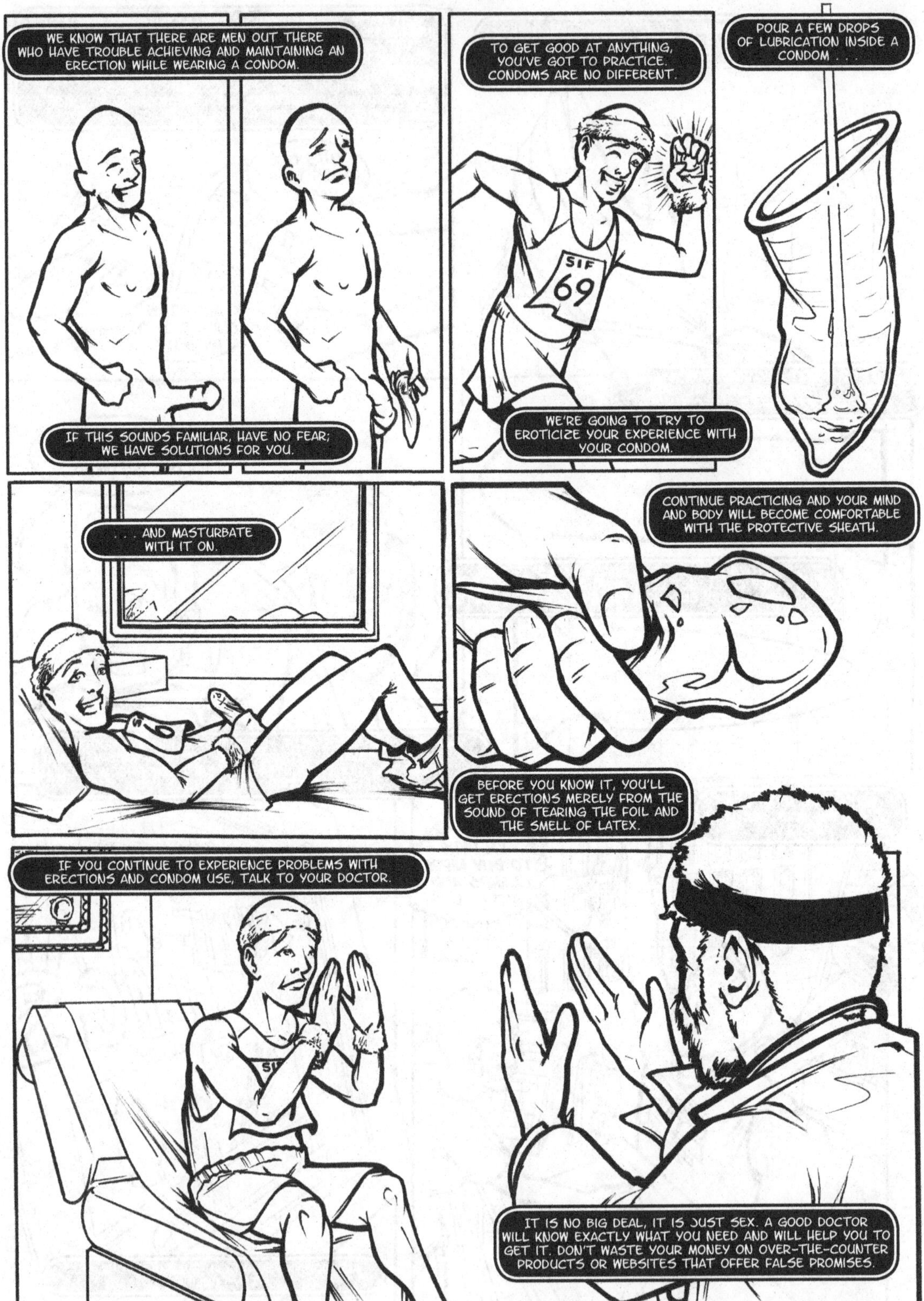
WE KNOW THAT THERE ARE MEN OUT THERE WHO HAVE TROUBLE ACHIEVING AND MAINTAINING AN ERECTION WHILE WEARING A CONDOM.
IF THIS SOUNDS FAMILIAR, HAVE NO FEAR; WE HAVE SOLUTIONS FOR YOU.
TO GET GOOD AT ANYTHING, YOU'VE GOT TO PRACTICE. CONDOMS ARE NO DIFFERENT.
SIF 69
WE'RE GOING TO TRY TO EROTICIZE YOUR EXPERIENCE WITH YOUR CONDOM.
POUR A FEW DROPS OF LUBRICATION INSIDE A CONDOM . . .
. . . AND MASTURBATE WITH IT ON.
CONTINUE PRACTICING AND YOUR MIND AND BODY WILL BECOME COMFORTABLE WITH THE PROTECTIVE SHEATH.
BEFORE YOU KNOW IT, YOU'LL GET ERECTIONS MERELY FROM THE SOUND OF TEARING THE FOIL AND THE SMELL OF LATEX.
IF YOU CONTINUE TO EXPERIENCE PROBLEMS WITH ERECTIONS AND CONDOM USE, TALK TO YOUR DOCTOR.
IT IS NO BIG DEAL, IT IS JUST SEX. A GOOD DOCTOR WILL KNOW EXACTLY WHAT YOU NEED AND WILL HELP YOU TO GET IT. DON'T WASTE YOUR MONEY ON OVER-THE-COUNTER PRODUCTS OR WEBSITES THAT OFFER FALSE PROMISES.

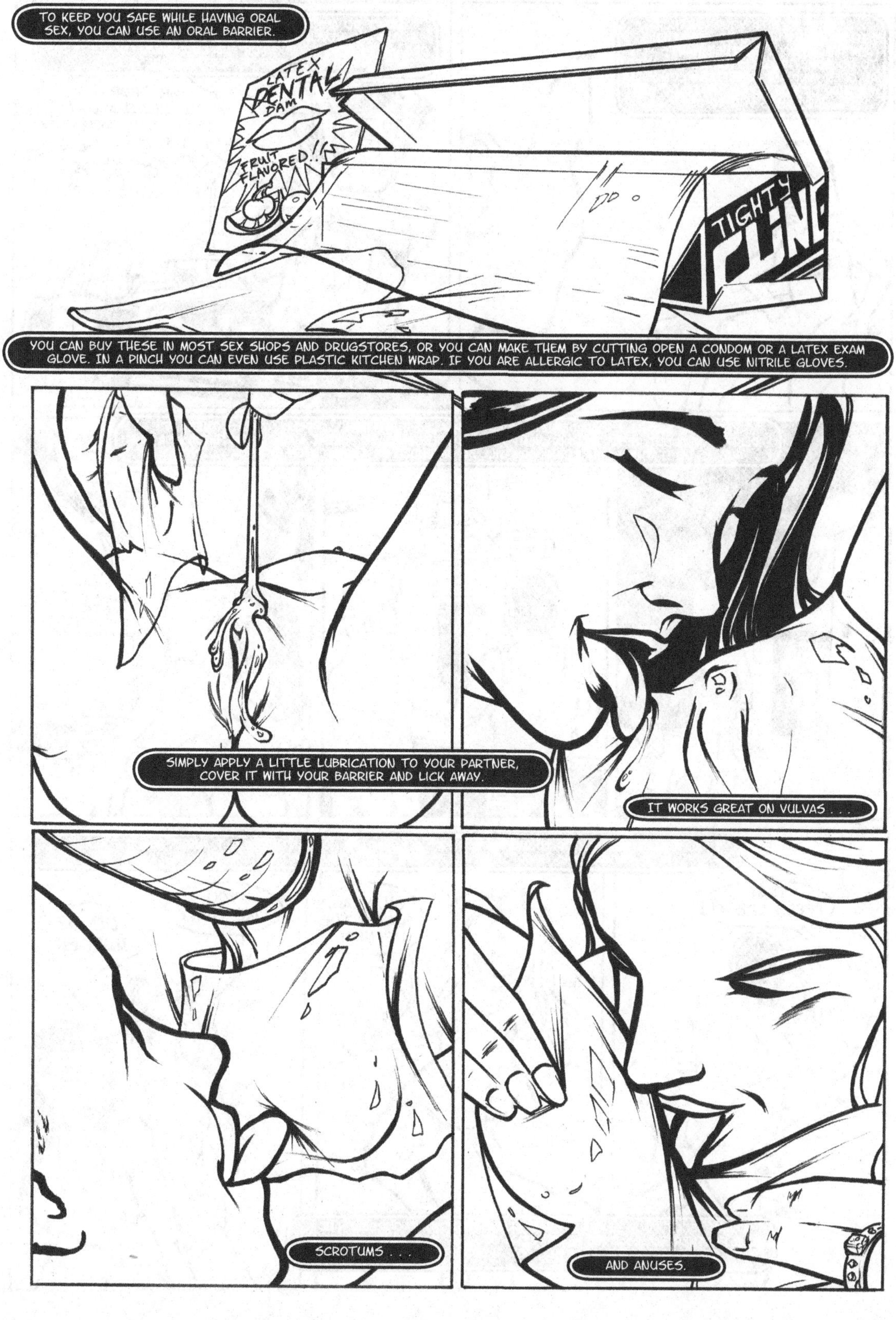
TO KEEP YOU SAFE WHILE HAVING ORAL SEX, YOU CAN USE AN ORAL BARRIER.
LATEX DENTAL DAM
FRUIT FLAVORED!!
TIGHTY
YOU CAN BUY THESE IN MOST SEX SHOPS AND DRUGSTORES, OR YOU CAN MAKE THEM BY CUTTING OPEN A CONDOM OR A LATEX EXAM GLOVE. IN A PINCH YOU CAN EVEN USE PLASTIC KITCHEN WRAP. IF YOU ARE ALLERGIC TO LATEX, YOU CAN USE NITRILE GLOVES.
SIMPLY APPLY A LITTLE LUBRICATION TO YOUR PARTNER, COVER IT WITH YOUR BARRIER AND LICK AWAY.
IT WORKS GREAT ON VULVAS . . .
SCROTUMS . . .
AND ANUSES.

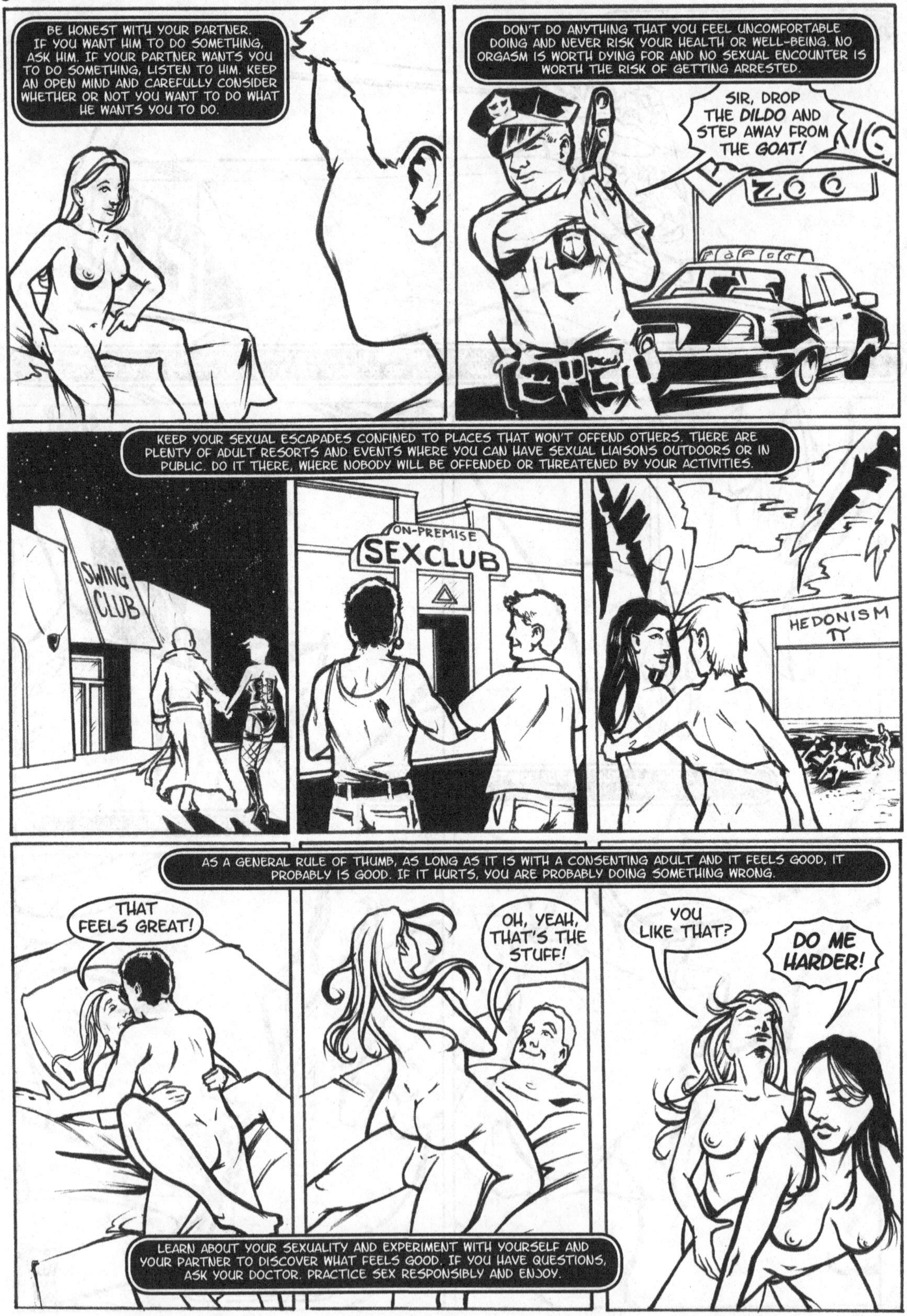
BE HONEST WITH YOUR PARTNER. IF YOU WANT HIM TO DO SOMETHING, ASK HIM. IF YOUR PARTNER WANTS YOU TO DO SOMETHING, LISTEN TO HIM. KEEP AN OPEN MIND AND CAREFULLY CONSIDER WHETHER OR NOT YOU WANT TO DO WHAT HE WANTS YOU TO DO.
DON'T DO ANYTHING THAT YOU FEEL UNCOMFORTABLE DOING AND NEVER RISK YOUR HEALTH OR WELL-BEING. NO ORGASM IS WORTH DYING FOR AND NO SEXUAL ENCOUNTER IS WORTH THE RISK OF GETTING ARRESTED.
SIR, DROP THE DILDO AND STEP AWAY FROM THE GOAT!
ZOO
KEEP YOUR SEXUAL ESCAPADES CONFINED TO PLACES THAT WON'T OFFEND OTHERS. THERE ARE PLENTY OF ADULT RESORTS AND EVENTS WHERE YOU CAN HAVE SEXUAL LIAISONS OUTDOORS OR IN PUBLIC. DO IT THERE, WHERE NOBODY WILL BE OFFENDED OR THREATENED BY YOUR ACTIVITIES.
SWING CLUB
ON-PREMISE
SEXCLUB
HEDONISM
AS A GENERAL RULE OF THUMB, AS LONG AS IT IS WITH A CONSENTING ADULT AND IT FEELS GOOD, IT PROBABLY IS GOOD. IF IT HURTS, YOU ARE PROBABLY DOING SOMETHING WRONG.
THAT FEELS GREAT!
OH, YEAH, THAT'S THE STUFF!
YOU LIKE THAT?
DO ME HARDER!
LEARN ABOUT YOUR SEXUALITY AND EXPERIMENT WITH YOURSELF AND YOUR PARTNER TO DISCOVER WHAT FEELS GOOD. IF YOU HAVE QUESTIONS, ASK YOUR DOCTOR. PRACTICE SEX RESPONSIBLY AND ENJOY.

CHAPTER 2

BEFORE THE FOREPLAY

MAKE SEX MORE ENJOYABLE FOR YOU AND YOUR PARTNER BY TAKING A LITTLE TIME TO PREPARE YOUR BODY FOR SEX PLAY.

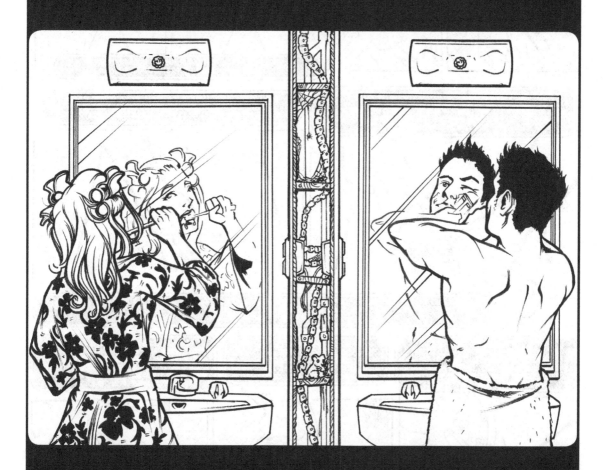

WHAT YOU'LL NEED . . . .

TOILETRIES

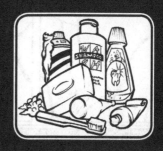

GOOD HYGIENE IS ESSENTIAL TO HAVING GREAT SEX. START WITH A SHOWER OR WARM BATH.

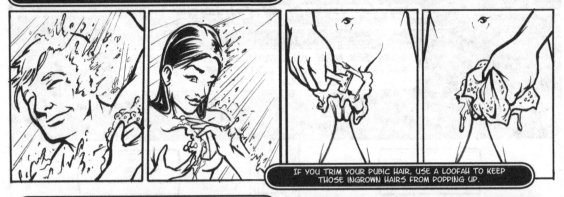

IF YOU TRIM YOUR PUBIC HAIR, USE A LOOFAH TO KEEP THOSE INGROWN HAIRS FROM POPPING UP.

YOU MIGHT WISH TO CONSIDER SHAVING THE FIRST QUARTER INCH OF PUBIC HAIR AROUND THE BASE OF YOUR PENIS. THIS CAN MAKE IT LOOK A LITTLE LONGER AND YOUR PARTNER MAY ENJOY THE WAY THE EXPOSED SKIN FEELS AGAINST THEM DURING ORAL SEX AND INTERCOURSE.

WASH YOUR PUBIC HAIR AND GIVE IT A GOOD TUG IN ALL DIRECTIONS TO GET RID OF ANY LOOSE HAIRS THAT MAY FALL OUT WHILE YOUR PARTNER IS PERFORMING ORAL SEX ON YOU.

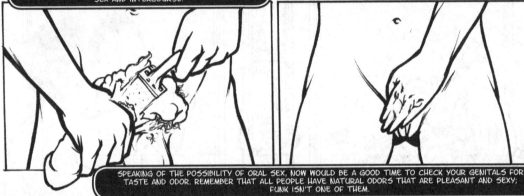

SPEAKING OF THE POSSIBILITY OF ORAL SEX, NOW WOULD BE A GOOD TIME TO CHECK YOUR GENITALS FOR TASTE AND ODOR. REMEMBER THAT ALL PEOPLE HAVE NATURAL ODORS THAT ARE PLEASANT AND SEXY; FUNK ISN'T ONE OF THEM.

TAKE A FINGER AND DRAW A CIRCLE AROUND YOUR SCROTUM. SMELL IT. IF IT SMELLS LIKE ANYTHING BUT AN IRISH SPRING, KEEP WASHING. IF YOU WANT YOUR PARTNER TO GO DOWN THERE, BE POLITE AND MAKE IT SMELL AND TASTE NICE.

YOU DON'T NEED TO FEEL SELF-CONSCIOUS ABOUT YOUR PARTNER GOING DOWN ON YOU. INSERT A FINGER INTO YOUR VAGINA. SMELL AND TASTE IT TO CHECK FOR ODOR.

WHILE YOU ARE AT IT, USE A LITTLE CONDITIONER IN YOUR PUBIC HAIR TO MAKE IT SOFT. CONSIDER SHAVING, OR EVEN PLUCKING THE HAIR OFF OF YOUR TESTICLES, AS IT WILL MAKE THEM MORE FUN TO TOUCH AND EVEN MORE FUN TO LICK.

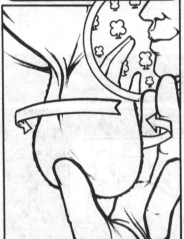 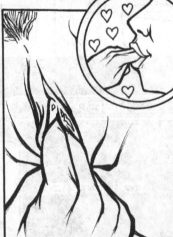 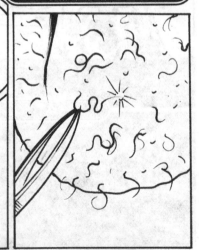

IF YOU SMELL SOMETHING THAT DOESN'T AGREE WITH YOU, WASH YOUR VAGINA WITH WATER. DON'T DOUCHE AND DON'T USE HAND SOAP! IF YOU FEEL THAT YOUR NATURAL ODOR HAS CHANGED, TALK TO YOUR DOCTOR.

NOW THAT YOU'VE WASHED EVERYWHERE, INCLUDING BEHIND YOUR EARS, YOU CAN CLEAN YOUR MOUTH.

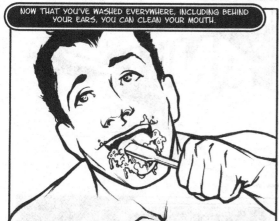

FLOSS YOUR TEETH AND SMELL THE FLOSS AFTER YOU PULL IT OUT FROM BETWEEN YOUR TEETH.

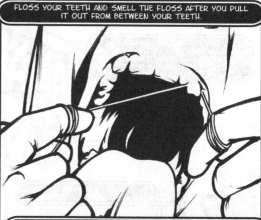

KISSING AND HEAVY BREATHING IS A BIG PART OF ENJOYABLE SEX. BRUSH YOUR TEETH AND YOUR TONGUE.

IF THE FLOSS SMELLS, SO DOES YOUR BREATH, AND THAT MEANS YOU NEED TO KEEP BRUSHING AND FLOSSING. AVOID USING MOUTHWASH THAT CONTAINS ALCOHOL, AS IT WILL DRY YOUR MOUTH, MAKING YOU LESS FUN TO KISS.

TRIM AND FILE YOUR FINGERNAILS. NOTHING KILLS THE MOOD LIKE CATCHING A HANGNAIL ON SENSITIVE SKIN.

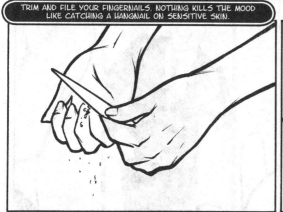

BEFORE YOU PUT ON YOUR SEXY OUTFIT, GIVE YOUR GENITALS A LITTLE WARM-UP.

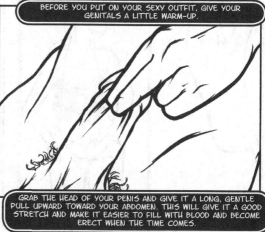

GRAB THE HEAD OF YOUR PENIS AND GIVE IT A LONG, GENTLE PULL UPWARD TOWARD YOUR ABDOMEN. THIS WILL GIVE IT A GOOD STRETCH AND MAKE IT EASIER TO FILL WITH BLOOD AND BECOME ERECT WHEN THE TIME COMES.

RUB YOUR LABIA AND CLITORIS; THIS WILL CAUSE YOUR GENITALS TO BECOME ENGORGED WITH BLOOD, MAKING THEM APPEAR FULL AND COLORFUL.

IF YOU HAVE A HARD TIME DELAYING YOUR ORGASM LONG ENOUGH TO PLEASE YOUR PARTNER, CONSIDER MASTURBATING A FEW HOURS BEFORE ENGAGING IN SEXUAL ACTIVITY.

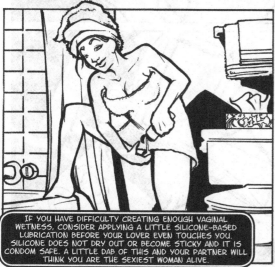

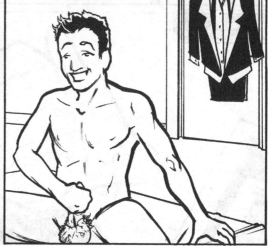

IF YOU HAVE DIFFICULTY CREATING ENOUGH VAGINAL WETNESS, CONSIDER APPLYING A LITTLE SILICONE-BASED LUBRICATION BEFORE YOUR LOVER EVEN TOUCHES YOU. SILICONE DOES NOT DRY OUT OR BECOME STICKY AND IT IS CONDOM SAFE. A LITTLE DAB OF THIS AND YOUR PARTNER WILL THINK YOU ARE THE SEXIEST WOMAN ALIVE.

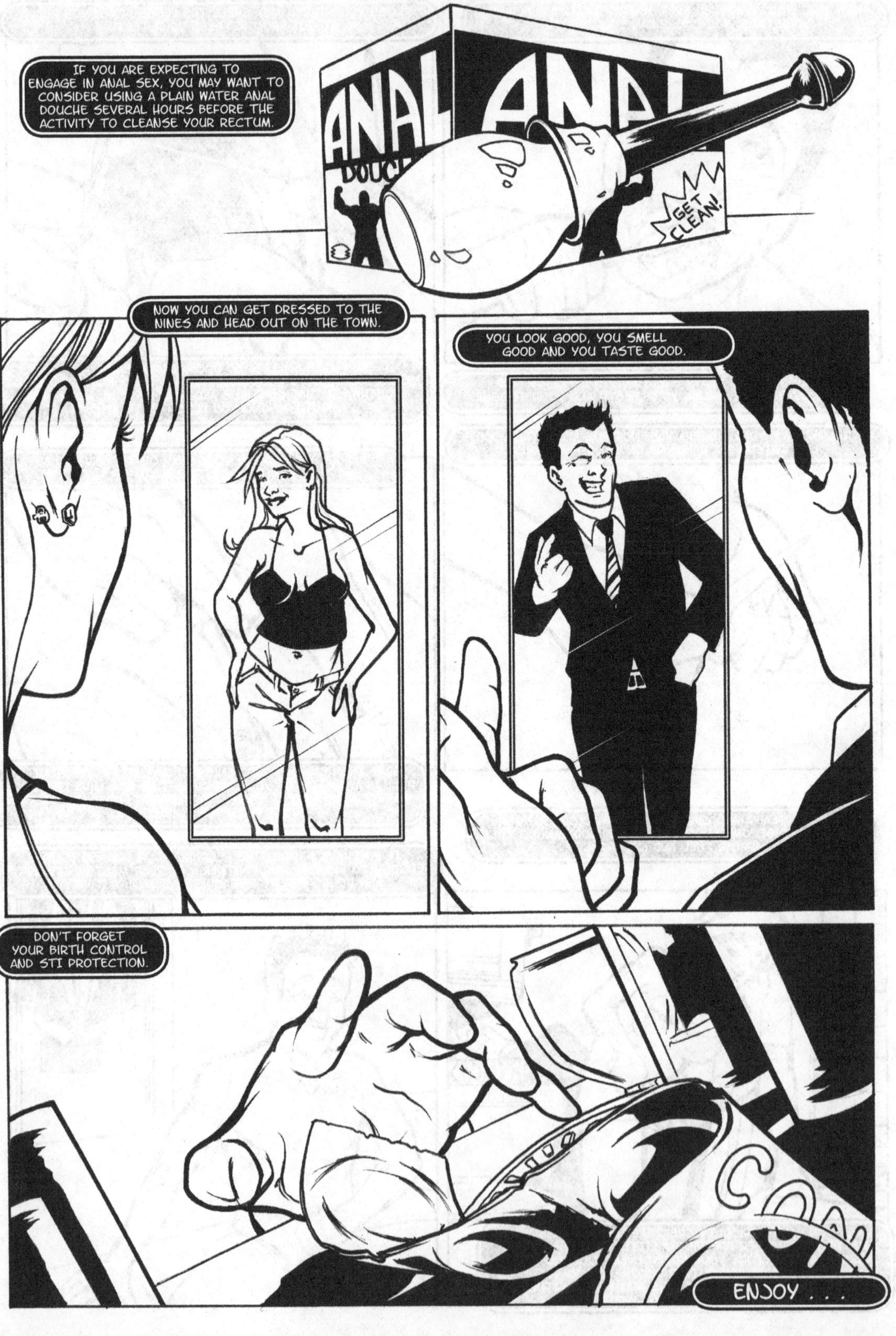
IF YOU ARE EXPECTING TO ENGAGE IN ANAL SEX, YOU MAY WANT TO CONSIDER USING A PLAIN WATER ANAL DOUCHE SEVERAL HOURS BEFORE THE ACTIVITY TO CLEANSE YOUR RECTUM.
ANAL ANAL
DOUCH
GET CLEAN!
NOW YOU CAN GET DRESSED TO THE NINES AND HEAD OUT ON THE TOWN.
YOU LOOK GOOD, YOU SMELL GOOD AND YOU TASTE GOOD.
DON'T FORGET YOUR BIRTH CONTROL AND STI PROTECTION.
ENJOY . . .

SEXUAL ANATOMY LESSON

TO BECOME A GREAT LOVER, IT IS NECESSARY TO UNDERSTAND ANATOMY AND SEXUAL FUNCTION.

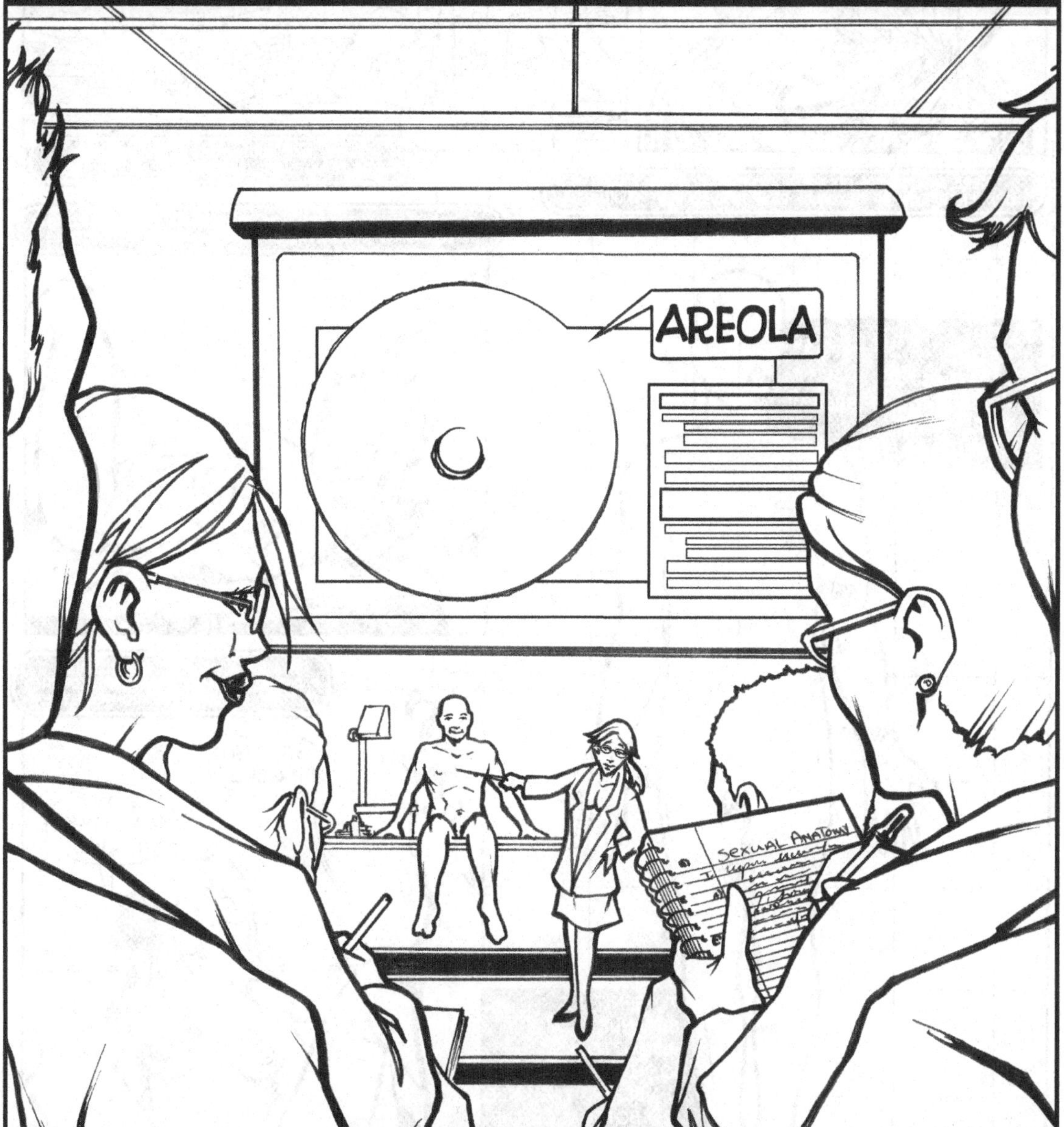
AREOLA
SEXUAL ANATOMY

WHAT YOU'LL NEED . . .

HANDHELD MIRROR

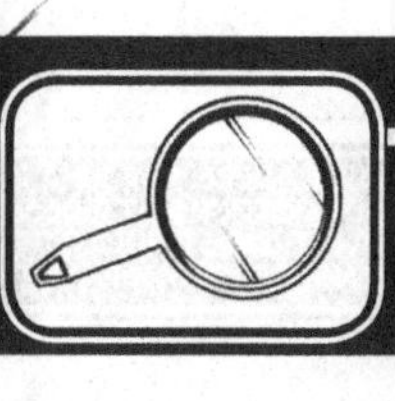

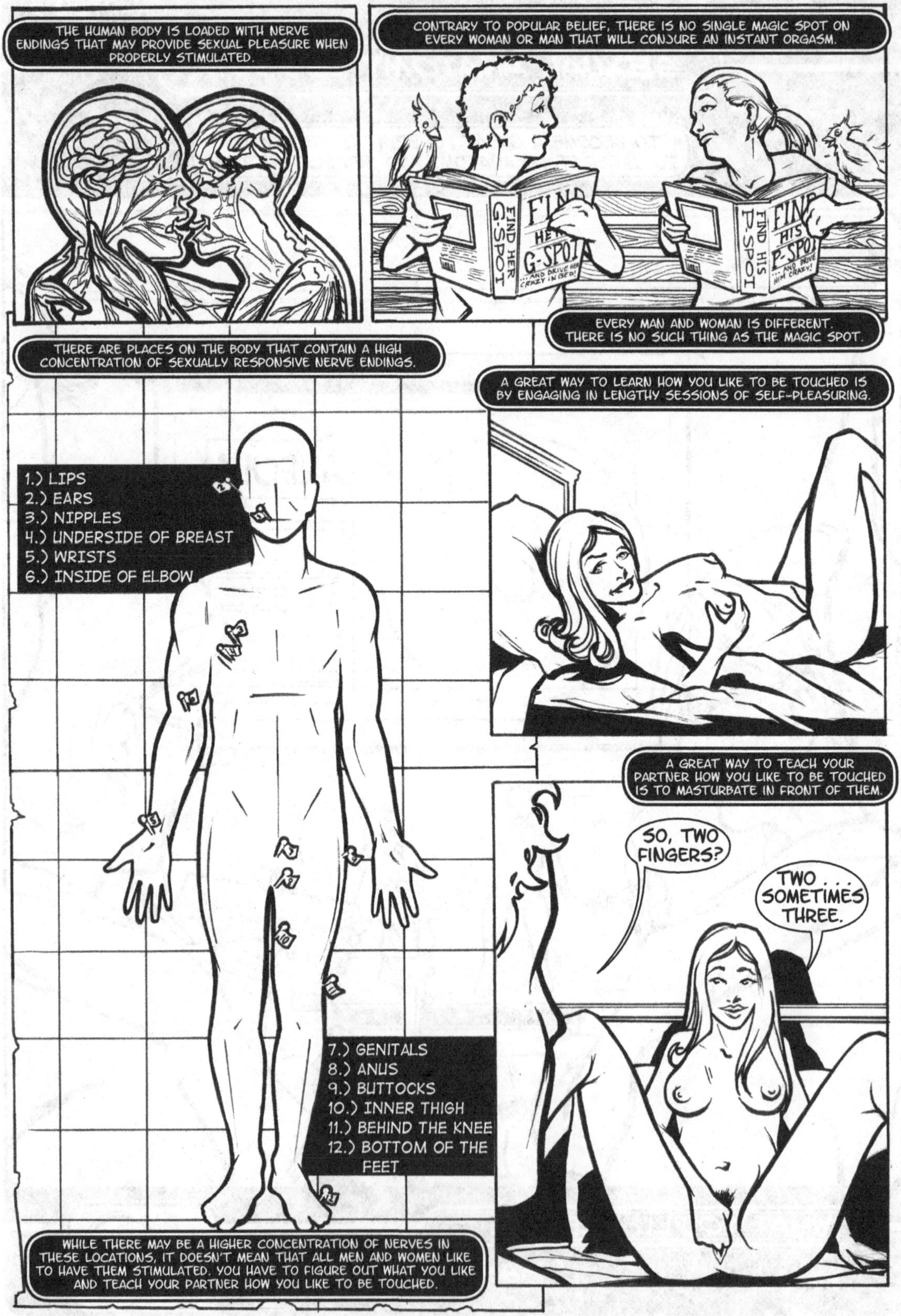
THE HUMAN BODY IS LOADED WITH NERVE ENDINGS THAT MAY PROVIDE SEXUAL PLEASURE WHEN PROPERLY STIMULATED.
CONTRARY TO POPULAR BELIEF, THERE IS NO SINGLE MAGIC SPOT ON EVERY WOMAN OR MAN THAT WILL CONJURE AN INSTANT ORGASM.
FIND HER G-SPOT
FIND HIS P-SPOT
EVERY MAN AND WOMAN IS DIFFERENT. THERE IS NO SUCH THING AS THE MAGIC SPOT.
THERE ARE PLACES ON THE BODY THAT CONTAIN A HIGH CONCENTRATION OF SEXUALLY RESPONSIVE NERVE ENDINGS.
1.) LIPS
2.) EARS
3.) NIPPLES
4.) UNDERSIDE OF BREAST
5.) WRISTS
6.) INSIDE OF ELBOW
7.) GENITALS
8.) ANUS
9.) BUTTOCKS
10.) INNER THIGH
11.) BEHIND THE KNEE
12.) BOTTOM OF THE FEET
WHILE THERE MAY BE A HIGHER CONCENTRATION OF NERVES IN THESE LOCATIONS, IT DOESN'T MEAN THAT ALL MEN AND WOMEN LIKE TO HAVE THEM STIMULATED. YOU HAVE TO FIGURE OUT WHAT YOU LIKE AND TEACH YOUR PARTNER HOW YOU LIKE TO BE TOUCHED.
A GREAT WAY TO LEARN HOW YOU LIKE TO BE TOUCHED IS BY ENGAGING IN LENGTHY SESSIONS OF SELF-PLEASURING.
A GREAT WAY TO TEACH YOUR PARTNER HOW YOU LIKE TO BE TOUCHED IS TO MASTURBATE IN FRONT OF THEM.
SO, TWO FINGERS?
TWO . . . SOMETIMES THREE.

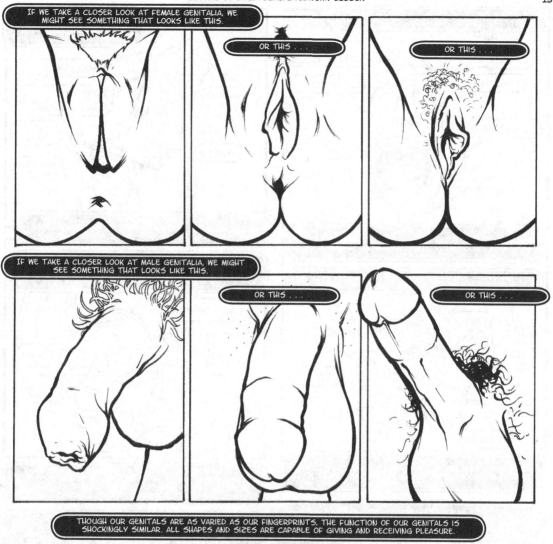

IF WE TAKE A CLOSER LOOK AT FEMALE GENITALIA, WE MIGHT SEE SOMETHING THAT LOOKS LIKE THIS.

OR THIS . . .

OR THIS . . .

IF WE TAKE A CLOSER LOOK AT MALE GENITALIA, WE MIGHT SEE SOMETHING THAT LOOKS LIKE THIS.

OR THIS . . .

OR THIS . . .

THOUGH OUR GENITALS ARE AS VARIED AS OUR FINGERPRINTS, THE FUNCTION OF OUR GENITALS IS SHOCKINGLY SIMILAR. ALL SHAPES AND SIZES ARE CAPABLE OF GIVING AND RECEIVING PLEASURE.

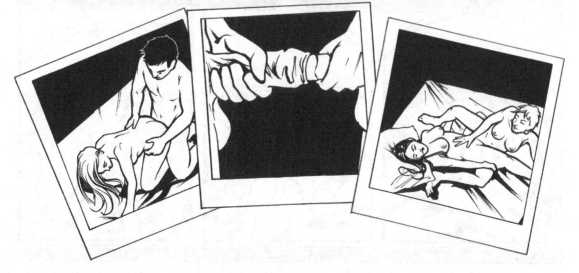

THE VISIBLE PARTS OF A WOMAN'S GENITALS ARE CALLED THE VULVA.

A MAN'S GENITALS CONSIST OF THE PENIS AND TESTICLES, SHOWN HERE INSIDE OF THE SCROTUM.

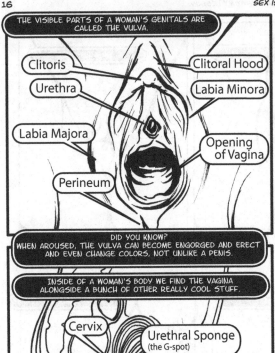

Clitoris
Urethra
Labia Majora
Perineum
Clitoral Hood
Labia Minora
Opening of Vagina

Frenulum
Shaft
Urethra
Glans Penis
Foreskin (may have been removed during circumcision)
Testicles (inside scrotum)
Scrotum

DID YOU KNOW? WHEN AROUSED, THE VULVA CAN BECOME ENGORGED AND ERECT AND EVEN CHANGE COLORS, NOT UNLIKE A PENIS.

DID YOU KNOW? WHEN AROUSED, THE PENIS CAN GROW TO MORE THAN TWICE ITS FLACCID SIZE, NOT UNLIKE A VAGINA.

INSIDE OF A WOMAN'S BODY WE FIND THE VAGINA ALONGSIDE A BUNCH OF OTHER REALLY COOL STUFF.

INSIDE OF A MAN WE SEE HOW THE PENIS AND TESTICLES ARE CONNECTED TO EACH OTHER. NOTICE HOW THE VAS DEFERENS PASSES THROUGH THE PROSTATE GLAND. WE'LL BE TALKING MORE ABOUT THIS LATER.

Cervix
Urethral Sponge (the G-spot)
Clitoris
Urethra
Rectum
Anus
Vagina

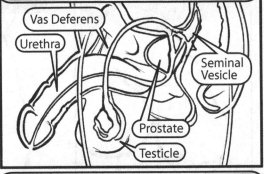

Vas Deferens
Urethra
Seminal Vesicle
Prostate
Testicle

DID YOU KNOW? MANY WOMEN CAN EJACULATE AND WHEN THEY DO SO IT LEAVES THEIR BODY THROUGH THEIR URETHRA IN MUCH THE SAME WAY A MAN EJACULATES.

DID YOU KNOW? THE AMOUNT OF FLUID PRODUCED DURING EJACULATION AVERAGES 1.5 ML TO 5 ML OF SEMEN. LESS THAN 1% OF THAT FLUID IS ACTUALLY SPERM. EACH TEASPOON OF EJACULATE CONTAINS ABOUT 6 CALORIES.

WHILE THE VAST MAJORITY OF WOMEN REACH CLIMAX THROUGH CLITORAL STIMULATION, IT IS NOT THE ONLY PART OF A WOMAN'S BODY THAT MAKES HER FEEL GOOD. MANY WOMEN CAN EXPERIENCE ORGASM FROM VAGINAL PENETRATION, ANAL STIMULATION, NIPPLE STIMULATION OR EVEN JUST THINKING ABOUT SEX.

MANY MEN ARE MOST SENSITIVE ON THE BOTTOM OF THEIR PENISES, JUST UNDERNEATH THE HEAD, BUT THEIR TESTICLES, PERINEUMS, ANUSES AND PROSTATE GLANDS MAY BE STIMULATED AND PRODUCE AS MUCH PLEASURE, IF NOT MORE.

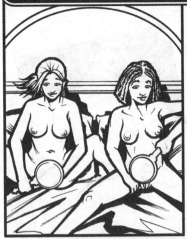 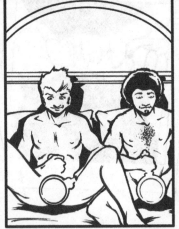 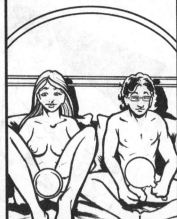

YOU MAY FIND IT MORE PLEASURABLE TO STIMULATE MULTIPLE PARTS OF YOUR BODY RATHER THAN FOCUSING ON ONLY ONE SPOT.

CHAPTER 4

SEX-TOY BUYER'S GUIDE

HOW TO FIND AND BUY THE BEST SEX ACCESSORIES

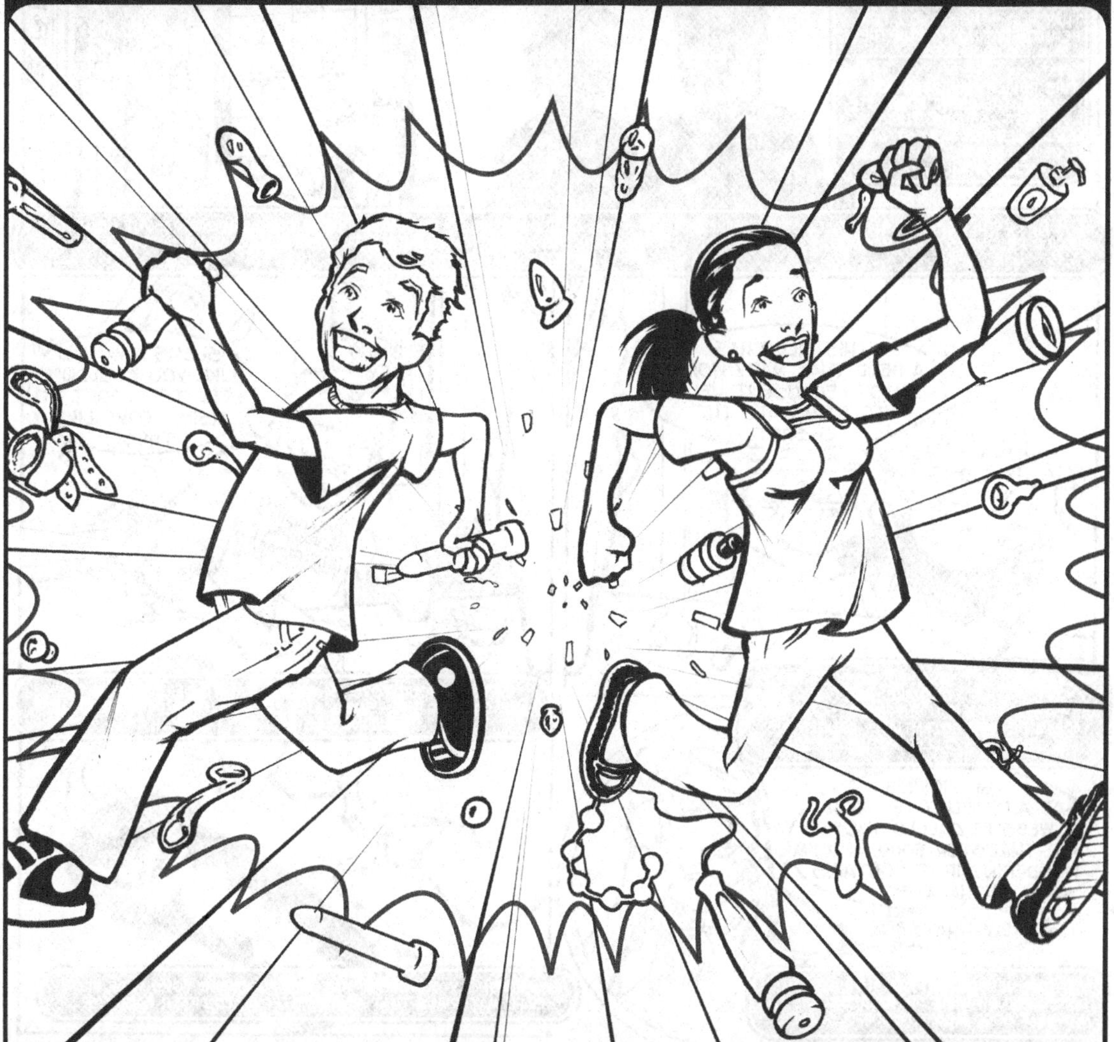

WHAT YOU'LL NEED . . .

MONEY

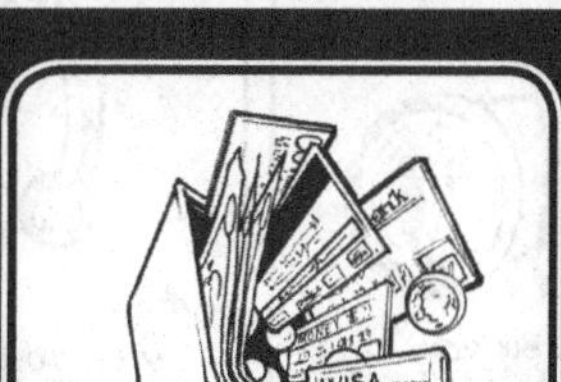
WISA

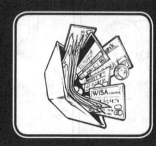

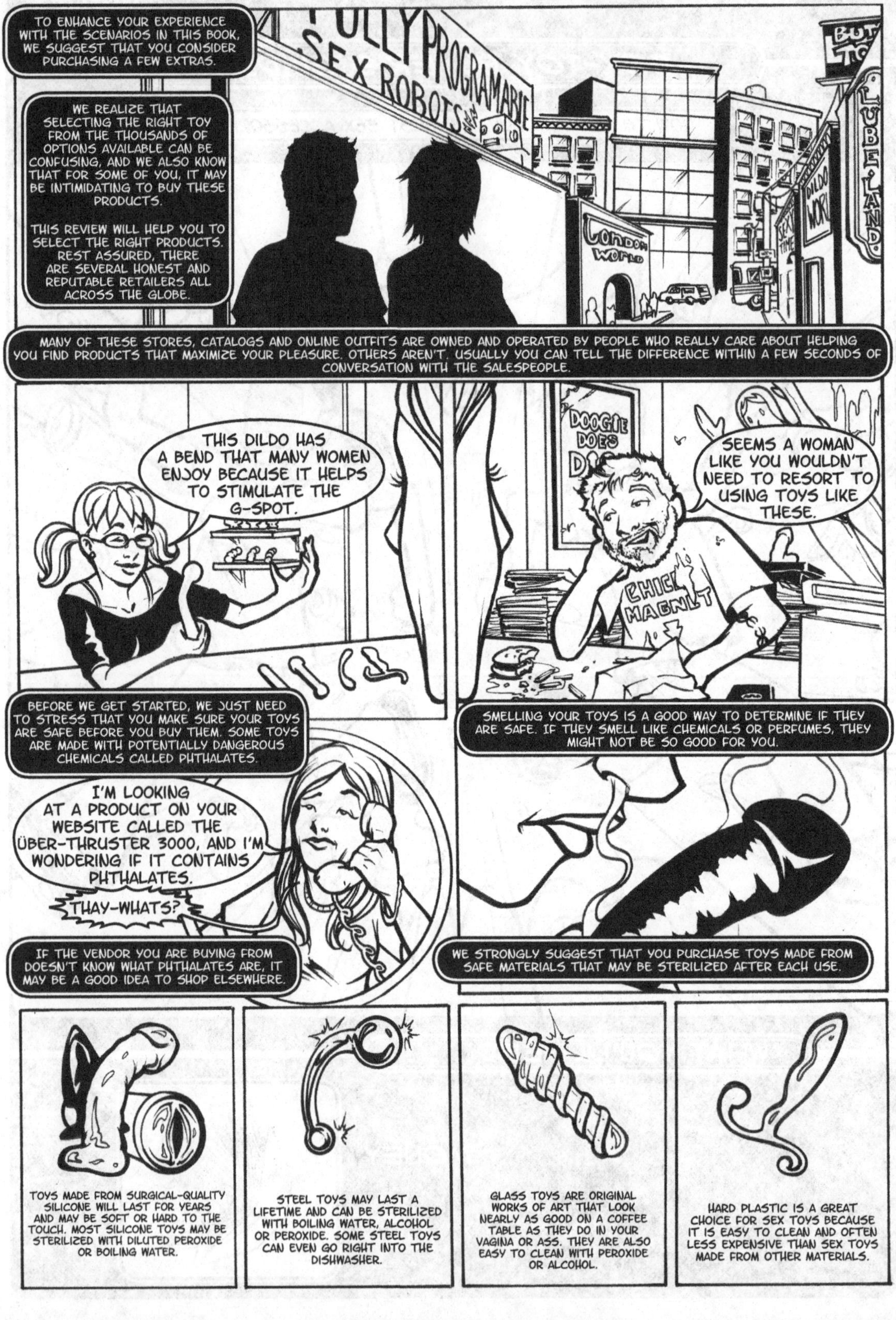

TO ENHANCE YOUR EXPERIENCE WITH THE SCENARIOS IN THIS BOOK, WE SUGGEST THAT YOU CONSIDER PURCHASING A FEW EXTRAS.
WE REALIZE THAT SELECTING THE RIGHT TOY FROM THE THOUSANDS OF OPTIONS AVAILABLE CAN BE CONFUSING, AND WE ALSO KNOW THAT FOR SOME OF YOU, IT MAY BE INTIMIDATING TO BUY THESE PRODUCTS.
THIS REVIEW WILL HELP YOU TO SELECT THE RIGHT PRODUCTS. REST ASSURED, THERE ARE SEVERAL HONEST AND REPUTABLE RETAILERS ALL ACROSS THE GLOBE.
SEX ROBOTS
CONDOM WORLD
LUBE LAND
MANY OF THESE STORES, CATALOGS AND ONLINE OUTFITS ARE OWNED AND OPERATED BY PEOPLE WHO REALLY CARE ABOUT HELPING YOU FIND PRODUCTS THAT MAXIMIZE YOUR PLEASURE. OTHERS AREN'T. USUALLY YOU CAN TELL THE DIFFERENCE WITHIN A FEW SECONDS OF CONVERSATION WITH THE SALESPEOPLE.
THIS DILDO HAS A BEND THAT MANY WOMEN ENJOY BECAUSE IT HELPS TO STIMULATE THE G-SPOT.
SEEMS A WOMAN LIKE YOU WOULDN'T NEED TO RESORT TO USING TOYS LIKE THESE.
BEFORE WE GET STARTED, WE JUST NEED TO STRESS THAT YOU MAKE SURE YOUR TOYS ARE SAFE BEFORE YOU BUY THEM. SOME TOYS ARE MADE WITH POTENTIALLY DANGEROUS CHEMICALS CALLED PHTHALATES.
I'M LOOKING AT A PRODUCT ON YOUR WEBSITE CALLED THE ÜBER-THRUSTER 3000, AND I'M WONDERING IF IT CONTAINS PHTHALATES.
THAY-WHATS?
IF THE VENDOR YOU ARE BUYING FROM DOESN'T KNOW WHAT PHTHALATES ARE, IT MAY BE A GOOD IDEA TO SHOP ELSEWHERE.
SMELLING YOUR TOYS IS A GOOD WAY TO DETERMINE IF THEY ARE SAFE. IF THEY SMELL LIKE CHEMICALS OR PERFUMES, THEY MIGHT NOT BE SO GOOD FOR YOU.
WE STRONGLY SUGGEST THAT YOU PURCHASE TOYS MADE FROM SAFE MATERIALS THAT MAY BE STERILIZED AFTER EACH USE.
TOYS MADE FROM SURGICAL-QUALITY SILICONE WILL LAST FOR YEARS AND MAY BE SOFT OR HARD TO THE TOUCH. MOST SILICONE TOYS MAY BE STERILIZED WITH DILUTED PEROXIDE OR BOILING WATER.
STEEL TOYS MAY LAST A LIFETIME AND CAN BE STERILIZED WITH BOILING WATER, ALCOHOL OR PEROXIDE. SOME STEEL TOYS CAN EVEN GO RIGHT INTO THE DISHWASHER.
GLASS TOYS ARE ORIGINAL WORKS OF ART THAT LOOK NEARLY AS GOOD ON A COFFEE TABLE AS THEY DO IN YOUR VAGINA OR ASS. THEY ARE ALSO EASY TO CLEAN WITH PEROXIDE OR ALCOHOL.
HARD PLASTIC IS A GREAT CHOICE FOR SEX TOYS BECAUSE IT IS EASY TO CLEAN AND OFTEN LESS EXPENSIVE THAN SEX TOYS MADE FROM OTHER MATERIALS.

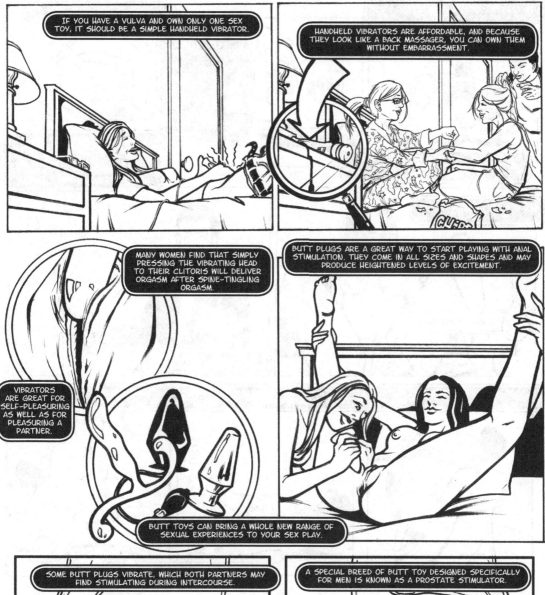

IF YOU HAVE A VULVA AND OWN ONLY ONE SEX TOY, IT SHOULD BE A SIMPLE HANDHELD VIBRATOR.

HANDHELD VIBRATORS ARE AFFORDABLE, AND BECAUSE THEY LOOK LIKE A BACK MASSAGER, YOU CAN OWN THEM WITHOUT EMBARRASSMENT.

MANY WOMEN FIND THAT SIMPLY PRESSING THE VIBRATING HEAD TO THEIR CLITORIS WILL DELIVER ORGASM AFTER SPINE-TINGLING ORGASM.

BUTT PLUGS ARE A GREAT WAY TO START PLAYING WITH ANAL STIMULATION. THEY COME IN ALL SIZES AND SHAPES AND MAY PRODUCE HEIGHTENED LEVELS OF EXCITEMENT.

VIBRATORS ARE GREAT FOR SELF-PLEASURING AS WELL AS FOR PLEASURING A PARTNER.

BUTT TOYS CAN BRING A WHOLE NEW RANGE OF SEXUAL EXPERIENCES TO YOUR SEX PLAY.

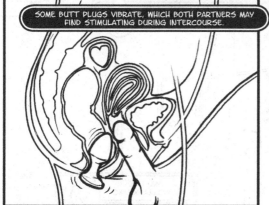

SOME BUTT PLUGS VIBRATE, WHICH BOTH PARTNERS MAY FIND STIMULATING DURING INTERCOURSE.

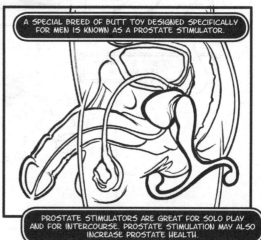

A SPECIAL BREED OF BUTT TOY DESIGNED SPECIFICALLY FOR MEN IS KNOWN AS A PROSTATE STIMULATOR.

PROSTATE STIMULATORS ARE GREAT FOR SOLO PLAY AND FOR INTERCOURSE. PROSTATE STIMULATION MAY ALSO INCREASE PROSTATE HEALTH.

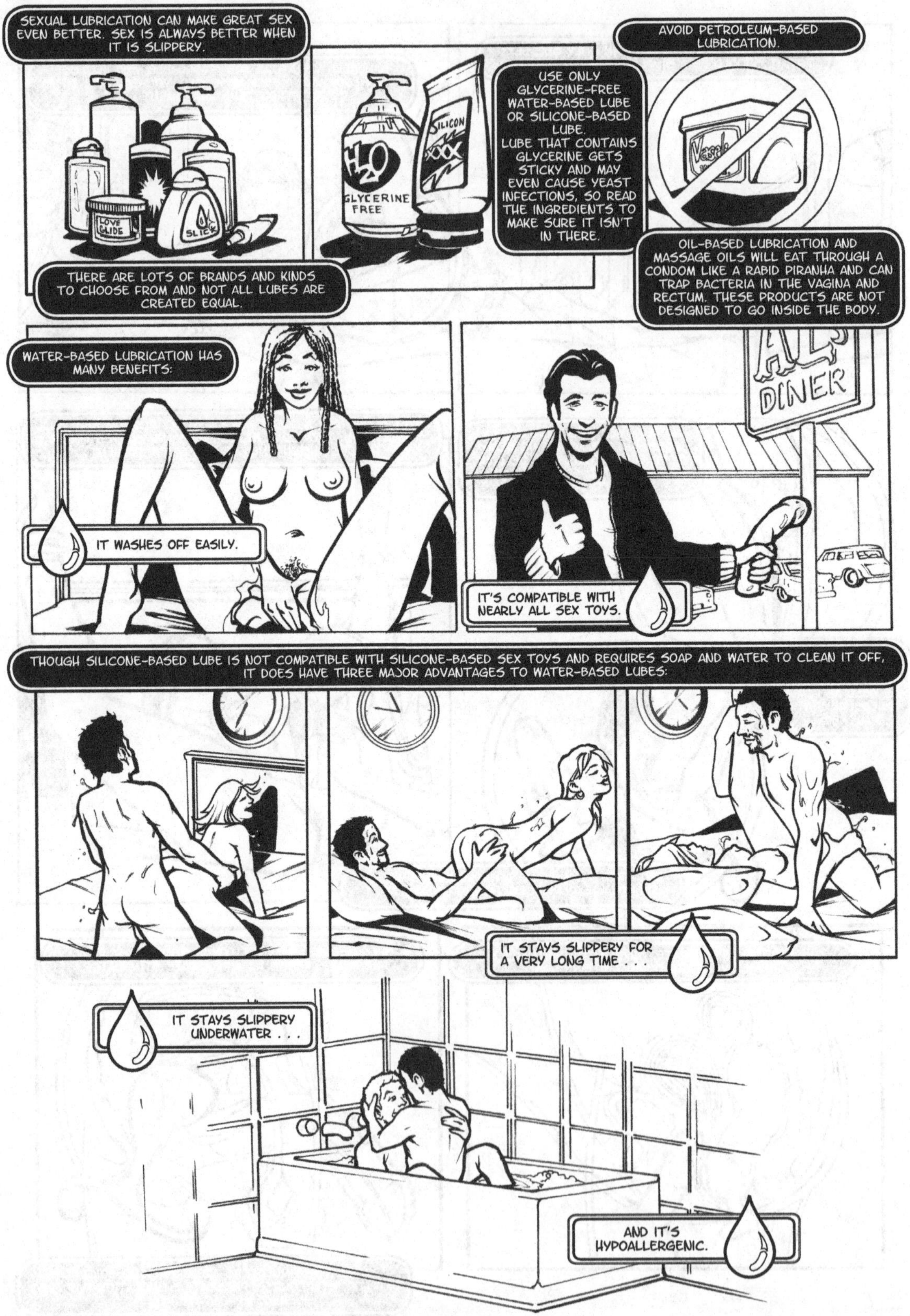

SEXUAL LUBRICATION CAN MAKE GREAT SEX EVEN BETTER. SEX IS ALWAYS BETTER WHEN IT IS SLIPPERY.
LOVE GLIDE
SLICK
THERE ARE LOTS OF BRANDS AND KINDS TO CHOOSE FROM AND NOT ALL LUBES ARE CREATED EQUAL.
GLYCERINE FREE
SILICON
XXX
USE ONLY GLYCERINE-FREE WATER-BASED LUBE OR SILICONE-BASED LUBE. LUBE THAT CONTAINS GLYCERINE GETS STICKY AND MAY EVEN CAUSE YEAST INFECTIONS, SO READ THE INGREDIENTS TO MAKE SURE IT ISN'T IN THERE.
AVOID PETROLEUM-BASED LUBRICATION.
OIL-BASED LUBRICATION AND MASSAGE OILS WILL EAT THROUGH A CONDOM LIKE A RABID PIRANHA AND CAN TRAP BACTERIA IN THE VAGINA AND RECTUM. THESE PRODUCTS ARE NOT DESIGNED TO GO INSIDE THE BODY.
WATER-BASED LUBRICATION HAS MANY BENEFITS:
IT WASHES OFF EASILY.
DINER
IT'S COMPATIBLE WITH NEARLY ALL SEX TOYS.
THOUGH SILICONE-BASED LUBE IS NOT COMPATIBLE WITH SILICONE-BASED SEX TOYS AND REQUIRES SOAP AND WATER TO CLEAN IT OFF, IT DOES HAVE THREE MAJOR ADVANTAGES TO WATER-BASED LUBES:
IT STAYS SLIPPERY FOR A VERY LONG TIME . . .
IT STAYS SLIPPERY UNDERWATER . . .
AND IT'S HYPOALLERGENIC.

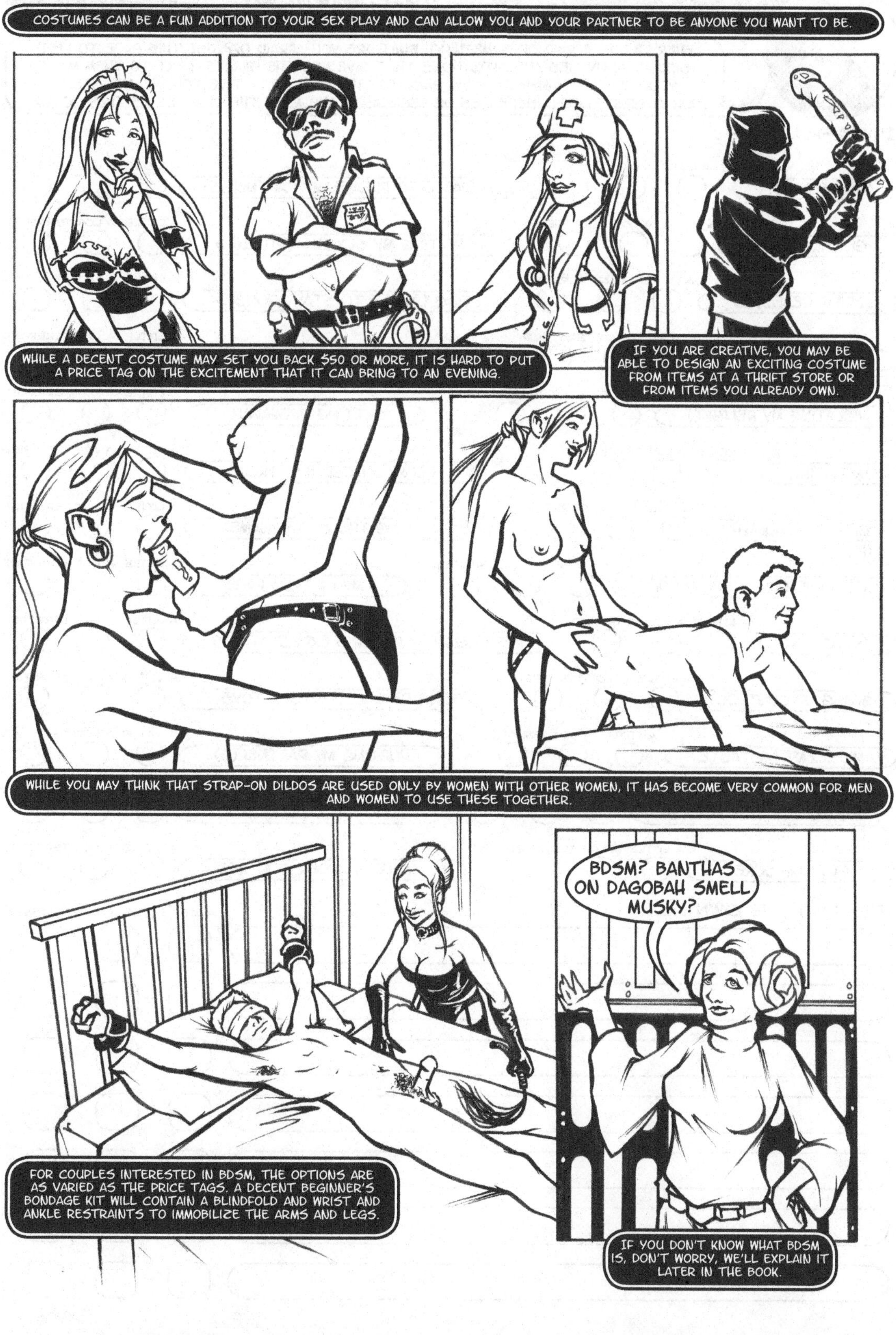
COSTUMES CAN BE A FUN ADDITION TO YOUR SEX PLAY AND CAN ALLOW YOU AND YOUR PARTNER TO BE ANYONE YOU WANT TO BE.
WHILE A DECENT COSTUME MAY SET YOU BACK $50 OR MORE, IT IS HARD TO PUT A PRICE TAG ON THE EXCITEMENT THAT IT CAN BRING TO AN EVENING.
IF YOU ARE CREATIVE, YOU MAY BE ABLE TO DESIGN AN EXCITING COSTUME FROM ITEMS AT A THRIFT STORE OR FROM ITEMS YOU ALREADY OWN.
WHILE YOU MAY THINK THAT STRAP-ON DILDOS ARE USED ONLY BY WOMEN WITH OTHER WOMEN, IT HAS BECOME VERY COMMON FOR MEN AND WOMEN TO USE THESE TOGETHER.
FOR COUPLES INTERESTED IN BDSM, THE OPTIONS ARE AS VARIED AS THE PRICE TAGS. A DECENT BEGINNER'S BONDAGE KIT WILL CONTAIN A BLINDFOLD AND WRIST AND ANKLE RESTRAINTS TO IMMOBILIZE THE ARMS AND LEGS.
BDSM? BANTHAS ON DAGOBAH SMELL MUSKY?
IF YOU DON'T KNOW WHAT BDSM IS, DON'T WORRY, WE'LL EXPLAIN IT LATER IN THE BOOK.

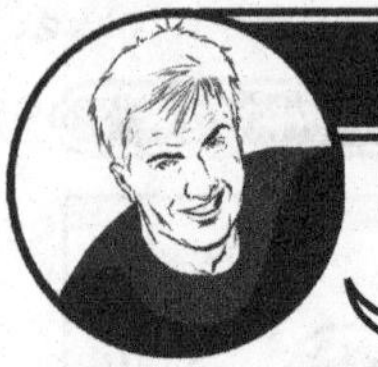

WHAT SCARES YOU?

EVERYONE IS AFRAID OF SOMETHING. WHAT ARE YOU AFRAID OF? USE THIS PAGE TO LIST SEXUAL ACTIVITIES AND SITUATIONS THAT GIVE YOU THE WILLIES. NEXT TO THEM MARK YOUR LEVEL OF ANXIETY. COME BACK TO THIS PAGE FROM TIME TO TIME AND SEE IF YOUR COMFORT LEVEL INCREASES OR DECREASES AND MARK THE CHANGES AS THEY OCCUR.

I'M AFRAID OF . . .

	A LITTLE	A LOT	TERRIFIED
ANAL SEX	◯	◯	◯
GETTING HURT	◯	◯	◯
BEING REJECTED	◯	◯	◯
LOSING CONTROL	◯	◯	◯
VIOLATING MY RELIGION	◯	◯	◯
INITIATING	◯	◯	◯
GETTING CAUGHT	◯	◯	◯
THE APPEARANCE OF MY BODY	◯	◯	◯
INFECTION	◯	◯	◯
GIVING UP CONTROL	◯	◯	◯
MY SCENT OR TASTE	◯	◯	◯
MAKING STRANGE NOISES	◯	◯	◯
GETTING SORE	◯	◯	◯
BEING UNABLE TO PLEASE MY PARTNER(S)	◯	◯	◯
ADMITTING MY SEXUAL FANTASIES	◯	◯	◯
BEING UNABLE TO STAY AROUSED	◯	◯	◯
MAKING A HORRIBLE STICKY MESS	◯	◯	◯
GETTING PREGNANT	◯	◯	◯
BEING JUDGED BY OTHERS	◯	◯	◯
SAYING THE WRONG NAME	◯	◯	◯
MY ORGASM FACE	◯	◯	◯
MEETING MY PARTNER'S EXPECTATIONS	◯	◯	◯
BEING REPLACED BY SEX TOYS	◯	◯	◯
HURTING MY PARTNER(S)	◯	◯	◯
CHOKING OR GAGGING	◯	◯	◯
LOSING BLADDER CONTROL	◯	◯	◯

FILL IN YOUR OWN . . .

	A LITTLE	A LOT	TERRIFIED
	☐	☐	☐
	☐	☐	☐
	☐	☐	☐
	☐	☐	☐
	☐	☐	☐
	☐	☐	☐
	☐	☐	☐

CHAPTER 5

TALKING DIRTY

SEXUAL AROUSAL THAT COMES FROM GREAT CONVERSATION CAN BE JUST AS POWERFUL AS THE FULL-CONTACT, LEGS-OVER-THE-SHOULDER VARIETY. IN THIS SCENARIO, WE'RE GOING TO TEACH YOU HOW TO FIND THE VERBIAGE THAT TURNS YOUR CRANK.

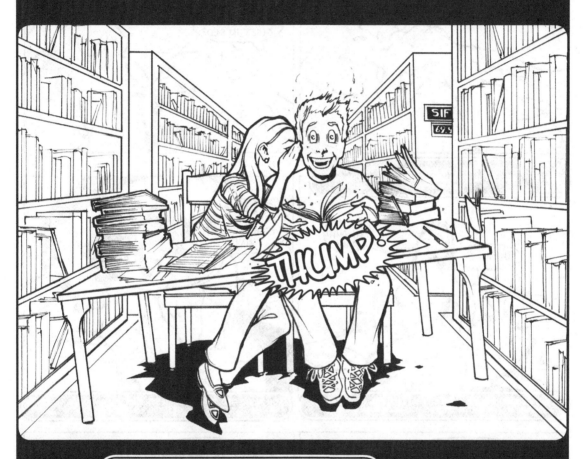

WHAT YOU'LL NEED . . .

WRITTEN EROTICA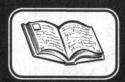

HANDHELD MIRROR

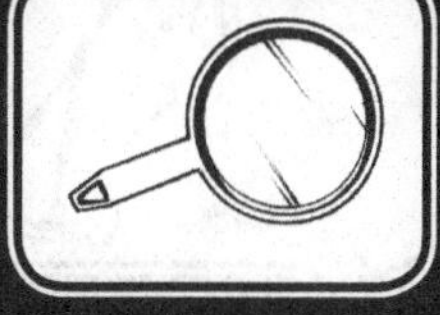

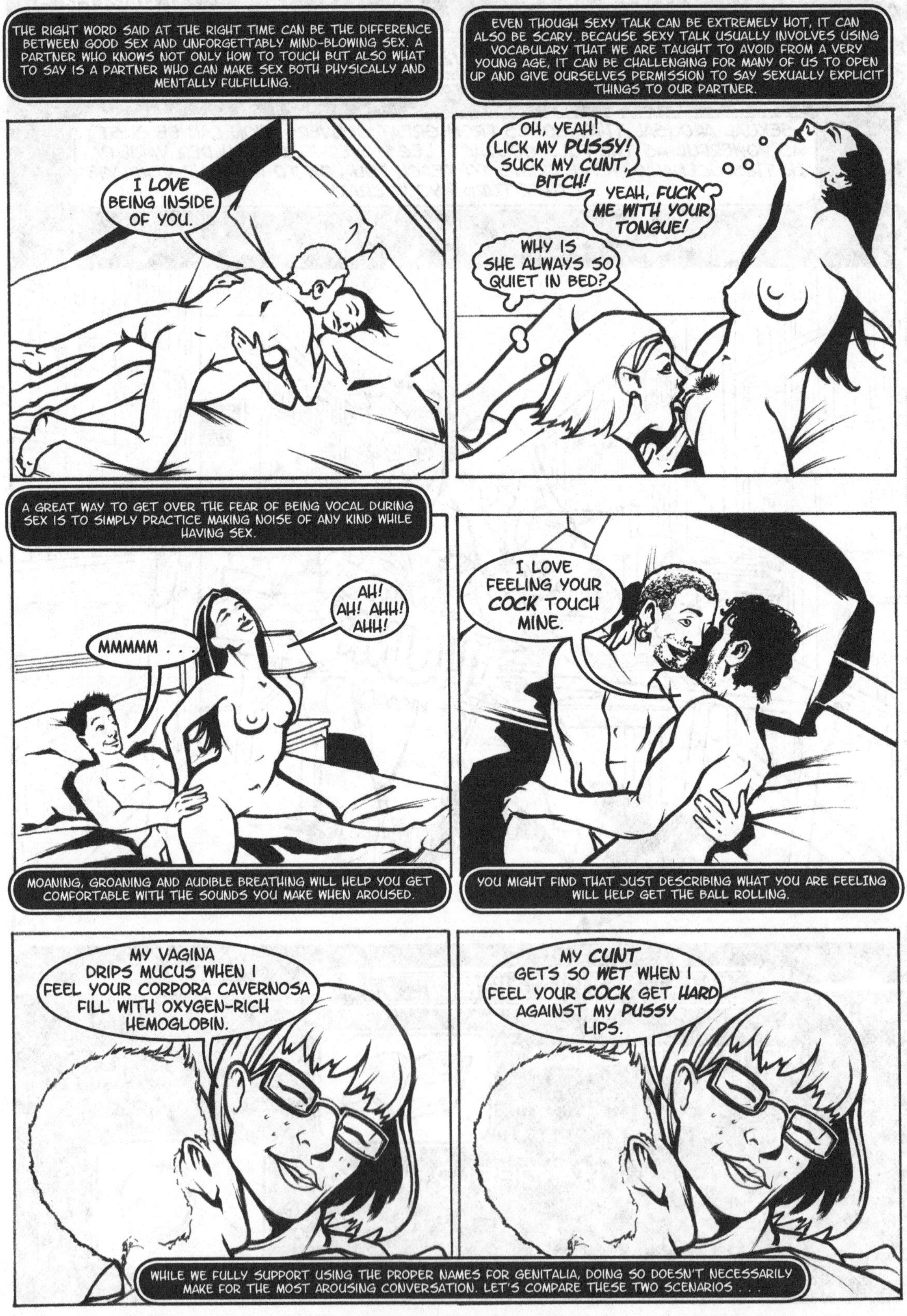
THE RIGHT WORD SAID AT THE RIGHT TIME CAN BE THE DIFFERENCE BETWEEN GOOD SEX AND UNFORGETTABLY MIND-BLOWING SEX. A PARTNER WHO KNOWS NOT ONLY HOW TO TOUCH BUT ALSO WHAT TO SAY IS A PARTNER WHO CAN MAKE SEX BOTH PHYSICALLY AND MENTALLY FULFILLING.
I LOVE BEING INSIDE OF YOU.
EVEN THOUGH SEXY TALK CAN BE EXTREMELY HOT, IT CAN ALSO BE SCARY. BECAUSE SEXY TALK USUALLY INVOLVES USING VOCABULARY THAT WE ARE TAUGHT TO AVOID FROM A VERY YOUNG AGE, IT CAN BE CHALLENGING FOR MANY OF US TO OPEN UP AND GIVE OURSELVES PERMISSION TO SAY SEXUALLY EXPLICIT THINGS TO OUR PARTNER.
OH, YEAH! LICK MY PUSSY! SUCK MY CUNT, BITCH!
YEAH, FUCK ME WITH YOUR TONGUE!
WHY IS SHE ALWAYS SO QUIET IN BED?
A GREAT WAY TO GET OVER THE FEAR OF BEING VOCAL DURING SEX IS TO SIMPLY PRACTICE MAKING NOISE OF ANY KIND WHILE HAVING SEX.
MMMMM . . .
AH! AH! AHH! AHH!
MOANING, GROANING AND AUDIBLE BREATHING WILL HELP YOU GET COMFORTABLE WITH THE SOUNDS YOU MAKE WHEN AROUSED.
I LOVE FEELING YOUR COCK TOUCH MINE.
YOU MIGHT FIND THAT JUST DESCRIBING WHAT YOU ARE FEELING WILL HELP GET THE BALL ROLLING.
MY VAGINA DRIPS MUCUS WHEN I FEEL YOUR CORPORA CAVERNOSA FILL WITH OXYGEN-RICH HEMOGLOBIN.
MY CUNT GETS SO WET WHEN I FEEL YOUR COCK GET HARD AGAINST MY PUSSY LIPS.
WHILE WE FULLY SUPPORT USING THE PROPER NAMES FOR GENITALIA, DOING SO DOESN'T NECESSARILY MAKE FOR THE MOST AROUSING CONVERSATION. LET'S COMPARE THESE TWO SCENARIOS . . .

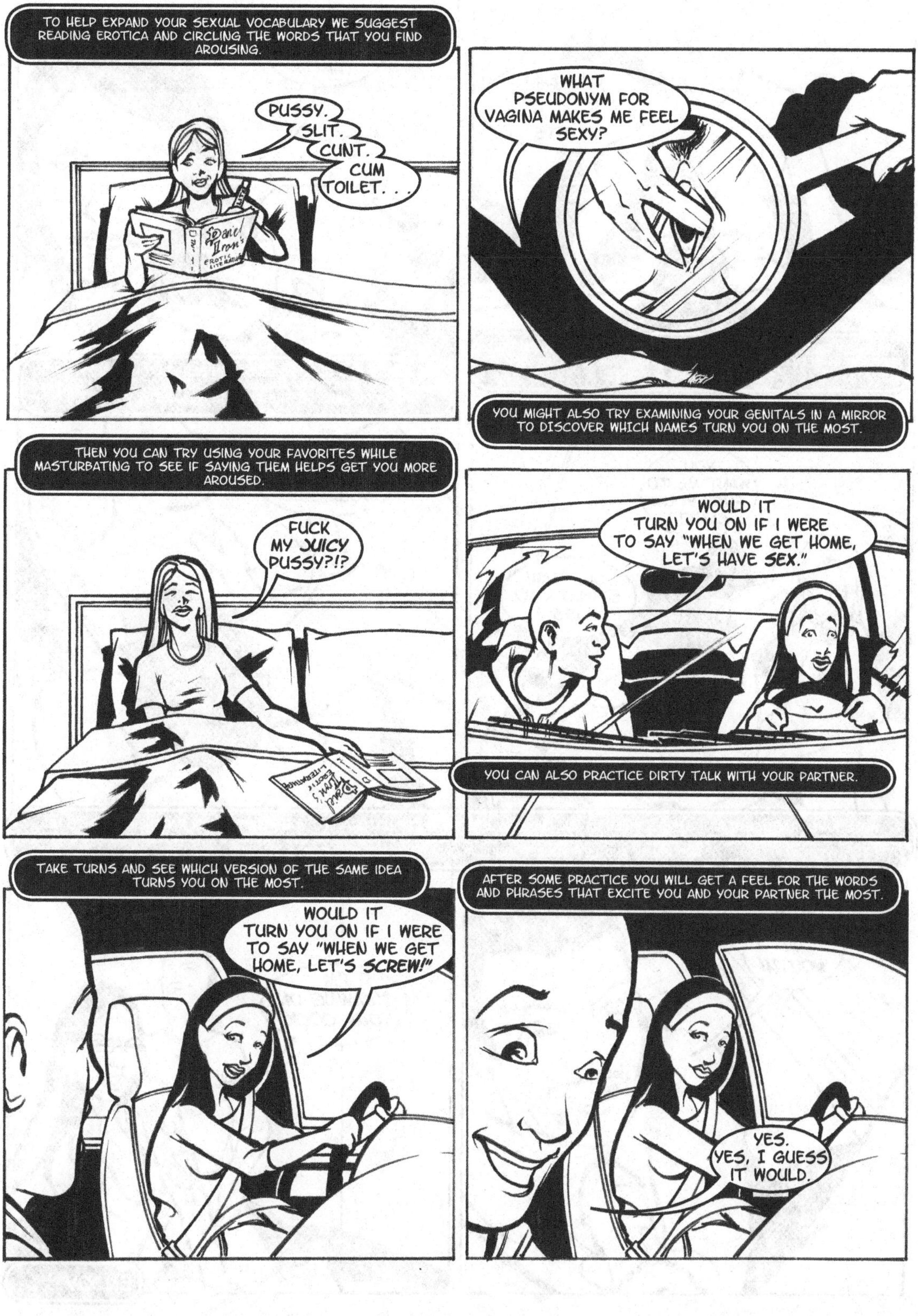
TO HELP EXPAND YOUR SEXUAL VOCABULARY WE SUGGEST READING EROTICA AND CIRCLING THE WORDS THAT YOU FIND AROUSING.
PUSSY.
SLIT.
CUNT.
CUM TOILET. . .
WHAT PSEUDONYM FOR VAGINA MAKES ME FEEL SEXY?
YOU MIGHT ALSO TRY EXAMINING YOUR GENITALS IN A MIRROR TO DISCOVER WHICH NAMES TURN YOU ON THE MOST.
THEN YOU CAN TRY USING YOUR FAVORITES WHILE MASTURBATING TO SEE IF SAYING THEM HELPS GET YOU MORE AROUSED.
FUCK MY JUICY PUSSY?!?
WOULD IT TURN YOU ON IF I WERE TO SAY "WHEN WE GET HOME, LET'S HAVE SEX."
YOU CAN ALSO PRACTICE DIRTY TALK WITH YOUR PARTNER.
TAKE TURNS AND SEE WHICH VERSION OF THE SAME IDEA TURNS YOU ON THE MOST.
WOULD IT TURN YOU ON IF I WERE TO SAY "WHEN WE GET HOME, LET'S SCREW!"
AFTER SOME PRACTICE YOU WILL GET A FEEL FOR THE WORDS AND PHRASES THAT EXCITE YOU AND YOUR PARTNER THE MOST.
YES. YES, I GUESS IT WOULD.

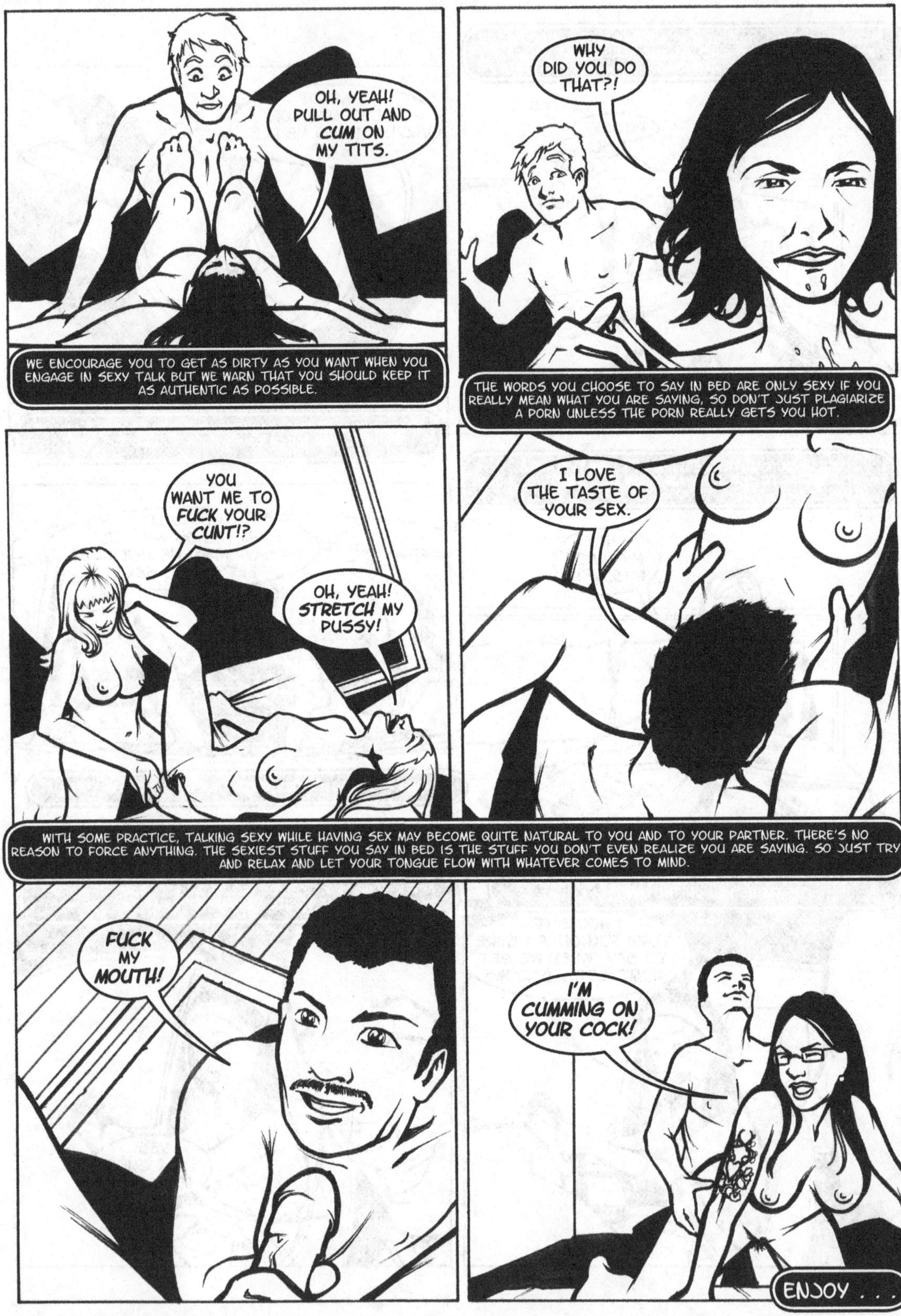
OH, YEAH! PULL OUT AND CUM ON MY TITS.
WE ENCOURAGE YOU TO GET AS DIRTY AS YOU WANT WHEN YOU ENGAGE IN SEXY TALK BUT WE WARN THAT YOU SHOULD KEEP IT AS AUTHENTIC AS POSSIBLE.
WHY DID YOU DO THAT?!
THE WORDS YOU CHOOSE TO SAY IN BED ARE ONLY SEXY IF YOU REALLY MEAN WHAT YOU ARE SAYING, SO DON'T JUST PLAGIARIZE A PORN UNLESS THE PORN REALLY GETS YOU HOT.
YOU WANT ME TO FUCK YOUR CUNT!?
OH, YEAH! STRETCH MY PUSSY!
I LOVE THE TASTE OF YOUR SEX.
WITH SOME PRACTICE, TALKING SEXY WHILE HAVING SEX MAY BECOME QUITE NATURAL TO YOU AND TO YOUR PARTNER. THERE'S NO REASON TO FORCE ANYTHING. THE SEXIEST STUFF YOU SAY IN BED IS THE STUFF YOU DON'T EVEN REALIZE YOU ARE SAYING. SO JUST TRY AND RELAX AND LET YOUR TONGUE FLOW WITH WHATEVER COMES TO MIND.
FUCK MY MOUTH!
I'M CUMMING ON YOUR COCK!
ENJOY . . .

CHAPTER 6

HOW TO WRITE A SEXY LETTER

SOME PEOPLE RESPOND TO VISUAL STIMULATION; OTHERS LOVE THE WRITTEN WORD. SO YOU ARE GOING TO WRITE YOUR PARTNER A DEVILISHLY SEXY LETTER AND WE'RE GOING TO HELP YOU WRITE IT.

THESAURUS
SHAKESPEARE FOR iDiOTS!
BIG BOOK OF POETRY
WEBSTER

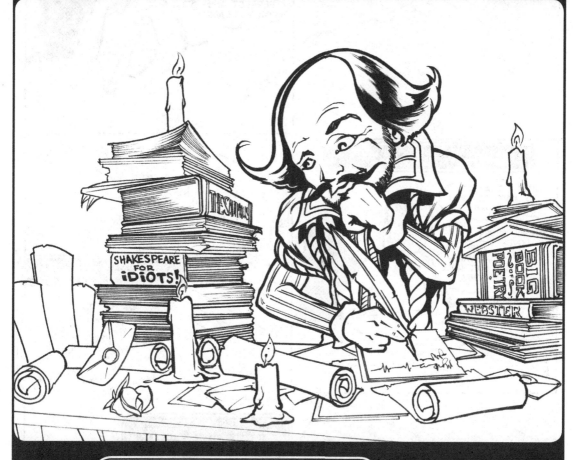

WHAT YOU'LL NEED . . .

PEN AND STATIONERY

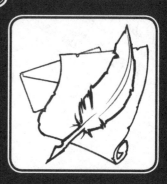

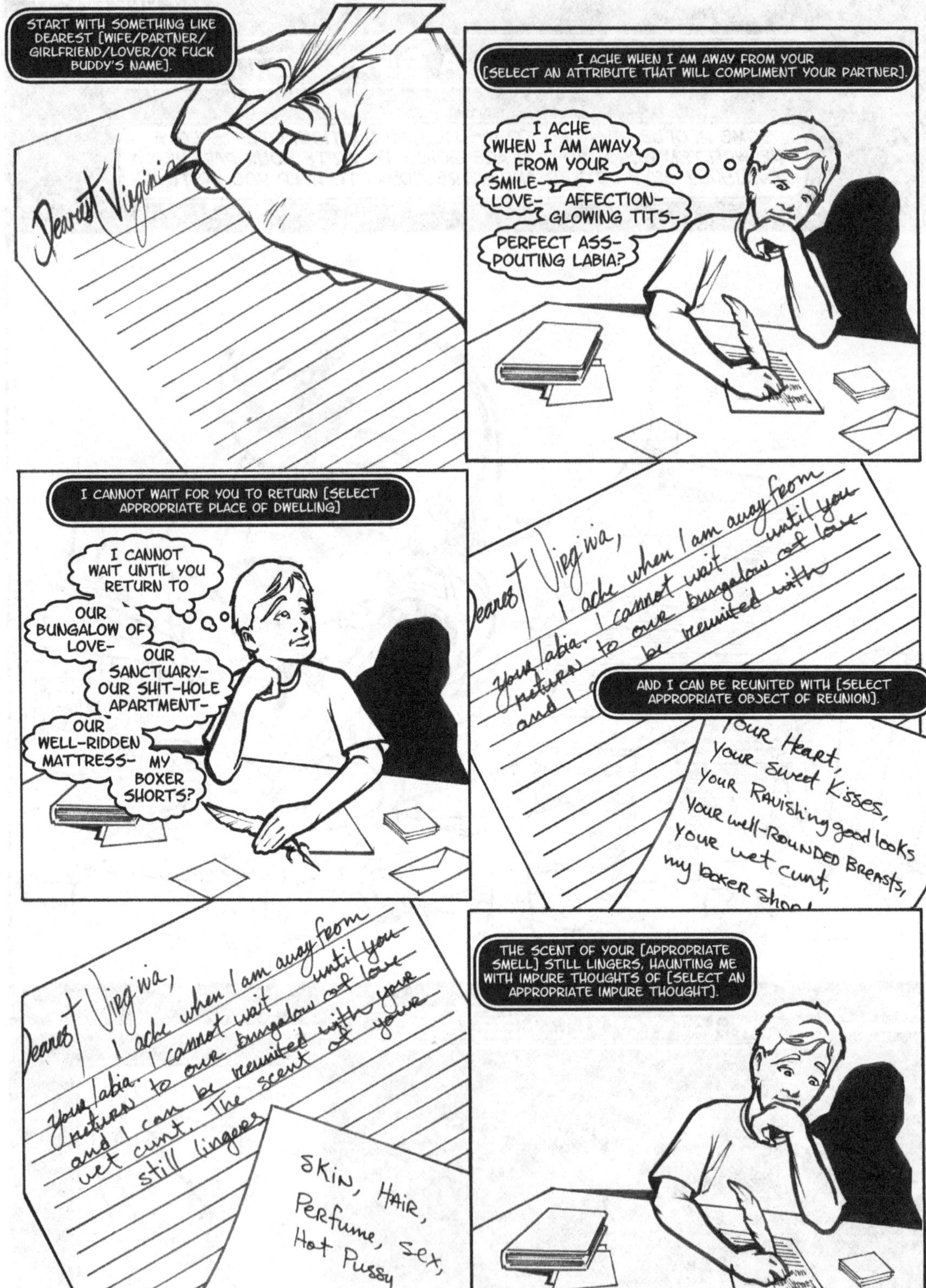
START WITH SOMETHING LIKE DEAREST [WIFE/PARTNER/ GIRLFRIEND/LOVER/OR FUCK BUDDY'S NAME].
Dearest Virginia
I ACHE WHEN I AM AWAY FROM YOUR [SELECT AN ATTRIBUTE THAT WILL COMPLIMENT YOUR PARTNER].
I ACHE WHEN I AM AWAY FROM YOUR
SMILE- LOVE- AFFECTION- GLOWING TITS-
PERFECT ASS- POUTING LABIA?
I CANNOT WAIT FOR YOU TO RETURN [SELECT APPROPRIATE PLACE OF DWELLING]
I CANNOT WAIT UNTIL YOU RETURN TO
OUR BUNGALOW OF LOVE-
OUR SANCTUARY- OUR SHIT-HOLE APARTMENT-
OUR WELL-RIDDEN MATTRESS-
MY BOXER SHORTS?
Dearest Virginia,
I ache when I am away from your labia. I cannot wait until you return to our bungalow of love and I can be reunited with
AND I CAN BE REUNITED WITH [SELECT APPROPRIATE OBJECT OF REUNION].
Your Heart, Your Sweet Kisses, Your Ravishing good looks Your well-Rounded Breasts, Your wet cunt, my boxer shor
Dearest Virginia,
I ache when I am away from your labia. I cannot wait until you return to our bungalow of love and I can be reunited with your wet cunt. The scent of your still lingers
SKIN, HAIR, Perfume, Sex, Hot Pussy
THE SCENT OF YOUR [APPROPRIATE SMELL] STILL LINGERS, HAUNTING ME WITH IMPURE THOUGHTS OF [SELECT AN APPROPRIATE IMPURE THOUGHT].

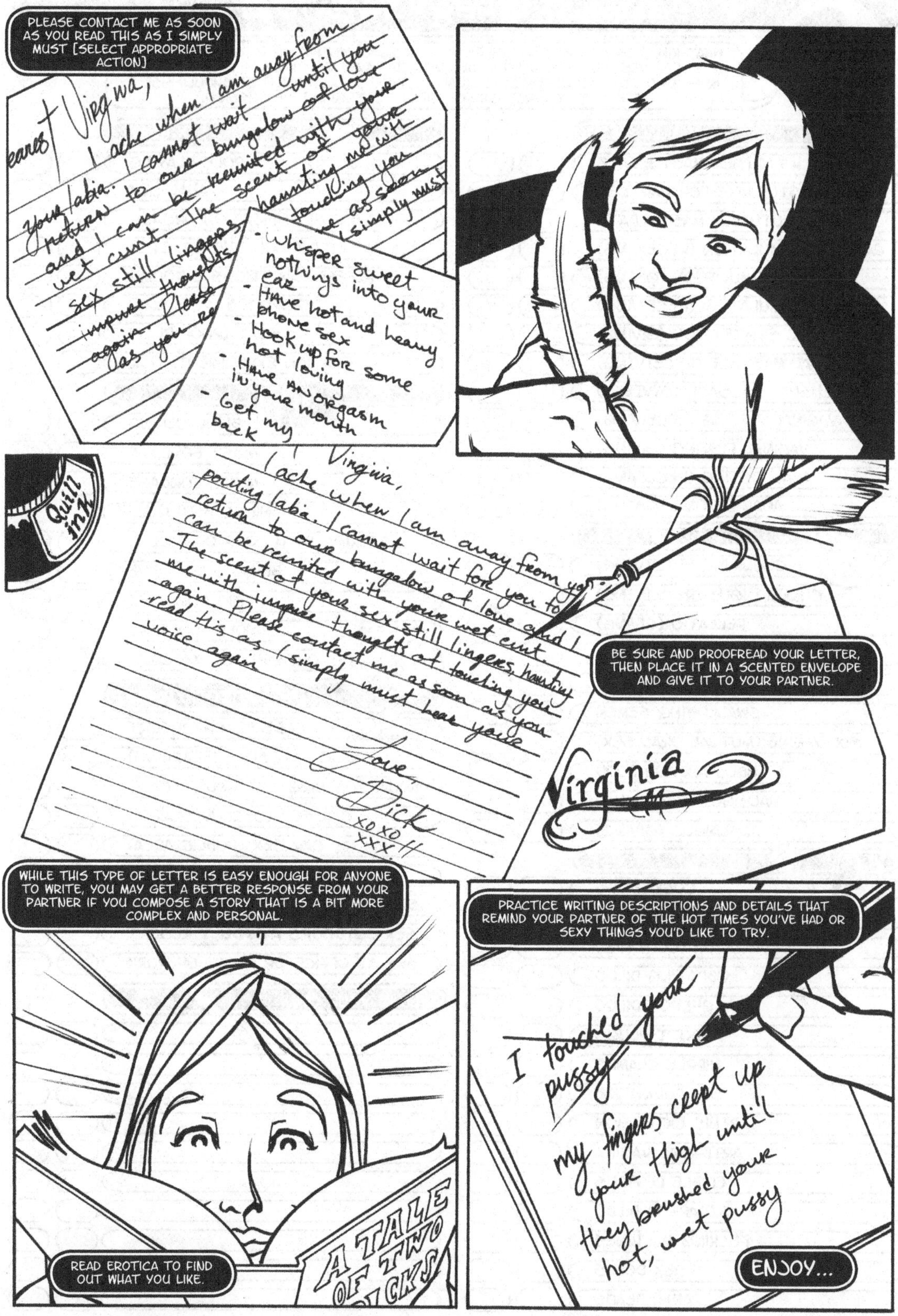
PLEASE CONTACT ME AS SOON AS YOU READ THIS AS I SIMPLY MUST [SELECT APPROPRIATE ACTION]
- Whisper sweet nothings into your ear
- Have hot and heavy phone sex
- Hook up for some hot loving
- Have an orgasm in your mouth
- Get my back
Quill ink
Virginia,
I ache when I am away from your pouting labia. I cannot wait for you to return to our bungalow of love and I can be reunited with your wet cunt. The scent of your sex still lingers, haunting me with impure thoughts of touching you again. Please contact me as soon as you read this as I simply must hear your voice again.
Love,
Dick
XOXO XXX!!
Virginia
BE SURE AND PROOFREAD YOUR LETTER, THEN PLACE IT IN A SCENTED ENVELOPE AND GIVE IT TO YOUR PARTNER.
WHILE THIS TYPE OF LETTER IS EASY ENOUGH FOR ANYONE TO WRITE, YOU MAY GET A BETTER RESPONSE FROM YOUR PARTNER IF YOU COMPOSE A STORY THAT IS A BIT MORE COMPLEX AND PERSONAL.
A TALE OF TWO
READ EROTICA TO FIND OUT WHAT YOU LIKE.
PRACTICE WRITING DESCRIPTIONS AND DETAILS THAT REMIND YOUR PARTNER OF THE HOT TIMES YOU'VE HAD OR SEXY THINGS YOU'D LIKE TO TRY.
I touched your pussy
my fingers crept up your thigh until they brushed your hot, wet pussy
ENJOY...

SEXUAL INTEREST INVENTORY

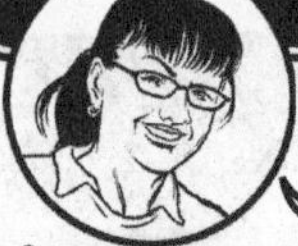

WHAT KINDS OF SEXUAL INTERESTS DO YOU SHARE WITH YOUR PARTNER(S)? WRITE A "Y" FOR YES, AN "N" FOR NO OR AN "M" FOR MAYBE TO INDICATE YOUR ATTITUDE IN REGARD TO EACH OF THESE SEXUAL ACTIVITIES. EACH PARTNER SHOULD USE A DIFFERENT COLORED INK FOR IDENTIFICATION AND DISCUSSION.

MANUAL SEX

- WATCH PARTNER MASTURBATE
- MASTURBATE FOR PARTNER
- MUTUALLY MASTURBATE
- GENITAL STIMULATION (RECEIVING)
- GENITAL STIMULATION (GIVING)
- ANAL STIMULATION (RECEIVING)
- ANAL STIMULATION (GIVING)
- SENSUAL MASSAGE (RECEIVING)
- SENSUAL MASSAGE (GIVING)
- VAGINAL FISTING (RECEIVING)
- VAGINAL FISTING (GIVING)
- ANAL FISTING (RECEIVING)
- ANAL FISTING (GIVING)

ORAL SEX

- CUNNILINGUS (GIVING)
- CUNNILINGUS (RECEIVING)
- FELLATIO (GIVING)
- FELLATIO (RECEIVING)
- SWALLOWING VAGINAL SECRETIONS
- SWALLOWING SEMEN
- SIXTY-NINE (MUTUAL ORAL SEX)
- EDIBLE LUBES AND/OR FOOD
- ANALINGUS (RECEIVING)
- ANALINGUS (GIVING)

TOYS

- COCK RINGS
- DILDO
- VIBRATOR (CLITORAL)
- VIBRATING DILDO
- G-SPOT DILDO
- BUTT PLUGS
- NIPPLE CLAMPS
- SEX FURNITURE
- PENIS EXTENSION
- ARTIFICIAL VAGINA
- EDIBLE LOTIONS
- STRAP-ON DILDO
- FUCKING MACHINES
- SEX DOLLS
- ANAL BEADS

SEX PLAY

- ROLE PLAYING
- ANAL SEX
- DELAYED-GRATIFICATION ORGASM
- SEX IN WATER (POOL, SHOWER, ETC.)
- DIFFERENT LOCATIONS & ROOMS
- WATERSPORTS (PEE PLAY)
- SCAT (POOP PLAY)
- POSITION EXPERIMENTATION

BDSM

- BLINDFOLDING
- WRIST BONDAGE
- ANKLE BONDAGE
- SPANKING WITH HAND
- SPANKING WITH CROP OR PADDLE
- BEING SUBMISSIVE
- BEING DOMINANT
- CANDLE-WAX PLAY
- ORGASM DELAY/DENIAL

OUTDOOR/PUBLIC

- NUDE BEACH/RESORT
- PUBLIC EXPOSURE (FLASHING)
- MANUAL FONDLING (E.G., UNDER TABLE)
- CAR SEX (SECLUDED AREA)
- CAR SEX (PUBLIC AREA)
- LOUD SEX IN HOTEL ROOM
- SEX OUTDOORS IN FOREST OR PARK
- SEX OUTDOORS AT ADULT RESORT
- SEX AT OFFICE OR PLACE OF WORK

FILL IN YOUR OWN

CHAPTER 7

HOW TO TAKE A SEXY PICTURE

WANT TO GIVE YOUR PARTNER SOMETHING REALLY SPECIAL? IN THIS SCENARIO, WE'LL HELP YOU TAKE AN EROTIC SELF-PORTRAIT.

Love Virginia
xoxo

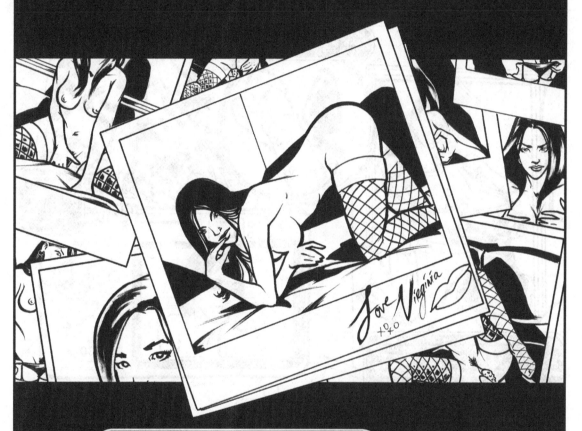

WHAT YOU'LL NEED . . .

DIGITAL CAMERA AND TRIPOD

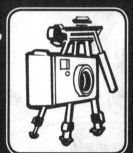

SEXY ACCESSORIES

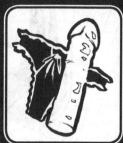

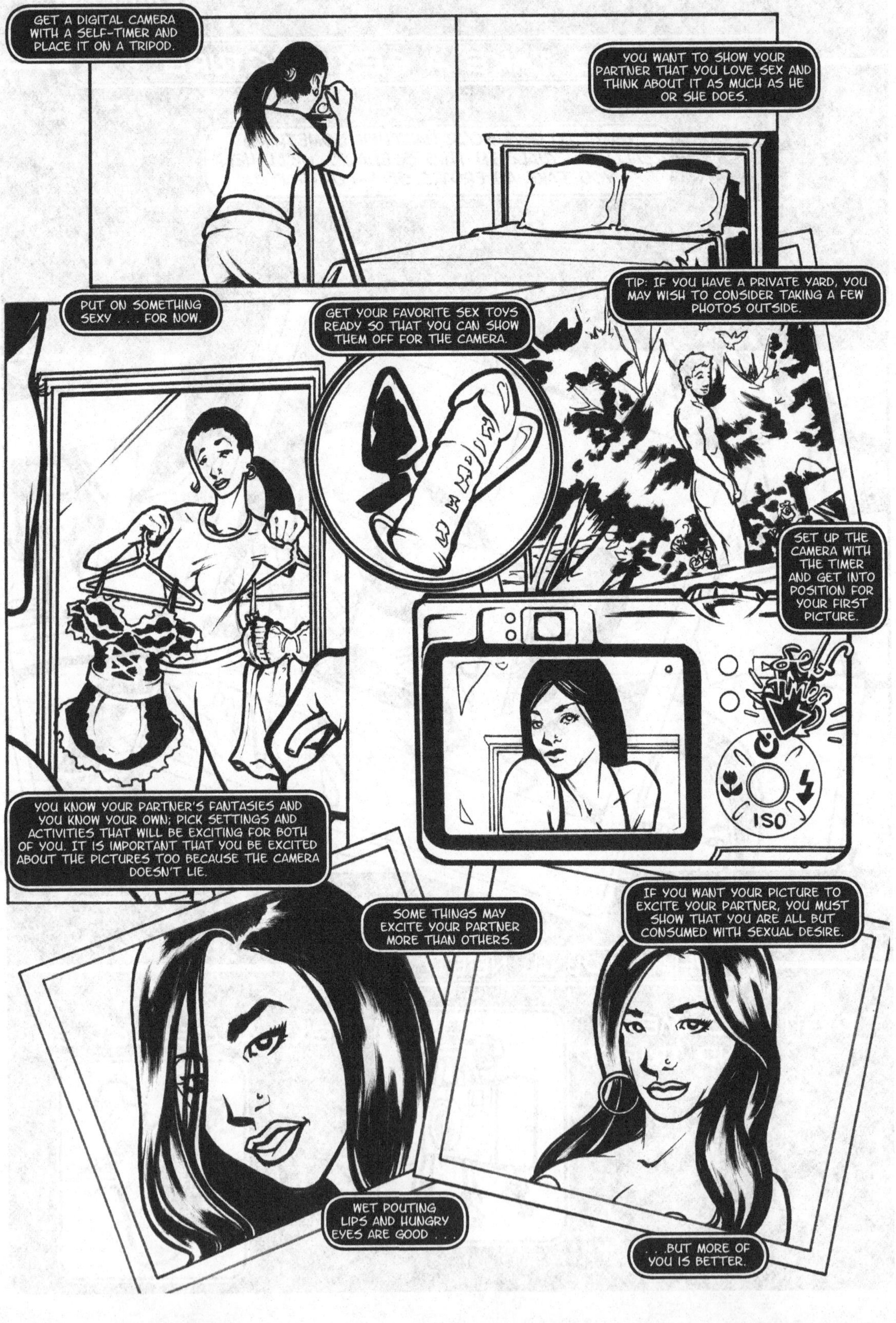
GET A DIGITAL CAMERA WITH A SELF-TIMER AND PLACE IT ON A TRIPOD.
YOU WANT TO SHOW YOUR PARTNER THAT YOU LOVE SEX AND THINK ABOUT IT AS MUCH AS HE OR SHE DOES.
PUT ON SOMETHING SEXY . . . FOR NOW.
GET YOUR FAVORITE SEX TOYS READY SO THAT YOU CAN SHOW THEM OFF FOR THE CAMERA.
TIP: IF YOU HAVE A PRIVATE YARD, YOU MAY WISH TO CONSIDER TAKING A FEW PHOTOS OUTSIDE.
SET UP THE CAMERA WITH THE TIMER AND GET INTO POSITION FOR YOUR FIRST PICTURE.
SELF TIMER
ISO
YOU KNOW YOUR PARTNER'S FANTASIES AND YOU KNOW YOUR OWN; PICK SETTINGS AND ACTIVITIES THAT WILL BE EXCITING FOR BOTH OF YOU. IT IS IMPORTANT THAT YOU BE EXCITED ABOUT THE PICTURES TOO BECAUSE THE CAMERA DOESN'T LIE.
SOME THINGS MAY EXCITE YOUR PARTNER MORE THAN OTHERS.
IF YOU WANT YOUR PICTURE TO EXCITE YOUR PARTNER, YOU MUST SHOW THAT YOU ARE ALL BUT CONSUMED WITH SEXUAL DESIRE.
WET POUTING LIPS AND HUNGRY EYES ARE GOOD . . .
. . .BUT MORE OF YOU IS BETTER.

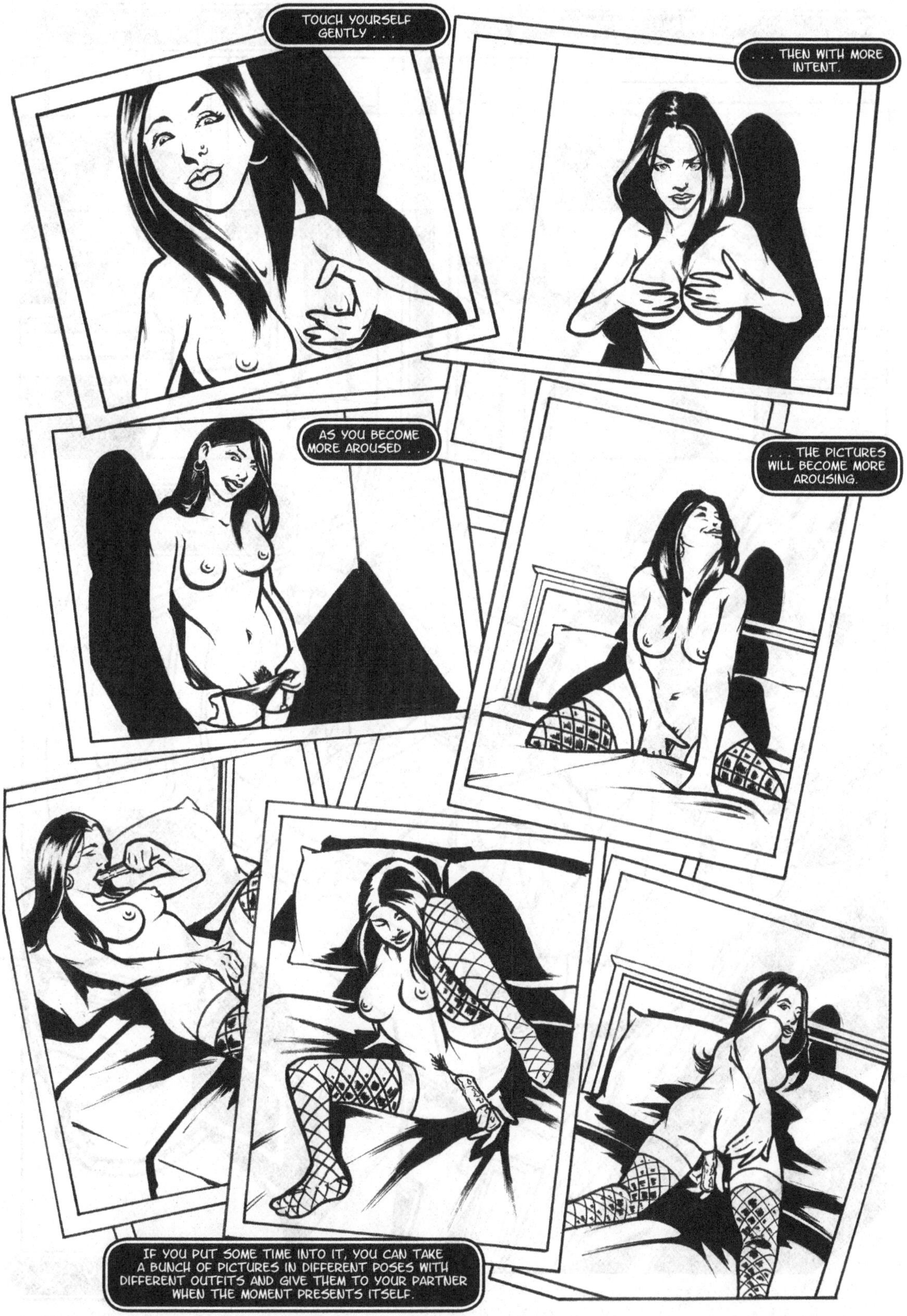
TOUCH YOURSELF GENTLY . . .
. . . THEN WITH MORE INTENT.
AS YOU BECOME MORE AROUSED . . .
. . . THE PICTURES WILL BECOME MORE AROUSING.
IF YOU PUT SOME TIME INTO IT, YOU CAN TAKE A BUNCH OF PICTURES IN DIFFERENT POSES WITH DIFFERENT OUTFITS AND GIVE THEM TO YOUR PARTNER WHEN THE MOMENT PRESENTS ITSELF.

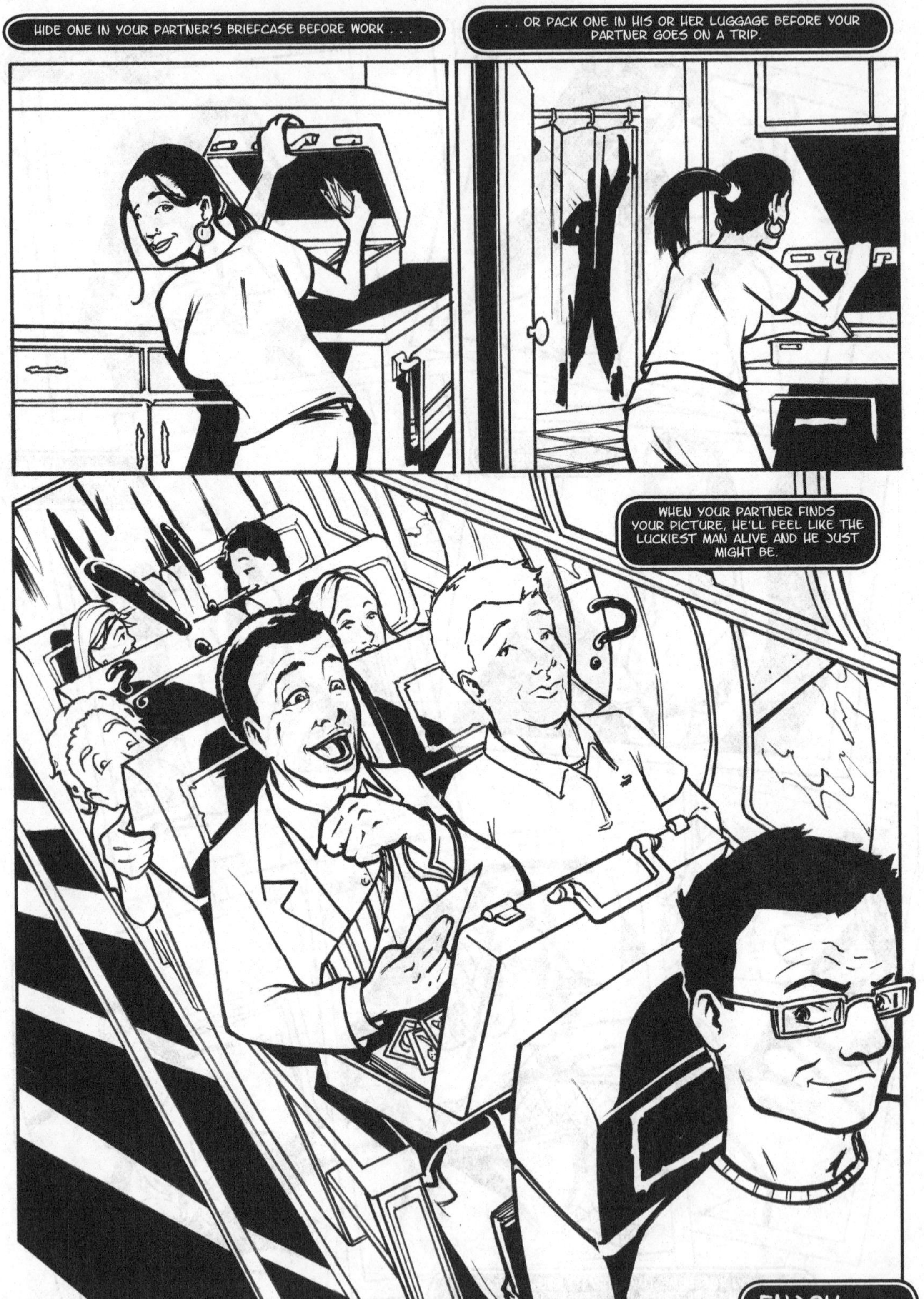
HIDE ONE IN YOUR PARTNER'S BRIEFCASE BEFORE WORK . . .
. . . OR PACK ONE IN HIS OR HER LUGGAGE BEFORE YOUR PARTNER GOES ON A TRIP.
WHEN YOUR PARTNER FINDS YOUR PICTURE, HE'LL FEEL LIKE THE LUCKIEST MAN ALIVE AND HE JUST MIGHT BE.
ENJOY . . .

CHAPTER 8

HOW TO MAKE A SEXY MOVIE

IN THIS SCENARIO, WE'LL SHOW YOU HOW TO MAKE A SUPER-LOW-BUDGET PORNOGRAPHIC MOVIE THAT IS SURE TO SEXUALLY EXCITE YOUR PARTNER.

FONY
INPUT 1
DVD
INSERT DISC
VIRGINIA'S VAGINA!

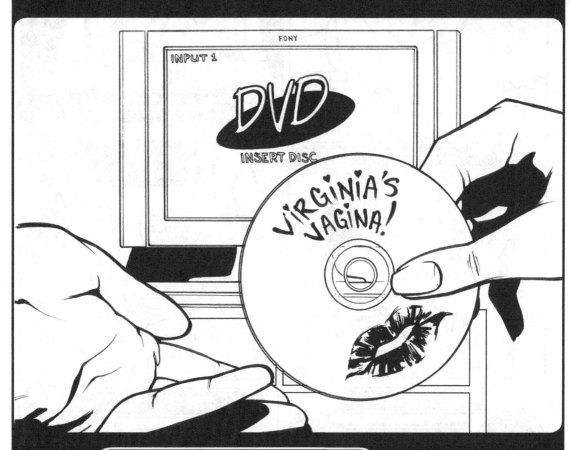

WHAT YOU'LL NEED . . .

DIGITAL VIDEO CAMERA AND TRIPOD

FONY

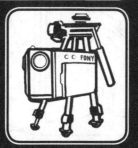

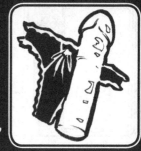

SEXY ACCESSORIES

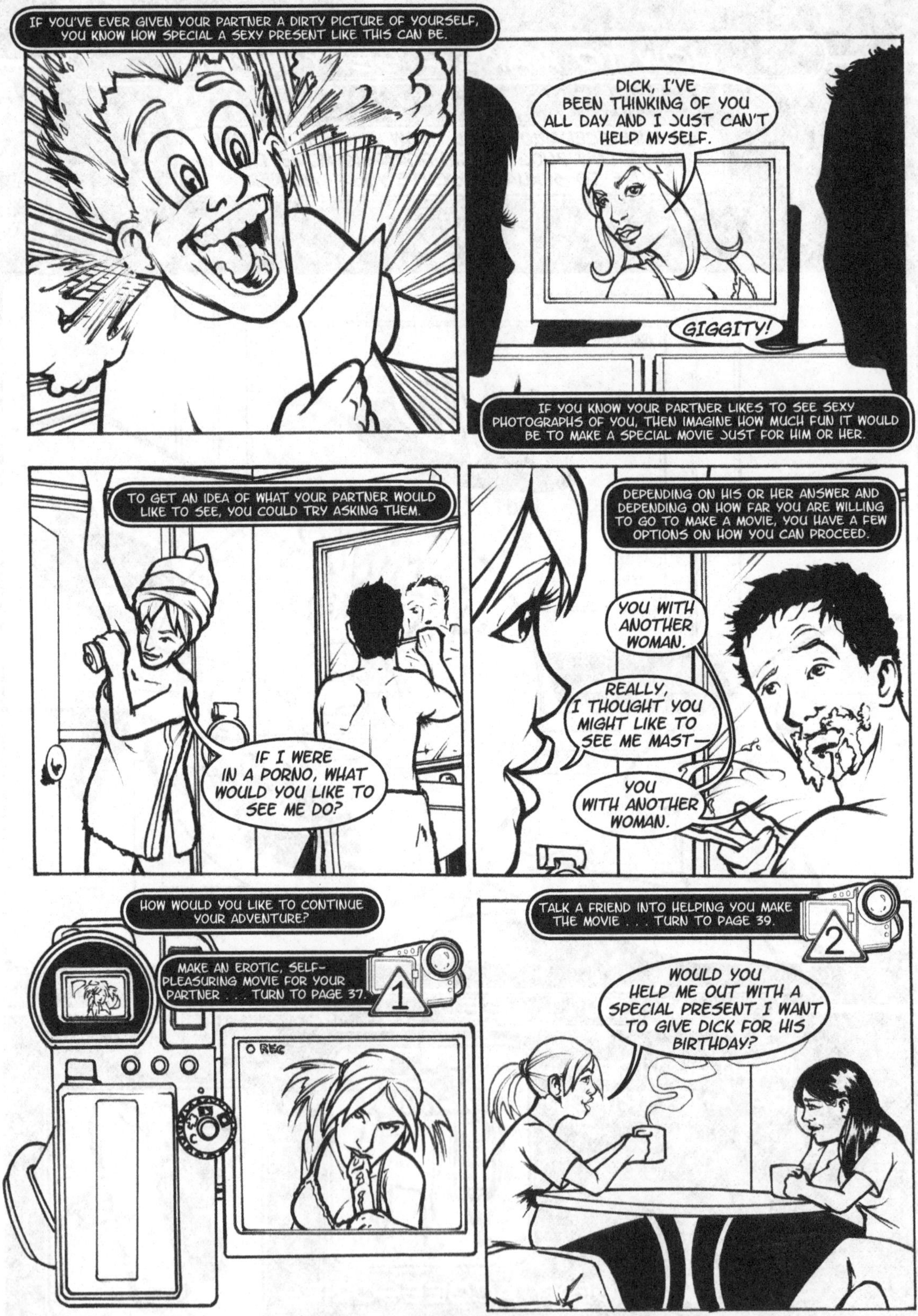
IF YOU'VE EVER GIVEN YOUR PARTNER A DIRTY PICTURE OF YOURSELF, YOU KNOW HOW SPECIAL A SEXY PRESENT LIKE THIS CAN BE.
DICK, I'VE BEEN THINKING OF YOU ALL DAY AND I JUST CAN'T HELP MYSELF.
GIGGITY!
IF YOU KNOW YOUR PARTNER LIKES TO SEE SEXY PHOTOGRAPHS OF YOU, THEN IMAGINE HOW MUCH FUN IT WOULD BE TO MAKE A SPECIAL MOVIE JUST FOR HIM OR HER.
TO GET AN IDEA OF WHAT YOUR PARTNER WOULD LIKE TO SEE, YOU COULD TRY ASKING THEM.
IF I WERE IN A PORNO, WHAT WOULD YOU LIKE TO SEE ME DO?
DEPENDING ON HIS OR HER ANSWER AND DEPENDING ON HOW FAR YOU ARE WILLING TO GO TO MAKE A MOVIE, YOU HAVE A FEW OPTIONS ON HOW YOU CAN PROCEED.
YOU WITH ANOTHER WOMAN.
REALLY, I THOUGHT YOU MIGHT LIKE TO SEE ME MAST—
YOU WITH ANOTHER WOMAN.
HOW WOULD YOU LIKE TO CONTINUE YOUR ADVENTURE?
MAKE AN EROTIC, SELF-PLEASURING MOVIE FOR YOUR PARTNER . . . TURN TO PAGE 37.
1
O REC
TALK A FRIEND INTO HELPING YOU MAKE THE MOVIE . . . TURN TO PAGE 39.
2
WOULD YOU HELP ME OUT WITH A SPECIAL PRESENT I WANT TO GIVE DICK FOR HIS BIRTHDAY?

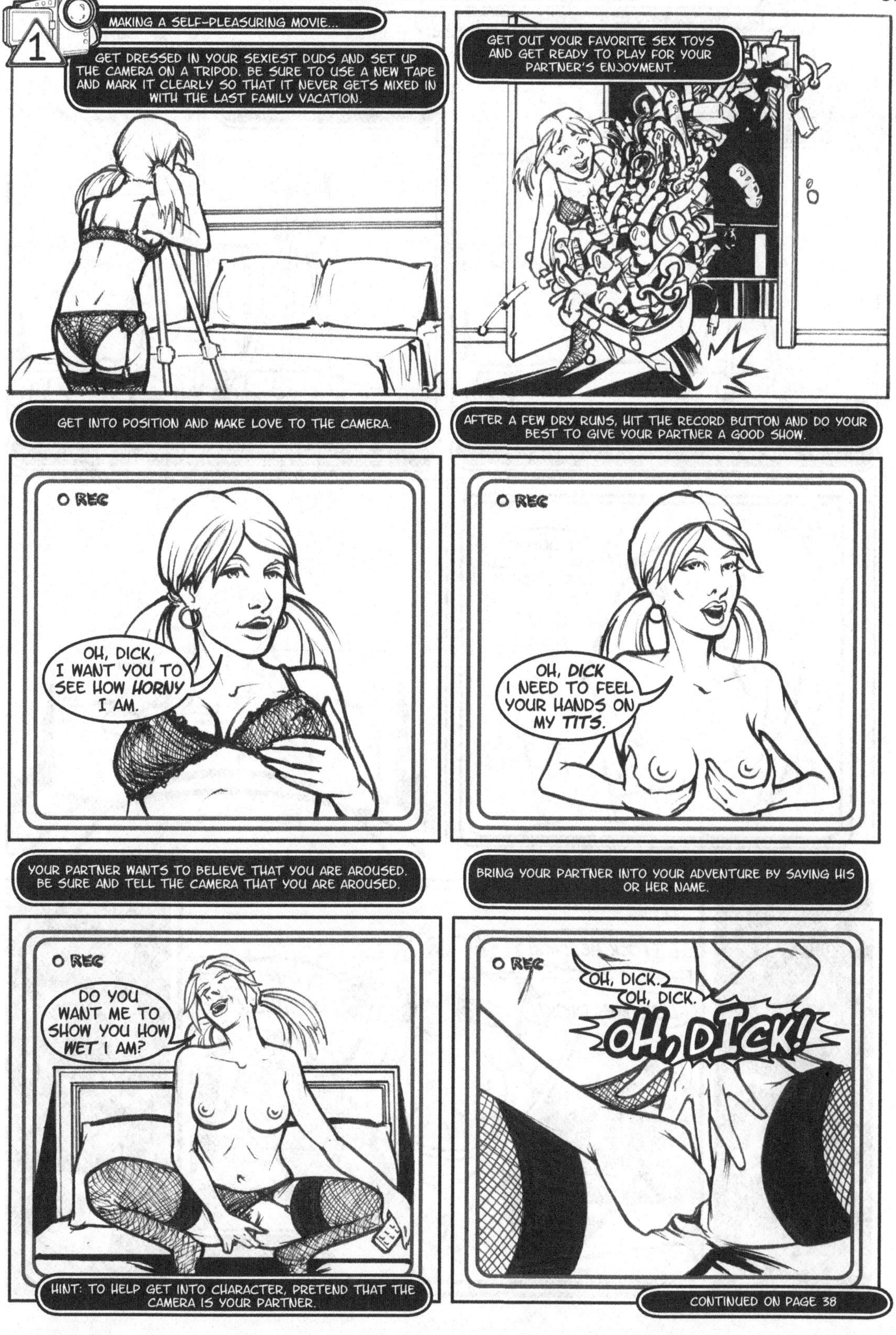
1
MAKING A SELF-PLEASURING MOVIE...
GET DRESSED IN YOUR SEXIEST DUDS AND SET UP THE CAMERA ON A TRIPOD. BE SURE TO USE A NEW TAPE AND MARK IT CLEARLY SO THAT IT NEVER GETS MIXED IN WITH THE LAST FAMILY VACATION.
GET OUT YOUR FAVORITE SEX TOYS AND GET READY TO PLAY FOR YOUR PARTNER'S ENJOYMENT.
GET INTO POSITION AND MAKE LOVE TO THE CAMERA.
AFTER A FEW DRY RUNS, HIT THE RECORD BUTTON AND DO YOUR BEST TO GIVE YOUR PARTNER A GOOD SHOW.
O REC
OH, DICK, I WANT YOU TO SEE HOW HORNY I AM.
O REC
OH, DICK I NEED TO FEEL YOUR HANDS ON MY TITS.
YOUR PARTNER WANTS TO BELIEVE THAT YOU ARE AROUSED. BE SURE AND TELL THE CAMERA THAT YOU ARE AROUSED.
BRING YOUR PARTNER INTO YOUR ADVENTURE BY SAYING HIS OR HER NAME.
O REC
DO YOU WANT ME TO SHOW YOU HOW WET I AM?
HINT: TO HELP GET INTO CHARACTER, PRETEND THAT THE CAMERA IS YOUR PARTNER.
O REC
OH, DICK.
OH, DICK.
OH, DICK!

CONTINUED ON PAGE 38

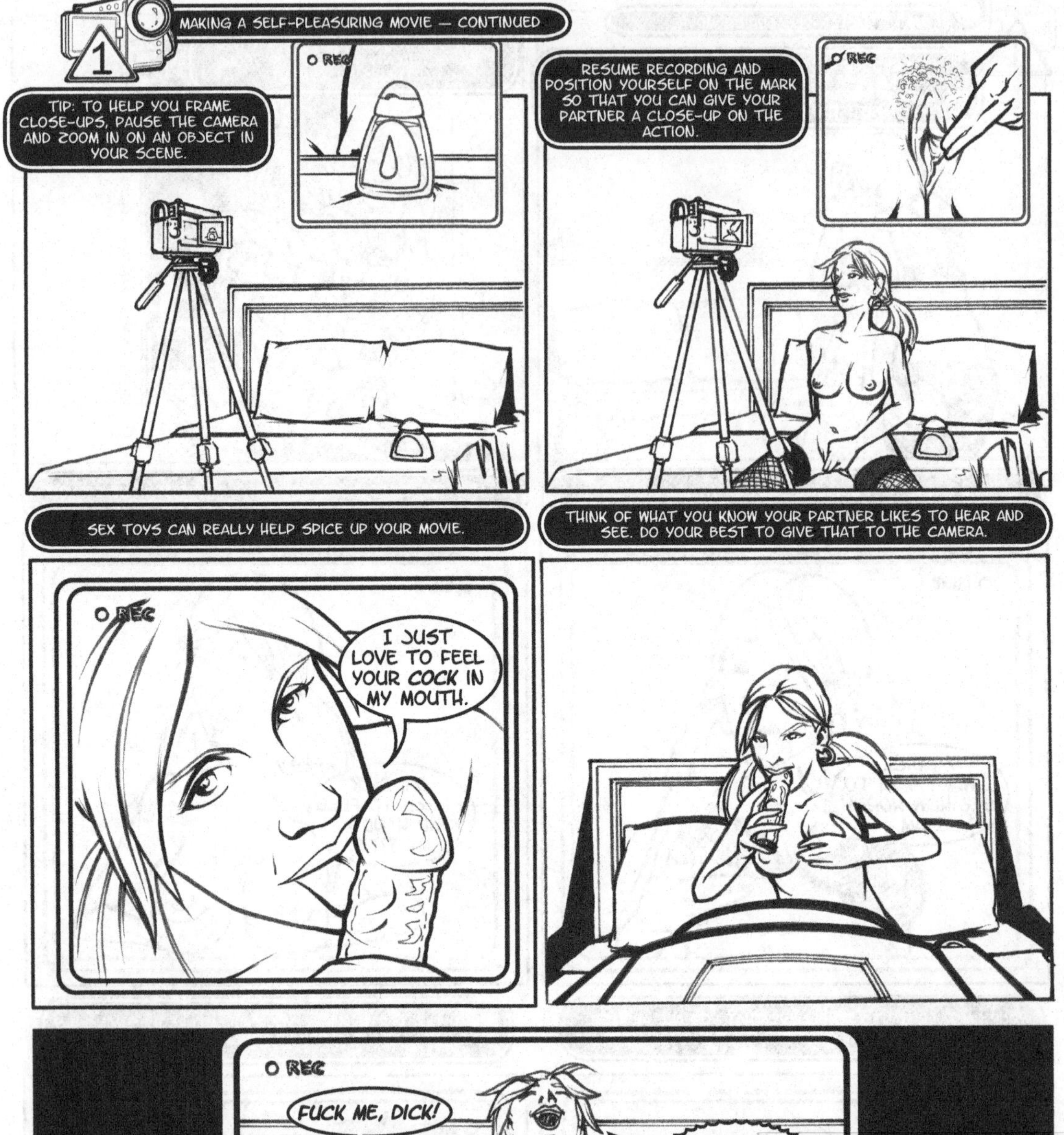
MAKING A SELF-PLEASURING MOVIE — CONTINUED
1
TIP: TO HELP YOU FRAME CLOSE-UPS, PAUSE THE CAMERA AND ZOOM IN ON AN OBJECT IN YOUR SCENE.
O REC
RESUME RECORDING AND POSITION YOURSELF ON THE MARK SO THAT YOU CAN GIVE YOUR PARTNER A CLOSE-UP ON THE ACTION.
O REC
SEX TOYS CAN REALLY HELP SPICE UP YOUR MOVIE.
O REC
I JUST LOVE TO FEEL YOUR COCK IN MY MOUTH.
THINK OF WHAT YOU KNOW YOUR PARTNER LIKES TO HEAR AND SEE. DO YOUR BEST TO GIVE THAT TO THE CAMERA.
O REC
FUCK ME, DICK!
FUCK ME, DICK!!
FUCK ME, DIIIIIIICK!!
CONTINUED ON PAGE 40

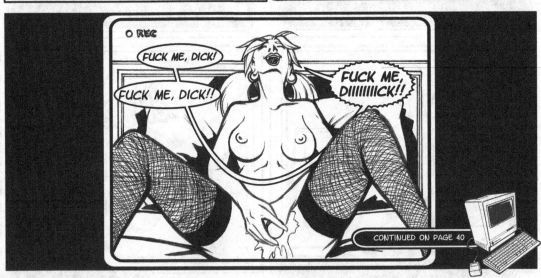

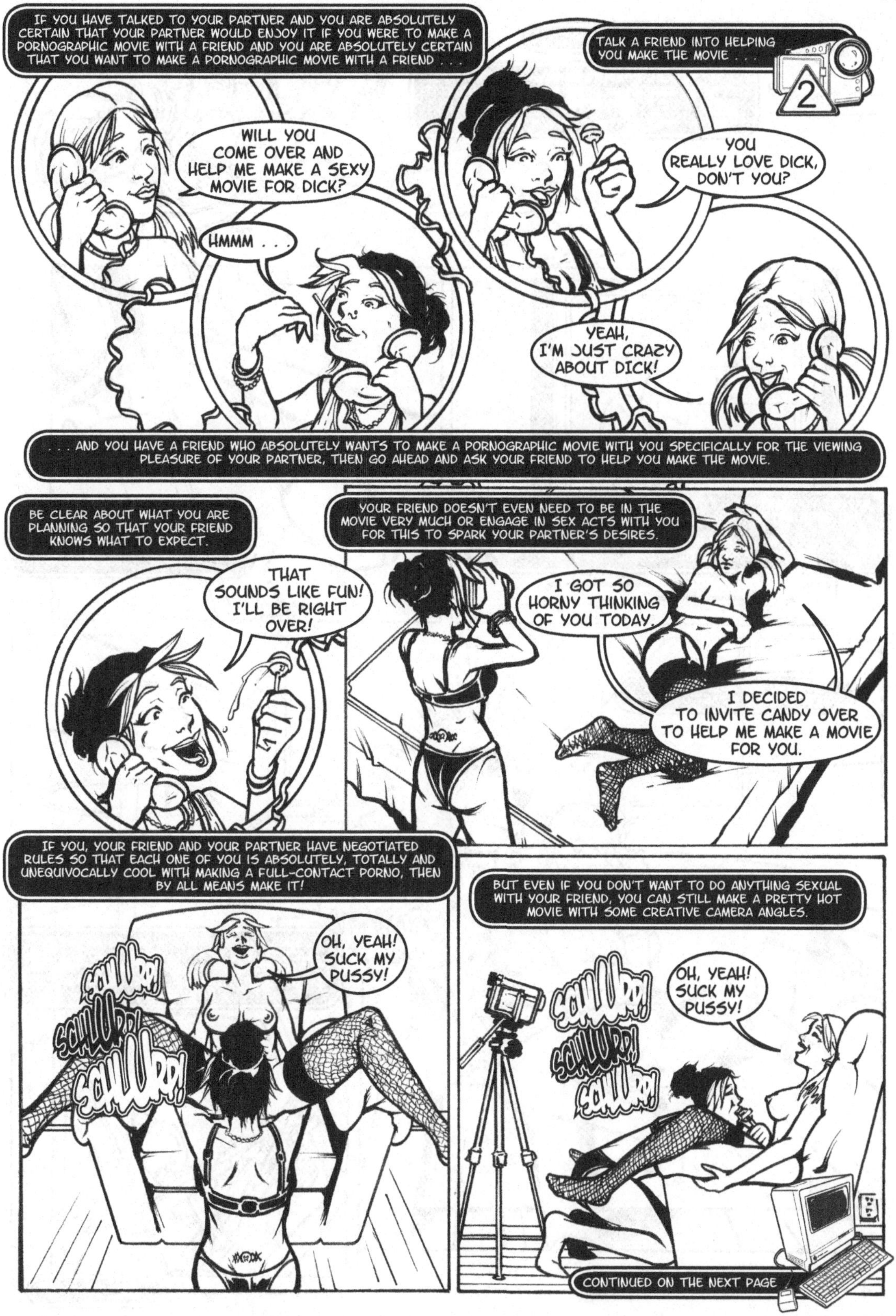
IF YOU HAVE TALKED TO YOUR PARTNER AND YOU ARE ABSOLUTELY CERTAIN THAT YOUR PARTNER WOULD ENJOY IT IF YOU WERE TO MAKE A PORNOGRAPHIC MOVIE WITH A FRIEND AND YOU ARE ABSOLUTELY CERTAIN THAT YOU WANT TO MAKE A PORNOGRAPHIC MOVIE WITH A FRIEND . . .
WILL YOU COME OVER AND HELP ME MAKE A SEXY MOVIE FOR DICK?
HMMM . . .
TALK A FRIEND INTO HELPING YOU MAKE THE MOVIE . . .
2
YOU REALLY LOVE DICK, DON'T YOU?
YEAH, I'M JUST CRAZY ABOUT DICK!
. . . AND YOU HAVE A FRIEND WHO ABSOLUTELY WANTS TO MAKE A PORNOGRAPHIC MOVIE WITH YOU SPECIFICALLY FOR THE VIEWING PLEASURE OF YOUR PARTNER, THEN GO AHEAD AND ASK YOUR FRIEND TO HELP YOU MAKE THE MOVIE.
BE CLEAR ABOUT WHAT YOU ARE PLANNING SO THAT YOUR FRIEND KNOWS WHAT TO EXPECT.
THAT SOUNDS LIKE FUN! I'LL BE RIGHT OVER!
YOUR FRIEND DOESN'T EVEN NEED TO BE IN THE MOVIE VERY MUCH OR ENGAGE IN SEX ACTS WITH YOU FOR THIS TO SPARK YOUR PARTNER'S DESIRES.
I GOT SO HORNY THINKING OF YOU TODAY.
I DECIDED TO INVITE CANDY OVER TO HELP ME MAKE A MOVIE FOR YOU.
IF YOU, YOUR FRIEND AND YOUR PARTNER HAVE NEGOTIATED RULES SO THAT EACH ONE OF YOU IS ABSOLUTELY, TOTALLY AND UNEQUIVOCALLY COOL WITH MAKING A FULL-CONTACT PORNO, THEN BY ALL MEANS MAKE IT!
OH, YEAH! SUCK MY PUSSY!
BUT EVEN IF YOU DON'T WANT TO DO ANYTHING SEXUAL WITH YOUR FRIEND, YOU CAN STILL MAKE A PRETTY HOT MOVIE WITH SOME CREATIVE CAMERA ANGLES.
OH, YEAH! SUCK MY PUSSY!
CONTINUED ON THE NEXT PAGE

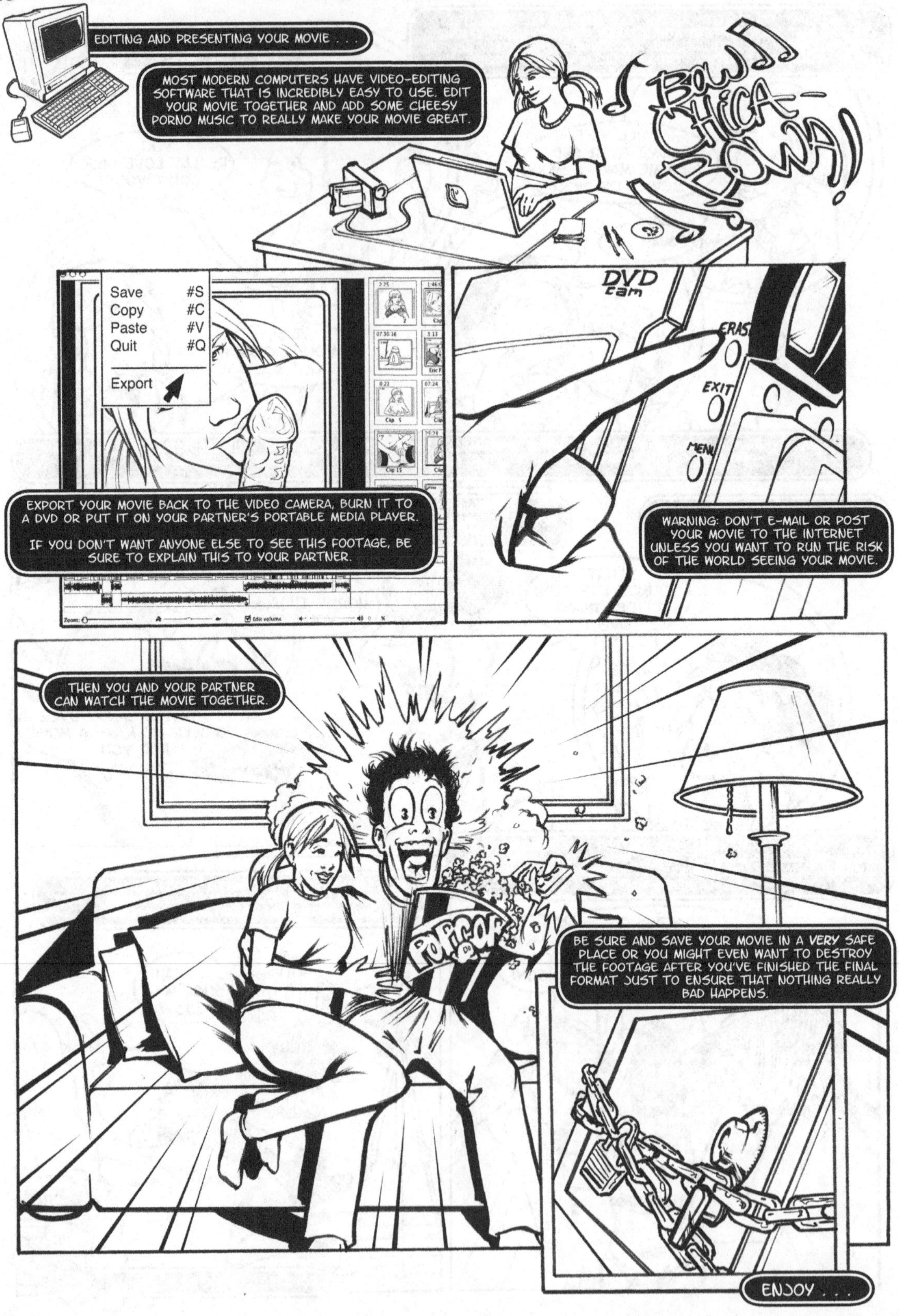
EDITING AND PRESENTING YOUR MOVIE . . .
MOST MODERN COMPUTERS HAVE VIDEO-EDITING SOFTWARE THAT IS INCREDIBLY EASY TO USE. EDIT YOUR MOVIE TOGETHER AND ADD SOME CHEESY PORNO MUSIC TO REALLY MAKE YOUR MOVIE GREAT.
BOW CHICA-BOWA!
Save #S
Copy #C
Paste #V
Quit #Q
Export
DVD cam
ERASE
EXIT
MENU
EXPORT YOUR MOVIE BACK TO THE VIDEO CAMERA, BURN IT TO A DVD OR PUT IT ON YOUR PARTNER'S PORTABLE MEDIA PLAYER.
IF YOU DON'T WANT ANYONE ELSE TO SEE THIS FOOTAGE, BE SURE TO EXPLAIN THIS TO YOUR PARTNER.
WARNING: DON'T E-MAIL OR POST YOUR MOVIE TO THE INTERNET UNLESS YOU WANT TO RUN THE RISK OF THE WORLD SEEING YOUR MOVIE.
THEN YOU AND YOUR PARTNER CAN WATCH THE MOVIE TOGETHER.
POPCORN
BE SURE AND SAVE YOUR MOVIE IN A VERY SAFE PLACE OR YOU MIGHT EVEN WANT TO DESTROY THE FOOTAGE AFTER YOU'VE FINISHED THE FINAL FORMAT JUST TO ENSURE THAT NOTHING REALLY BAD HAPPENS.
ENJOY . . .

CHAPTER 9

LEARNING HOW TO TOUCH YOUR PARTNER

BECAUSE EACH PERSON IS DIFFERENT, THERE IS NO SINGLE WAY TO KNOW WHERE OR HOW SOMEONE LIKES TO BE TOUCHED. A LOT OF THE FUN OF SEX IS LEARNING HOW TO GIVE YOUR PARTNER PLEASURE, AND IN THIS SCENARIO WE'LL SHOW YOU HOW TO FIND OUT WHERE AND HOW YOUR PARTNER LIKES TO BE TOUCHED.

KISS
SUCK
TOUCH
SEXPERATION
a sif game
©2008

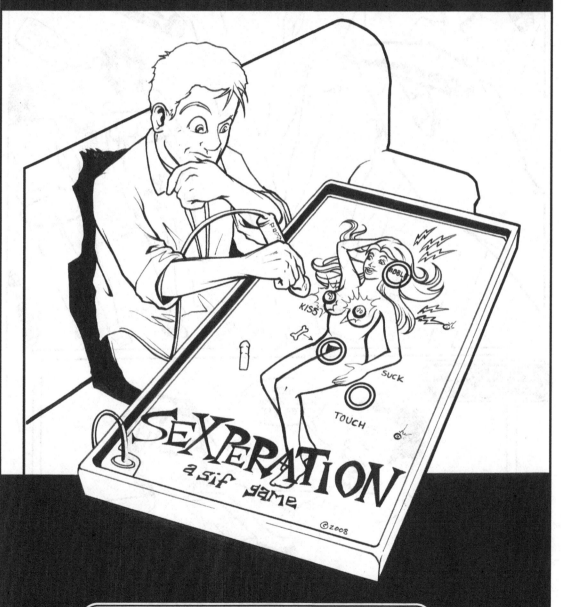

WE'LL SHOW YOU HOW . . .

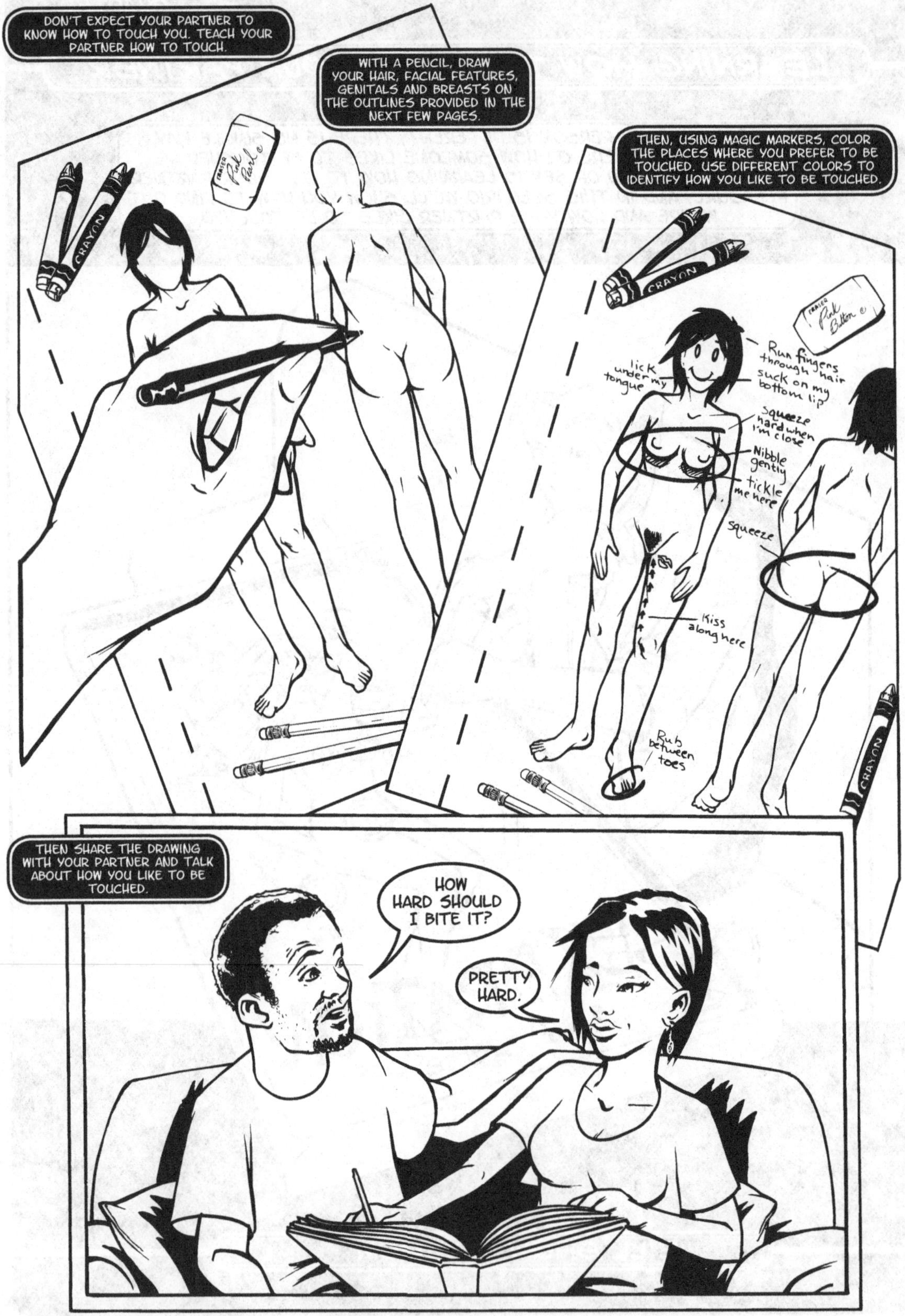
DON'T EXPECT YOUR PARTNER TO KNOW HOW TO TOUCH YOU. TEACH YOUR PARTNER HOW TO TOUCH.
WITH A PENCIL, DRAW YOUR HAIR, FACIAL FEATURES, GENITALS AND BREASTS ON THE OUTLINES PROVIDED IN THE NEXT FEW PAGES.
ERASER Pink Pearl
CRAYON
THEN, USING MAGIC MARKERS, COLOR THE PLACES WHERE YOU PREFER TO BE TOUCHED. USE DIFFERENT COLORS TO IDENTIFY HOW YOU LIKE TO BE TOUCHED.
CRAYON
ERASER Pink Button
Run fingers through hair
lick under my tongue
suck on my bottom lip
squeeze hard when I'm close
Nibble gently
tickle me here
squeeze
Kiss along here
Rub between toes
CRAYON
THEN SHARE THE DRAWING WITH YOUR PARTNER AND TALK ABOUT HOW YOU LIKE TO BE TOUCHED.
HOW HARD SHOULD I BITE IT?
PRETTY HARD.

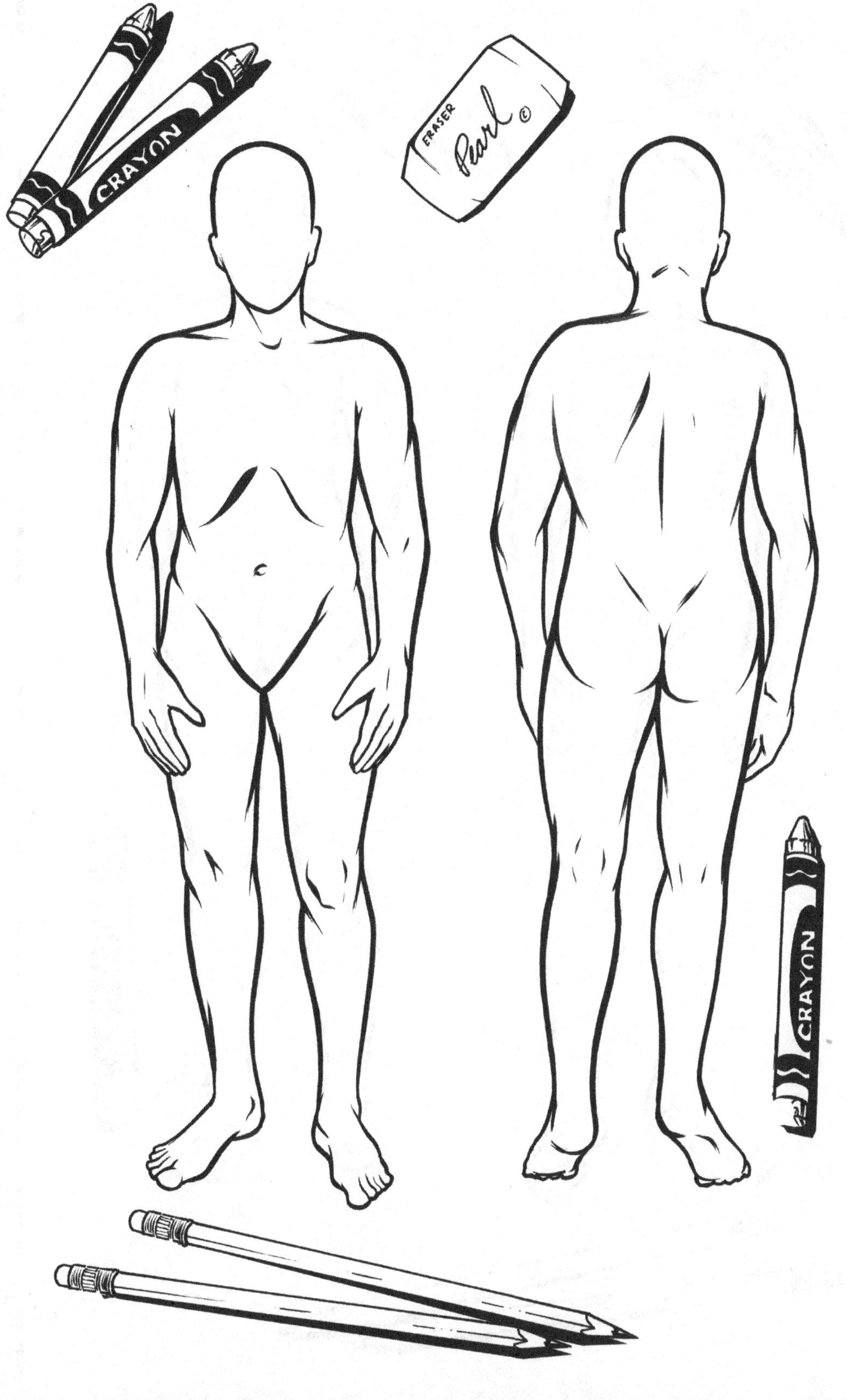
CRAYON
CRAYON
ERASER
Pearl
CRAYON

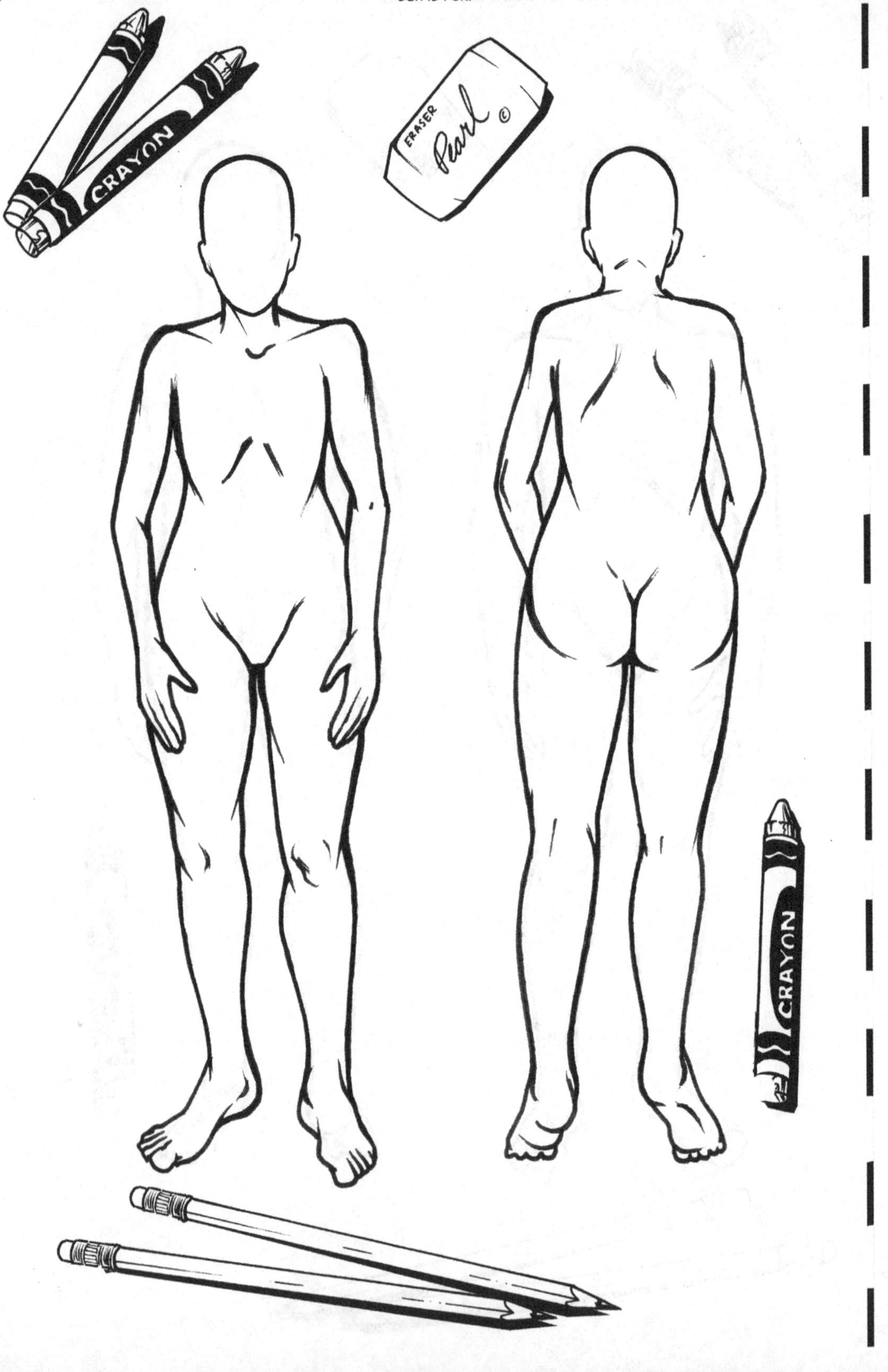
CRAYON
CRAYON
ERASER
Pearl ©
CRAYON

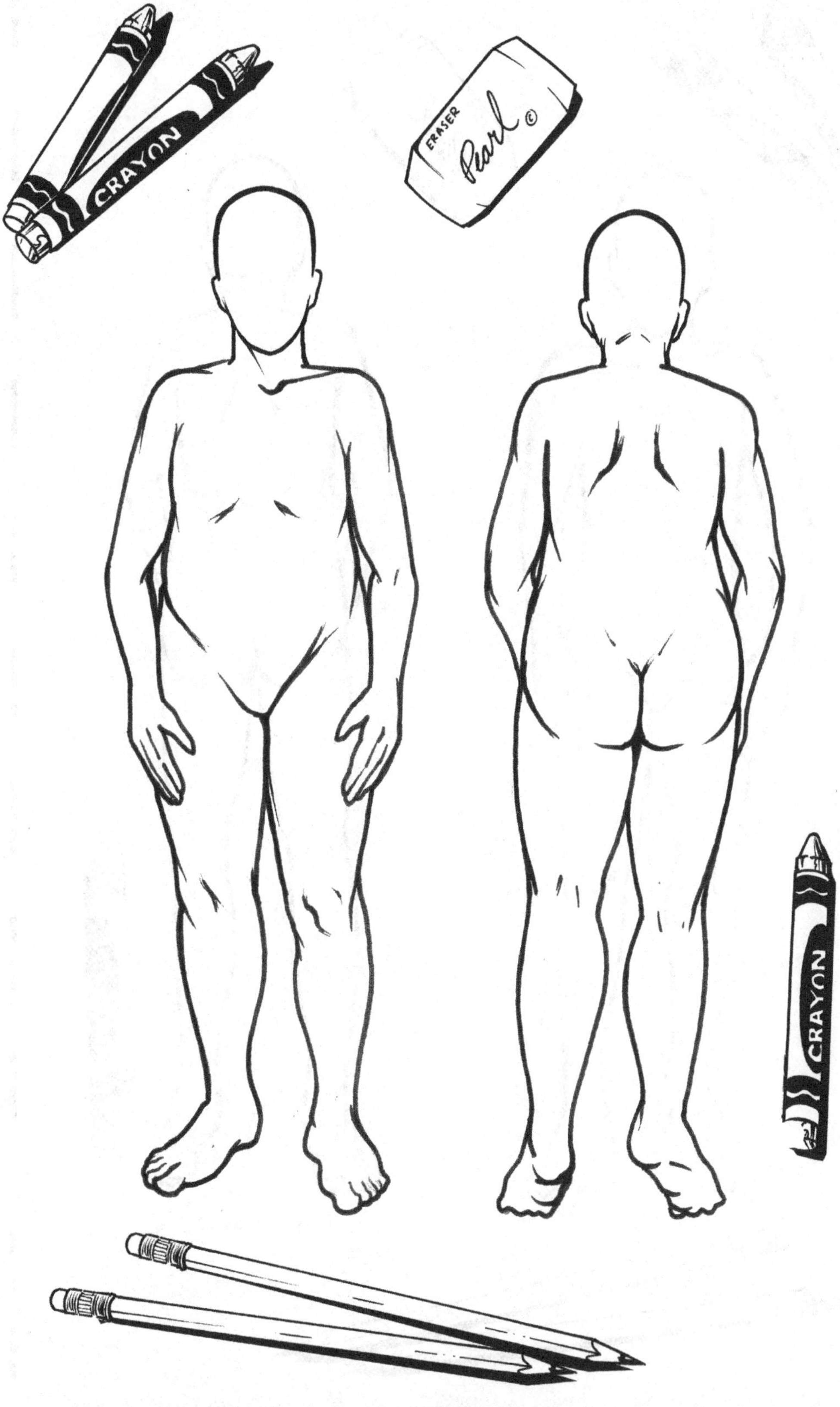
CRAYON
CRAYON
ERASER
Pearl ©
CRAYON

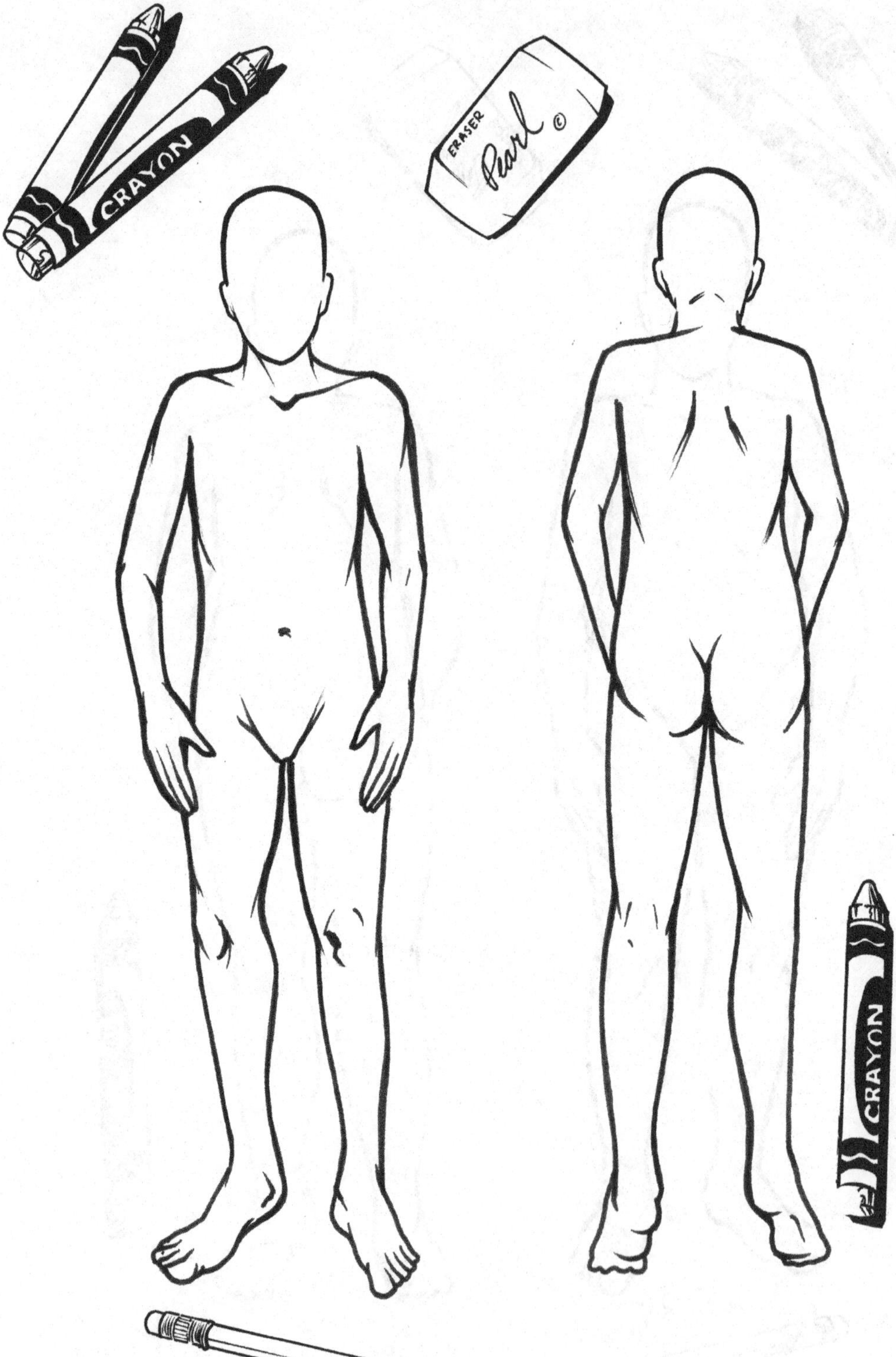
CRAYON
ERASER
Pearl
©
CRAYON

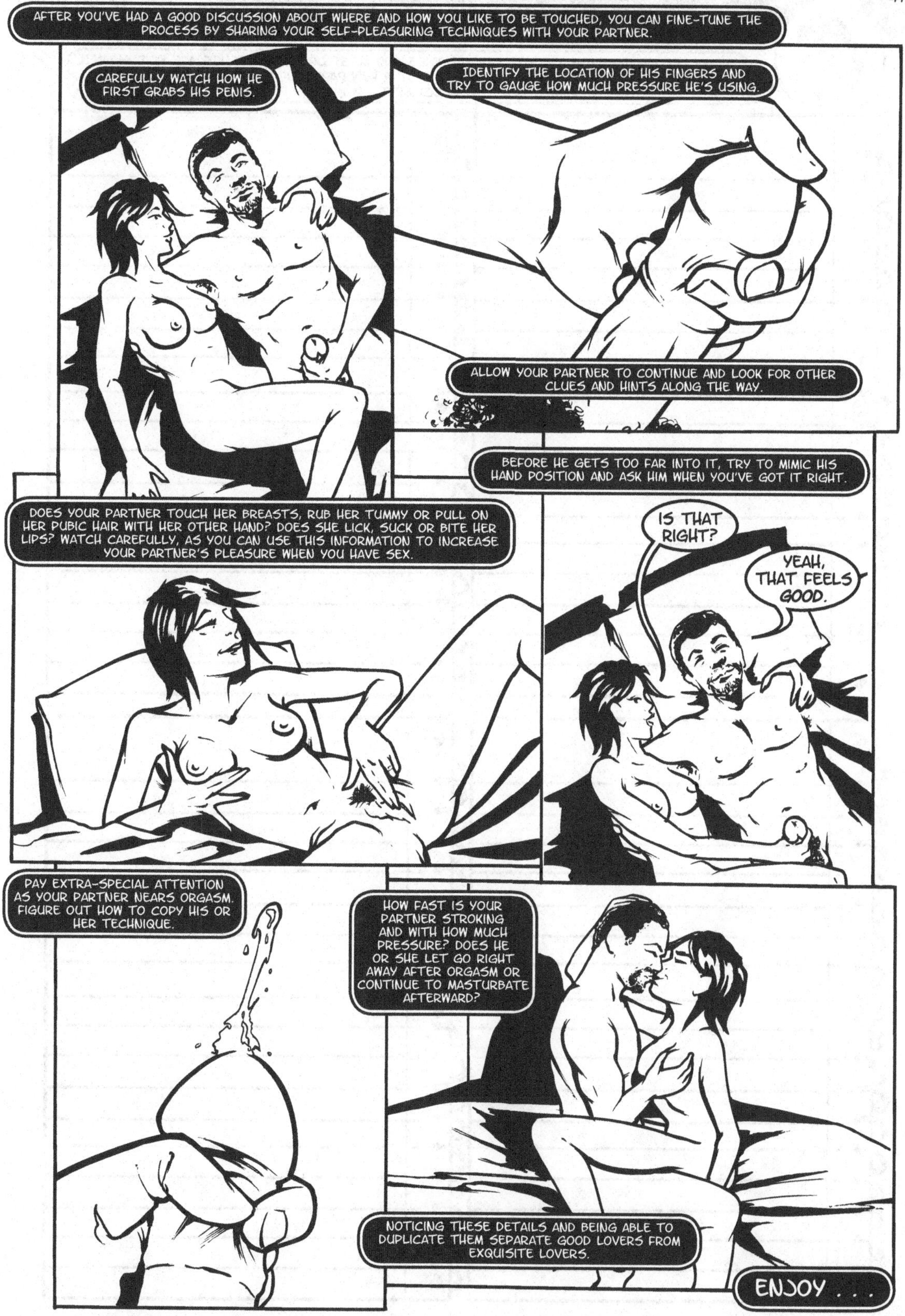
AFTER YOU'VE HAD A GOOD DISCUSSION ABOUT WHERE AND HOW YOU LIKE TO BE TOUCHED, YOU CAN FINE-TUNE THE PROCESS BY SHARING YOUR SELF-PLEASURING TECHNIQUES WITH YOUR PARTNER.
CAREFULLY WATCH HOW HE FIRST GRABS HIS PENIS.
IDENTIFY THE LOCATION OF HIS FINGERS AND TRY TO GAUGE HOW MUCH PRESSURE HE'S USING.
ALLOW YOUR PARTNER TO CONTINUE AND LOOK FOR OTHER CLUES AND HINTS ALONG THE WAY.
DOES YOUR PARTNER TOUCH HER BREASTS, RUB HER TUMMY OR PULL ON HER PUBIC HAIR WITH HER OTHER HAND? DOES SHE LICK, SUCK OR BITE HER LIPS? WATCH CAREFULLY, AS YOU CAN USE THIS INFORMATION TO INCREASE YOUR PARTNER'S PLEASURE WHEN YOU HAVE SEX.
BEFORE HE GETS TOO FAR INTO IT, TRY TO MIMIC HIS HAND POSITION AND ASK HIM WHEN YOU'VE GOT IT RIGHT.
IS THAT RIGHT?
YEAH, THAT FEELS GOOD.
PAY EXTRA-SPECIAL ATTENTION AS YOUR PARTNER NEARS ORGASM. FIGURE OUT HOW TO COPY HIS OR HER TECHNIQUE.
HOW FAST IS YOUR PARTNER STROKING AND WITH HOW MUCH PRESSURE? DOES HE OR SHE LET GO RIGHT AWAY AFTER ORGASM OR CONTINUE TO MASTURBATE AFTERWARD?
NOTICING THESE DETAILS AND BEING ABLE TO DUPLICATE THEM SEPARATE GOOD LOVERS FROM EXQUISITE LOVERS.
ENJOY . . .

BODY IMAGE

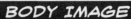

MOST PEOPLE HAVE ISSUES WITH THEIR BODIES AND MOST OF THESE ISSUES ARE NOT SHARED BY THEIR PARTNERS. IN THE SPACES BELOW, LIST A FEW PARTS OF YOUR PARTNER'S BODY THAT YOU ESPECIALLY LIKE AND DESCRIBE THEM IN ONLY POSITIVE TERMS.

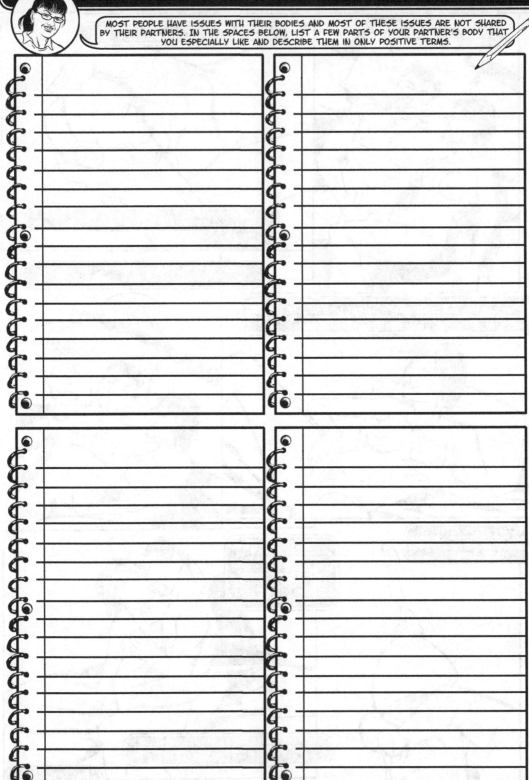

CHAPTER 10

FIFTEEN WAYS TO BE A GENEROUS LOVER
EVEN WHEN INTERCOURSE ISN'T AN OPTION

EVERYONE IS GOING TO EXPERIENCE AN EVENING WHEN YOUR PARTNER WANTS TO HAVE SEX BUT YOU CAN'T BECAUSE OF MEDICAL REASONS OR BECAUSE YOU AREN'T IN THE MOOD. THAT DOESN'T MEAN THAT YOU CAN'T HELP YOUR PARTNER OUT. IN THIS SCENARIO, WE'LL SHOW YOU FIFTEEN GREAT WAYS TO BE A GOOD, GIVING AND GENEROUS LOVER.

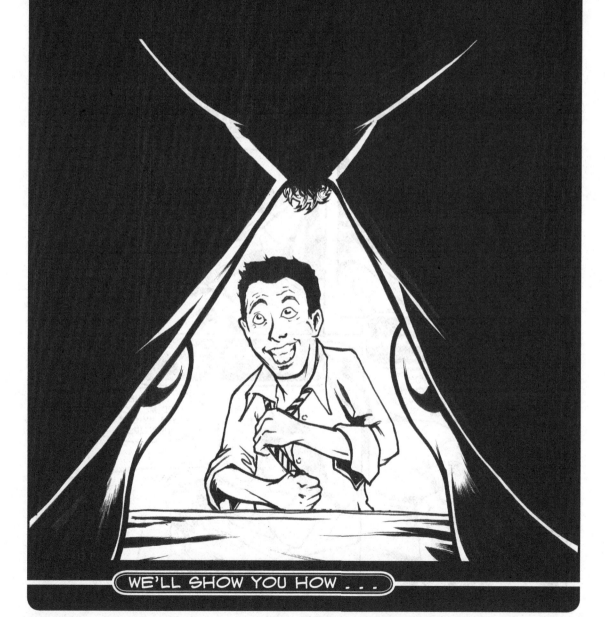

WE'LL SHOW YOU HOW . . .

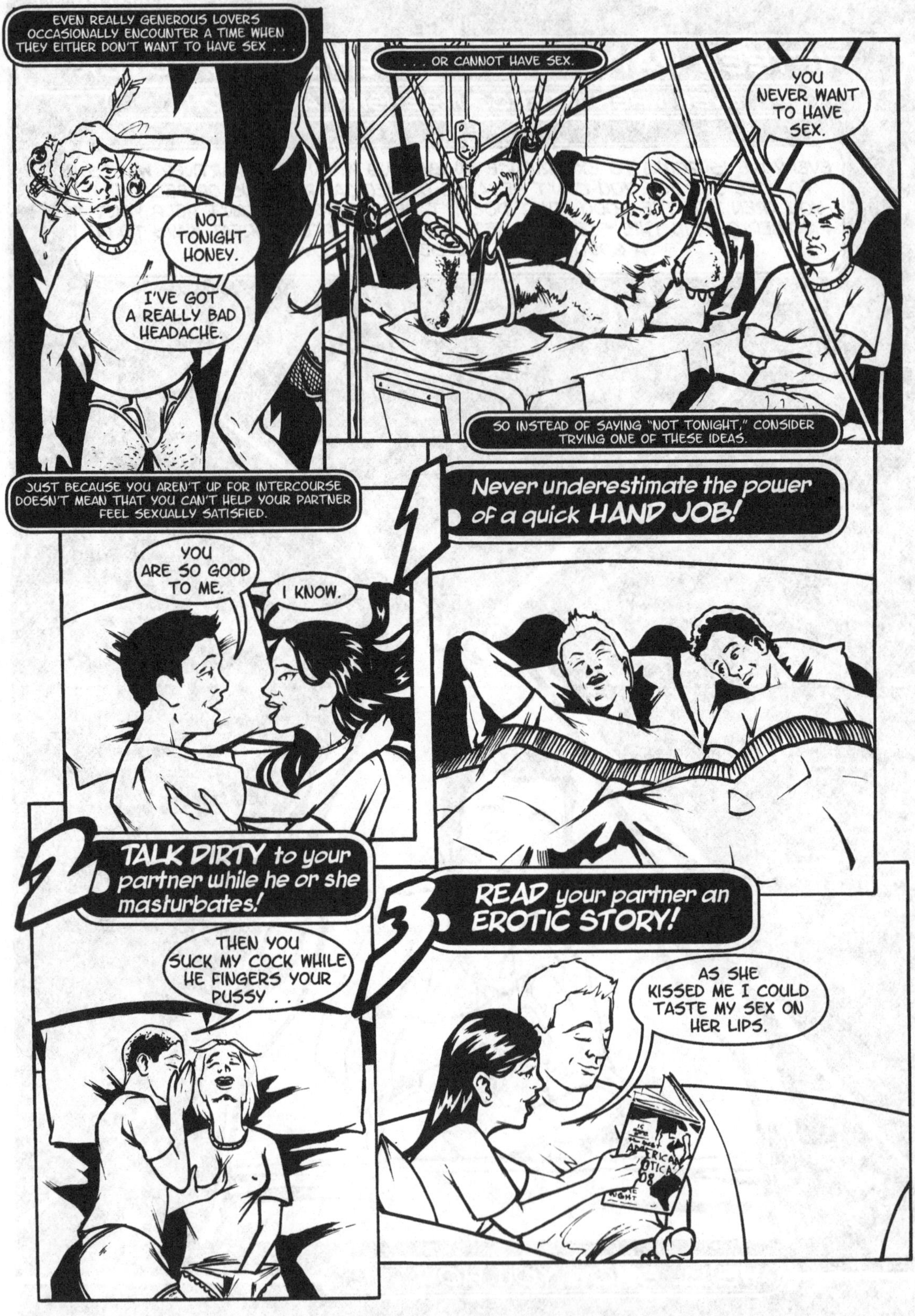
EVEN REALLY GENEROUS LOVERS OCCASIONALLY ENCOUNTER A TIME WHEN THEY EITHER DON'T WANT TO HAVE SEX . . .
NOT TONIGHT HONEY.
I'VE GOT A REALLY BAD HEADACHE.
. . . OR CANNOT HAVE SEX.
YOU NEVER WANT TO HAVE SEX.
SO INSTEAD OF SAYING "NOT TONIGHT," CONSIDER TRYING ONE OF THESE IDEAS.
JUST BECAUSE YOU AREN'T UP FOR INTERCOURSE DOESN'T MEAN THAT YOU CAN'T HELP YOUR PARTNER FEEL SEXUALLY SATISFIED.
1. Never underestimate the power of a quick HAND JOB!
YOU ARE SO GOOD TO ME.
I KNOW.
2. TALK DIRTY to your partner while he or she masturbates!
THEN YOU SUCK MY COCK WHILE HE FINGERS YOUR PUSSY . . .
3. READ your partner an EROTIC STORY!
AS SHE KISSED ME I COULD TASTE MY SEX ON HER LIPS.

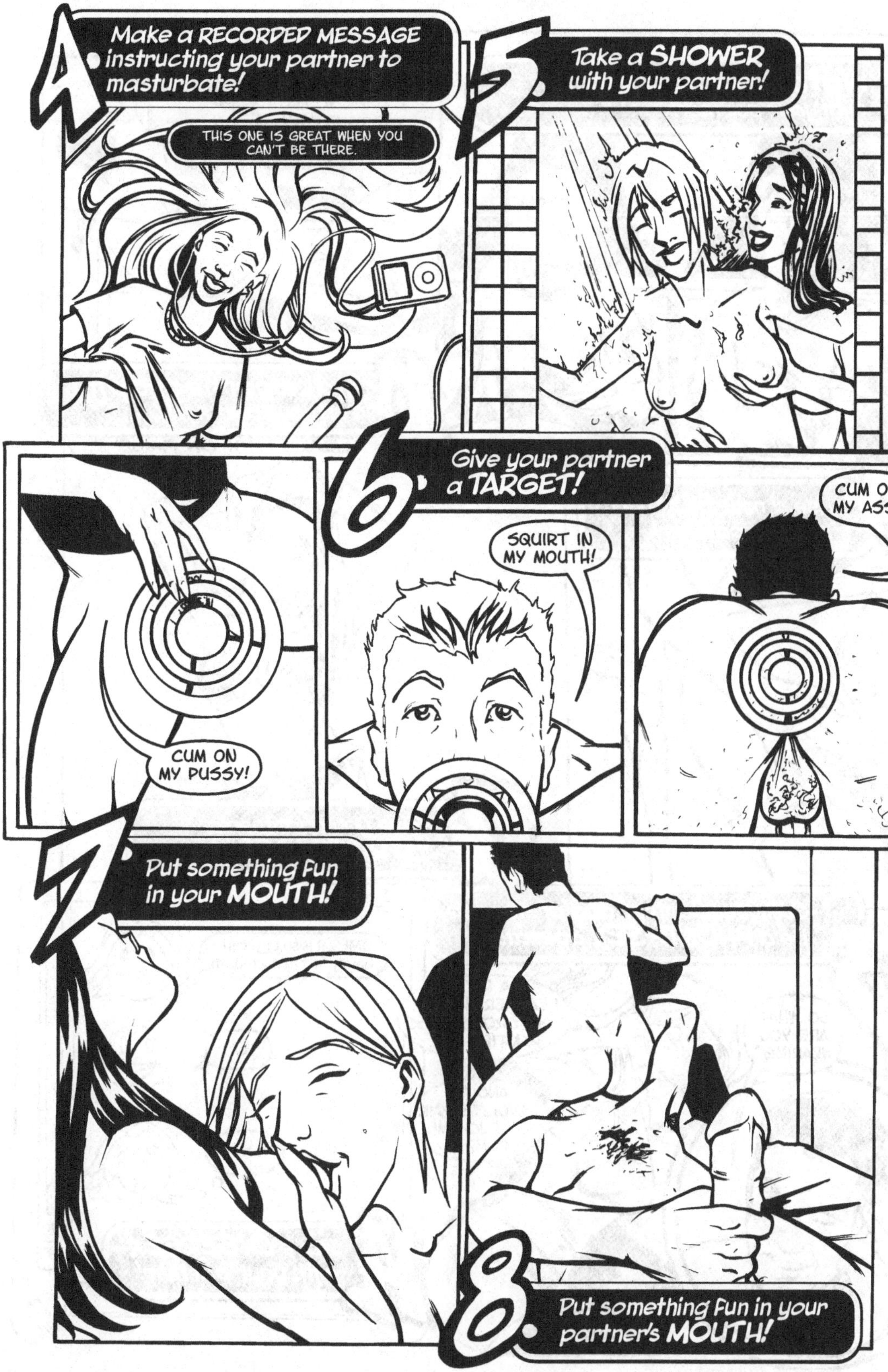
4. Make a RECORDED MESSAGE instructing your partner to masturbate!
THIS ONE IS GREAT WHEN YOU CAN'T BE THERE.
5. Take a SHOWER with your partner!
6. Give your partner a TARGET!
CUM ON MY PUSSY!
SQUIRT IN MY MOUTH!
CUM ON MY ASS!
7. Put something fun in your MOUTH!
8. Put something fun in your partner's MOUTH!

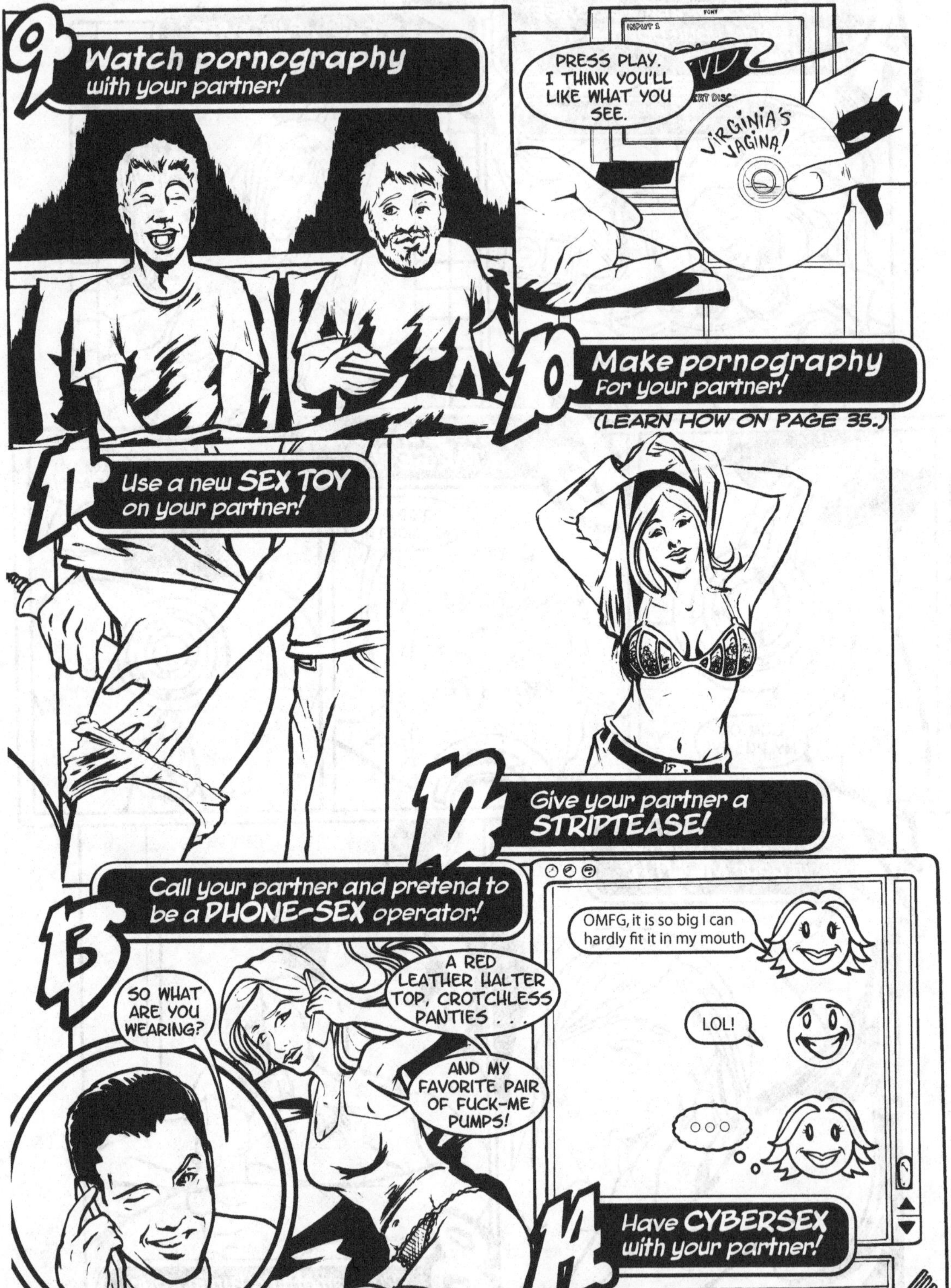
9
Watch pornography
with your partner!
PRESS PLAY. I THINK YOU'LL LIKE WHAT YOU SEE.
VIRGINIA'S VAGINA!
10
Make pornography
for your partner!
(LEARN HOW ON PAGE 35.)
11
Use a new SEX TOY
on your partner!
12
Give your partner a
STRIPTEASE!
13
Call your partner and pretend to
be a PHONE-SEX operator!
SO WHAT ARE YOU WEARING?
A RED LEATHER HALTER TOP, CROTCHLESS PANTIES . . .
AND MY FAVORITE PAIR OF FUCK-ME PUMPS!
OMFG, it is so big I can hardly fit it in my mouth
LOL!
OOO
14
Have CYBERSEX
with your partner!

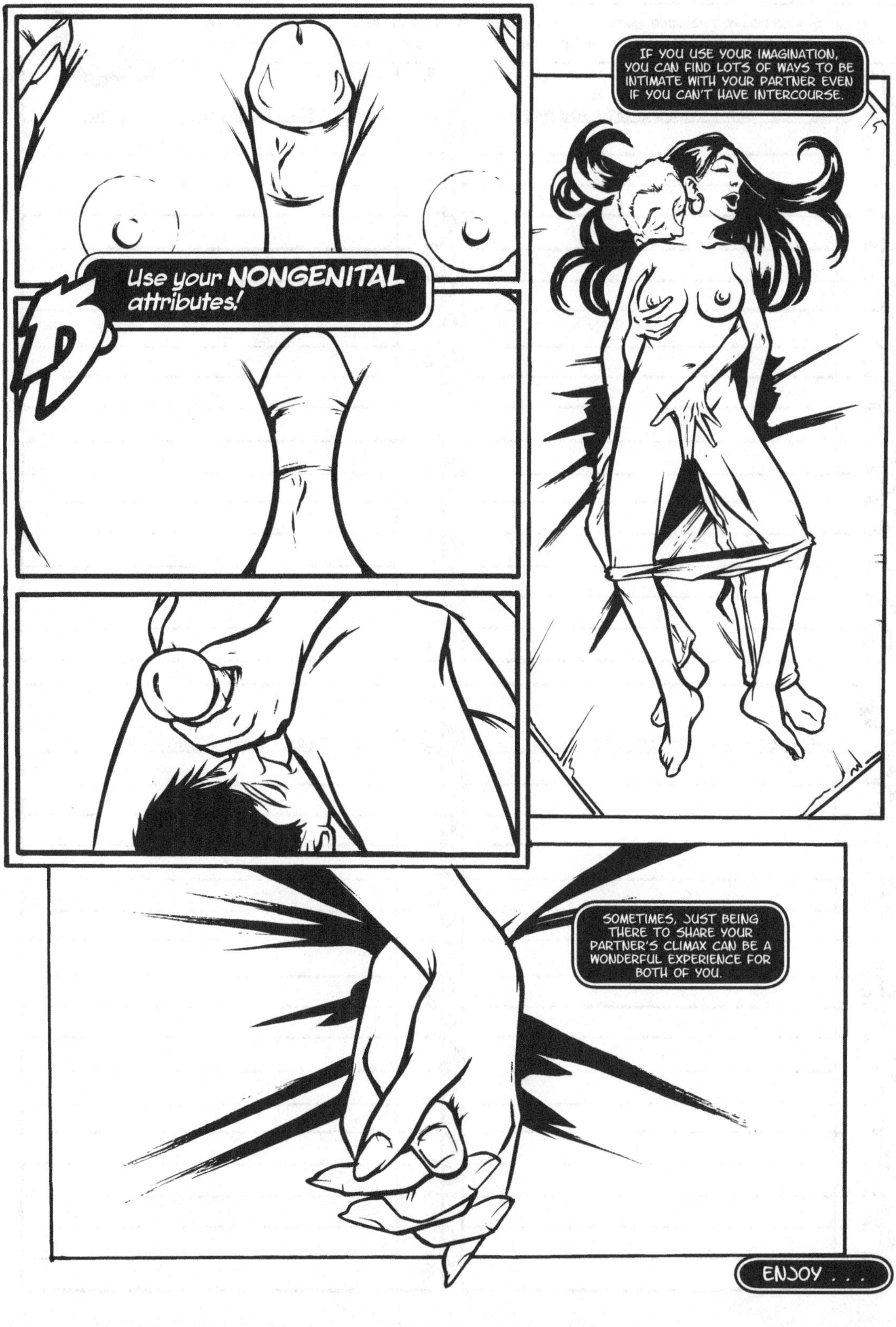
15
Use your NONGENITAL attributes!
IF YOU USE YOUR IMAGINATION, YOU CAN FIND LOTS OF WAYS TO BE INTIMATE WITH YOUR PARTNER EVEN IF YOU CAN'T HAVE INTERCOURSE.
SOMETIMES, JUST BEING THERE TO SHARE YOUR PARTNER'S CLIMAX CAN BE A WONDERFUL EXPERIENCE FOR BOTH OF YOU.
ENJOY . . .

MY FAVORITE SO FAR

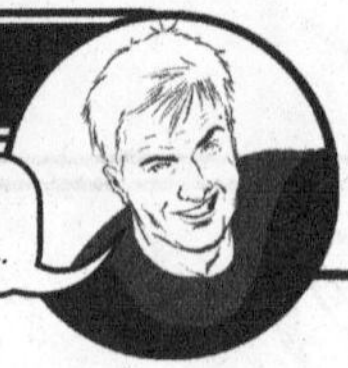

IN THE SPACES BELOW, TELL YOUR PARTNER(S) ABOUT THE BEST SEXUAL EXPERIENCE THAT YOU'VE HAD TOGETHER. REMIND YOUR PARTNER(S) ABOUT THE SITUATION AND TRY TO DESCRIBE WHY IT WAS SO ENJOYABLE.

THE BEST SEX I EVER HAD WITH YOU WAS . . .

THE BEST SEX I EVER HAD WITH YOU WAS . . .

THE BEST SEX I EVER HAD WITH YOU WAS . . .

THE BEST SEX I EVER HAD WITH YOU WAS . . .

CHAPTER 11

HOW TO GIVE AN EROTIC MASSAGE

EROTIC MASSAGE IS A GREAT WAY TO SELFLESSLY GIVE YOUR PARTNER PLEASURE AND PREPARE HIS OR HER BODY FOR SEX PLAY.

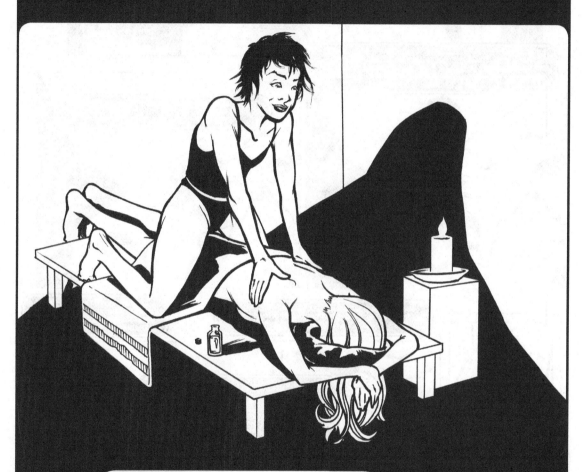

WHAT YOU'LL NEED . . .

LUBE AND MASSAGE OIL

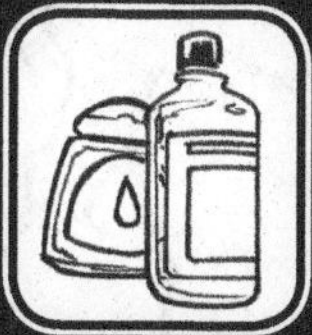

TOWELS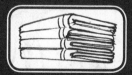

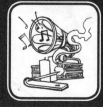 ITEMS TO HELP SET THE MOOD

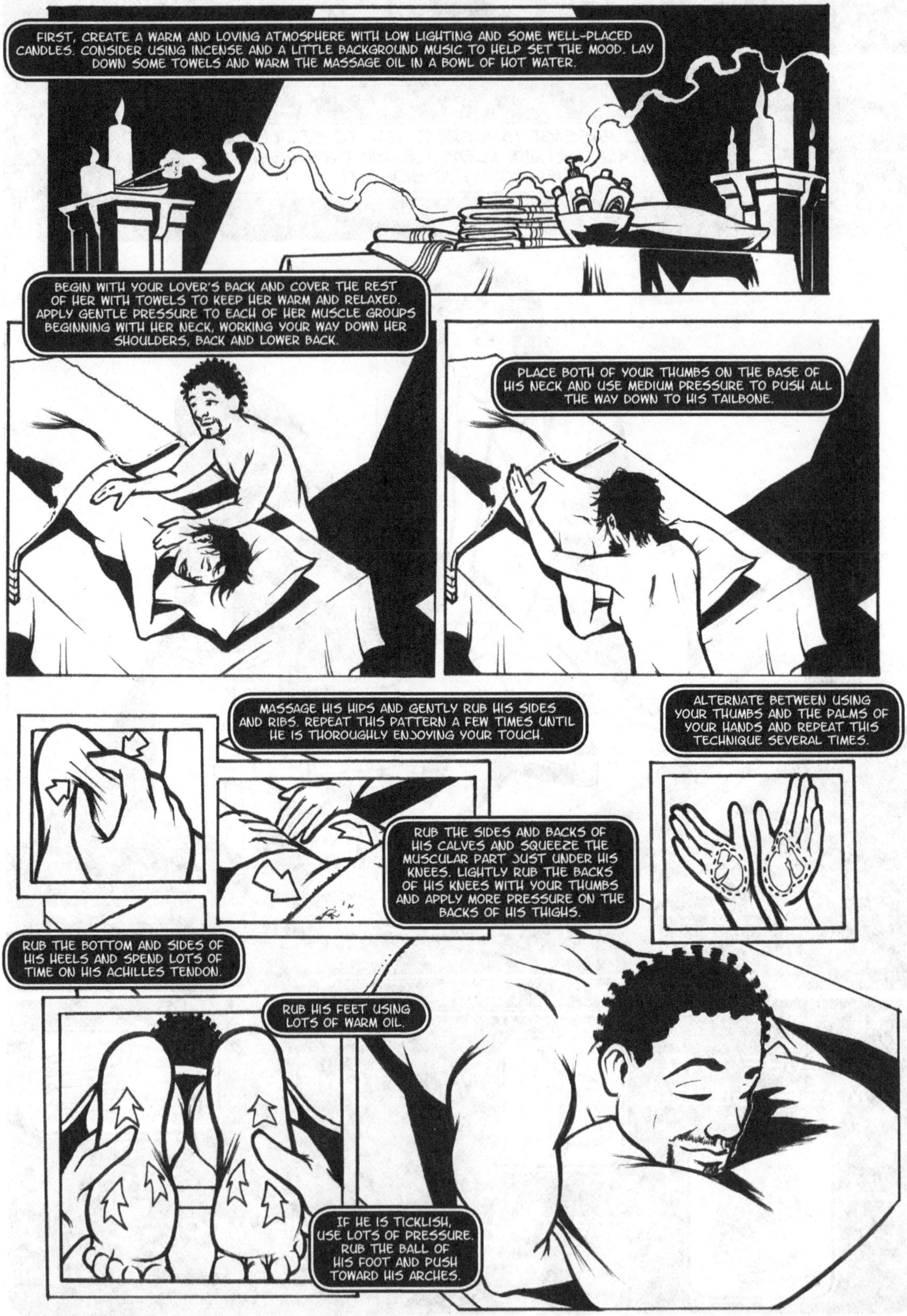
FIRST, CREATE A WARM AND LOVING ATMOSPHERE WITH LOW LIGHTING AND SOME WELL-PLACED CANDLES. CONSIDER USING INCENSE AND A LITTLE BACKGROUND MUSIC TO HELP SET THE MOOD. LAY DOWN SOME TOWELS AND WARM THE MASSAGE OIL IN A BOWL OF HOT WATER.
BEGIN WITH YOUR LOVER'S BACK AND COVER THE REST OF HER WITH TOWELS TO KEEP HER WARM AND RELAXED. APPLY GENTLE PRESSURE TO EACH OF HER MUSCLE GROUPS BEGINNING WITH HER NECK, WORKING YOUR WAY DOWN HER SHOULDERS, BACK AND LOWER BACK.
PLACE BOTH OF YOUR THUMBS ON THE BASE OF HIS NECK AND USE MEDIUM PRESSURE TO PUSH ALL THE WAY DOWN TO HIS TAILBONE.
MASSAGE HIS HIPS AND GENTLY RUB HIS SIDES AND RIBS. REPEAT THIS PATTERN A FEW TIMES UNTIL HE IS THOROUGHLY ENJOYING YOUR TOUCH.
ALTERNATE BETWEEN USING YOUR THUMBS AND THE PALMS OF YOUR HANDS AND REPEAT THIS TECHNIQUE SEVERAL TIMES.
RUB THE SIDES AND BACKS OF HIS CALVES AND SQUEEZE THE MUSCULAR PART JUST UNDER HIS KNEES. LIGHTLY RUB THE BACKS OF HIS KNEES WITH YOUR THUMBS AND APPLY MORE PRESSURE ON THE BACKS OF HIS THIGHS.
RUB THE BOTTOM AND SIDES OF HIS HEELS AND SPEND LOTS OF TIME ON HIS ACHILLES TENDON.
RUB HIS FEET USING LOTS OF WARM OIL.
IF HE IS TICKLISH, USE LOTS OF PRESSURE. RUB THE BALL OF HIS FOOT AND PUSH TOWARD HIS ARCHES.

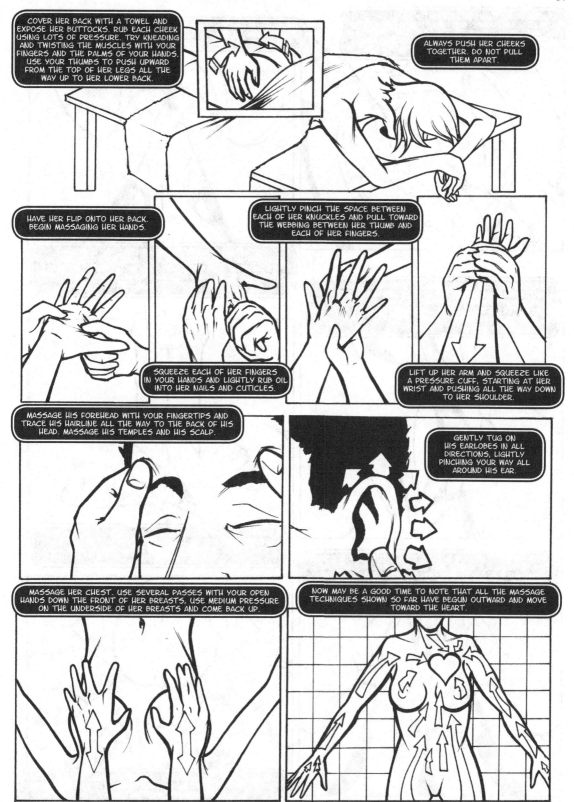

COVER HER BACK WITH A TOWEL AND EXPOSE HER BUTTOCKS. RUB EACH CHEEK USING LOTS OF PRESSURE. TRY KNEADING AND TWISTING THE MUSCLES WITH YOUR FINGERS AND THE PALMS OF YOUR HANDS. USE YOUR THUMBS TO PUSH UPWARD FROM THE TOP OF HER LEGS ALL THE WAY UP TO HER LOWER BACK.

ALWAYS PUSH HER CHEEKS TOGETHER. DO NOT PULL THEM APART.

HAVE HER FLIP ONTO HER BACK. BEGIN MASSAGING HER HANDS.

LIGHTLY PINCH THE SPACE BETWEEN EACH OF HER KNUCKLES AND PULL TOWARD THE WEBBING BETWEEN HER THUMB AND EACH OF HER FINGERS.

SQUEEZE EACH OF HER FINGERS IN YOUR HANDS AND LIGHTLY RUB OIL INTO HER NAILS AND CUTICLES.

LIFT UP HER ARM AND SQUEEZE LIKE A PRESSURE CUFF, STARTING AT HER WRIST AND PUSHING ALL THE WAY DOWN TO HER SHOULDER.

MASSAGE HIS FOREHEAD WITH YOUR FINGERTIPS AND TRACE HIS HAIRLINE ALL THE WAY TO THE BACK OF HIS HEAD. MASSAGE HIS TEMPLES AND HIS SCALP.

GENTLY TUG ON HIS EARLOBES IN ALL DIRECTIONS, LIGHTLY PINCHING YOUR WAY ALL AROUND HIS EAR.

MASSAGE HER CHEST. USE SEVERAL PASSES WITH YOUR OPEN HANDS DOWN THE FRONT OF HER BREASTS, USE MEDIUM PRESSURE ON THE UNDERSIDE OF HER BREASTS AND COME BACK UP.

NOW MAY BE A GOOD TIME TO NOTE THAT ALL THE MASSAGE TECHNIQUES SHOWN SO FAR HAVE BEGUN OUTWARD AND MOVE TOWARD THE HEART.

TOUCHING ONLY THE AREOLA, LIGHTLY PINCH THE SKIN BETWEEN YOUR THUMBS AND FOREFINGERS AND GENTLY PULL AWAY FROM THE NIPPLE. IMAGINE THAT THERE IS A CLOCK AROUND THE NIPPLE AND PINCH AT 12:00 & 6:00, 1:00 & 7:00, 2:00 & 8:00, 3:00 & 9:00 AND SO ON.

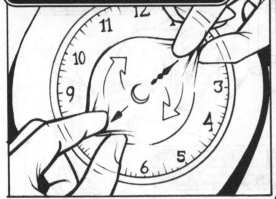

BEFORE YOU BEGIN MASSAGING YOUR PARTNER'S GENITALS, IT MAY BE WISE TO WASH THE MASSAGE OIL OFF OF YOUR HANDS AND SWITCH TO USING SILICONE-BASED LUBRICATION TO AVOID INFECTIONS.

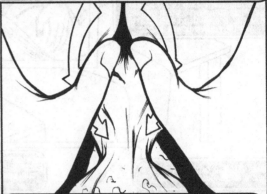

POSITION YOURSELF BETWEEN HIS LEGS AND GIVE HIM A PERINEUM MASSAGE. PLACE YOUR THUMBS ON EITHER SIDE OF HIS ANUS AND RUB ALL THE WAY UP TO THE BOTTOM OF HIS SCROTUM. USE AS MUCH PRESSURE AS HE FINDS COMFORTABLE AND REPEAT SEVERAL TIMES.

GENTLY PINCH HER OUTER LABIA BETWEEN YOUR THUMB AND FOREFINGERS. START AT THE BOTTOM AND WORK YOUR WAY TO THE TOP. AVOID TOUCHING HER CLITORIS AND ALTERNATE BETWEEN THE LEFT AND RIGHT LABIA SEVERAL TIMES. THEN DO THE SAME THING TO HER INNER LABIA BY GENTLY TUGGING THE FOLD OF SKIN OUTWARD.

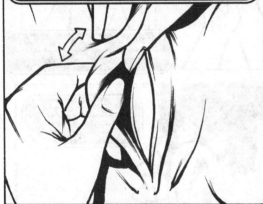

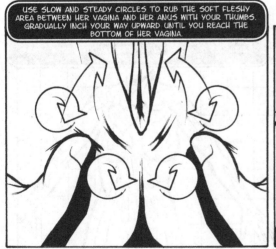

USE SLOW AND STEADY CIRCLES TO RUB THE SOFT FLESHY AREA BETWEEN HER VAGINA AND HER ANUS WITH YOUR THUMBS. GRADUALLY INCH YOUR WAY UPWARD UNTIL YOU REACH THE BOTTOM OF HER VAGINA.

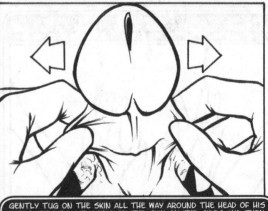

LIGHTLY PINCH THE CENTER OF HIS SCROTUM, AND SLOWLY WORK YOUR WAY UP THE MIDDLE UNTIL YOU REACH THE FORESKIN OF HIS PENIS. WORK YOUR WAY BACK DOWN AND REPEAT THIS SEVERAL TIMES.

STOP

GENTLY TUG ON THE SKIN ALL THE WAY AROUND THE HEAD OF HIS PENIS. START BY TUGGING ON THE SKIN ON THE SIDES AND THEN ON THE TOP AND THE BOTTOM.

USING ONLY YOUR FIRST TWO FINGERS, GENTLY RUB, USING SEVERAL DOWNWARD STROKES OVER YOUR PARTNER'S CLITORIS.

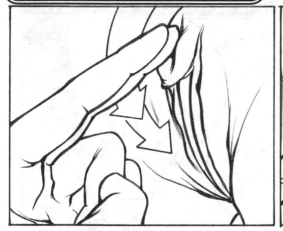

IF YOUR PARTNER IS NOT YET FULLY ERECT, MASSAGE HIS PERINEUM AND TESTICLES BY PRESSING THE PALM OF YOUR HAND FIRMLY INTO THE SOFT FLESHY AREA JUST ABOVE HIS ANUS AND PUSHING UPWARD TOWARD HIS PENIS. DO THIS FOR SEVERAL MINUTES OR UNTIL HE BECOMES ERECT.

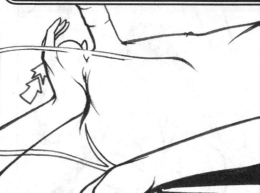

AFTER SPENDING SEVERAL MINUTES USING DOWNWARD STROKES, REVERSE THE MOTION AND GO UPWARD.

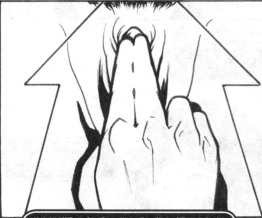

YOU MIGHT ALSO TRY SIDE-TO-SIDE STROKES AND MOVING IN CIRCLES.

PLACE ONE HAND AT THE BASE OF HIS SHAFT AND THE OTHER TOWARD THE TOP AND GENTLY ROTATE YOUR HANDS IN OPPOSITE DIRECTIONS.

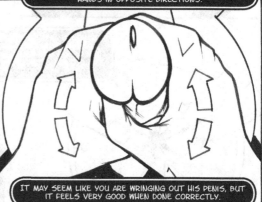

IT MAY SEEM LIKE YOU ARE WRINGING OUT HIS PENIS, BUT IT FEELS VERY GOOD WHEN DONE CORRECTLY.

REAPPLY LUBRICATION AND MASSAGE THE OPENING OF HER VAGINA WITH YOUR FINGERS. INSERT ONE OR TWO FINGERS SLOWLY AND PUSH UPWARD GENTLY.

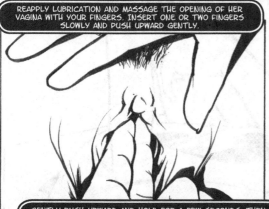

GENTLY PUSH UPWARD AND HOLD FOR A FEW SECONDS. THEN RELEASE WITHOUT PULLING BACK OUT. CONTINUE SEVERAL TIMES.

REAPPLY LOTS OF LUBRICATION AND PLACE YOUR FISTS ONE ON TOP OF THE OTHER AT THE TIP OF HIS PENIS. SLIDE YOUR FIST DOWNWARD TO THE BASE OF HIS SHAFT AND REPEAT THIS MOVEMENT WITH YOUR OTHER HAND. CONTINUE THIS MOTION SEVERAL TIMES.

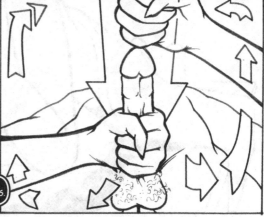

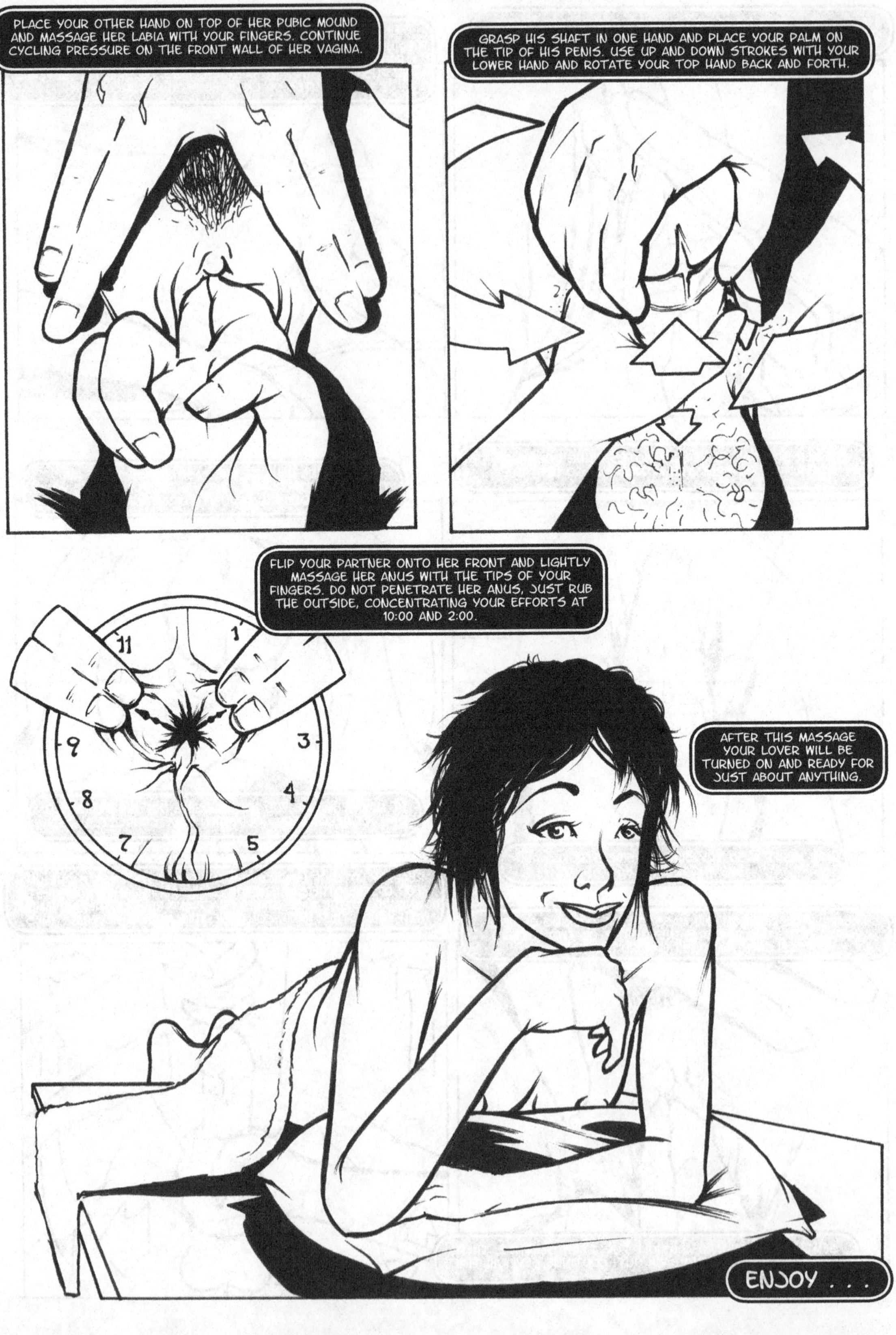
PLACE YOUR OTHER HAND ON TOP OF HER PUBIC MOUND AND MASSAGE HER LABIA WITH YOUR FINGERS. CONTINUE CYCLING PRESSURE ON THE FRONT WALL OF HER VAGINA.
GRASP HIS SHAFT IN ONE HAND AND PLACE YOUR PALM ON THE TIP OF HIS PENIS. USE UP AND DOWN STROKES WITH YOUR LOWER HAND AND ROTATE YOUR TOP HAND BACK AND FORTH.
FLIP YOUR PARTNER ONTO HER FRONT AND LIGHTLY MASSAGE HER ANUS WITH THE TIPS OF YOUR FINGERS. DO NOT PENETRATE HER ANUS, JUST RUB THE OUTSIDE, CONCENTRATING YOUR EFFORTS AT 10:00 AND 2:00.
AFTER THIS MASSAGE YOUR LOVER WILL BE TURNED ON AND READY FOR JUST ABOUT ANYTHING.
ENJOY . . .

CHAPTER 12

HOW TO FIND AND STIMULATE HER G-SPOT

EVER SINCE DR. ERNEST GRAFENBERG RELEASED HIS FINDING TO THE WORLD, THE G-SPOT HAS BEEN A TARGET OF GREAT INTEREST AND SKEPTICISM. IN THIS SCENARIO, WE'LL SHOW YOU HOW TO FIND THE G-SPOT AND PROPERLY STIMULATE IT FOR MAXIMUM PLEASURE.

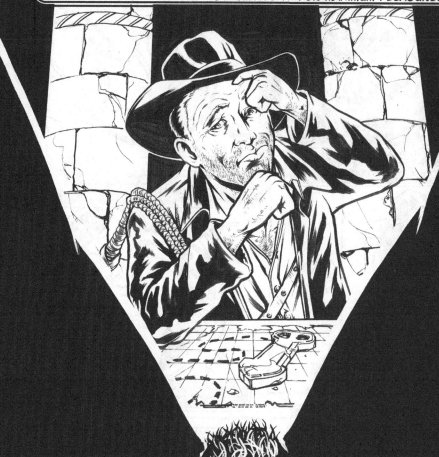

WHAT YOU'LL NEED . . .

LUBRICATION

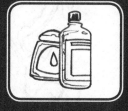

YOU MAY WISH TO TRY AN ANGLED G-SPOT-SEEKING TOY

WE HIGHLY RECOMMEND THAT YOU GIVE HER AN EROTIC MASSAGE AS DESCRIBED IN CHAPTER 11 TO RELAX HER BEFORE TRYING THIS SCENARIO.

THE G-SPOT IS A MASS OF ERECTILE TISSUE LOCATED IN THE FRONT WALL OF HER VAGINA.

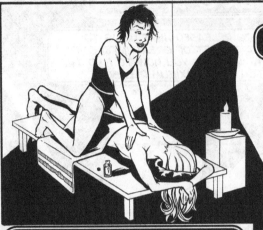

IT IS IMPORTANT TO REALIZE THAT THIS ERECTILE TISSUE MAY CHANGE ITS SIZE AND SHAPE DEPENDING ON A WOMAN'S AGE, STAGE OF HER MENSTRUAL CYCLE AND HER LEVEL OF AROUSAL.

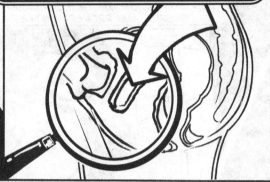

BECAUSE HER G-SPOT WILL BECOME ENGORGED AND PUT PRESSURE ON HER URETHRA AND BLADDER, MAKE SURE THAT SHE EMPTIES HER BLADDER BEFORE YOU BEGIN.

AS YOUR G-SPOT IS BEING STIMULATED, YOU MIGHT FEEL THE NEED TO URINATE. THIS FEELING IS CAUSED BY YOUR URETHRAL SPONGE BECOMING ENGORGED.

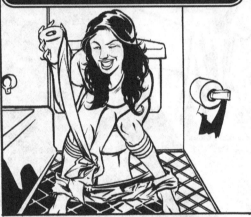

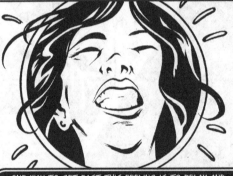

ONE WAY TO GET PAST THIS FEELING IS TO RELAX AND ACTUALLY TRY AND PEE. IF YOU JUST EMPTIED YOUR BLADDER BEFORE YOU BEGAN, YOU SHOULD HAVE LITTLE TO FEAR.

BEGINNING WITH HER ON HER BACK AND HER KNEES BENT, INSERT ONE OR TWO WELL-LUBRICATED FINGERS INTO HER VAGINA.

CURL YOUR FINGERS UPWARD IN A "COME HITHER" MOTION.

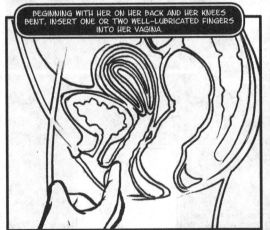

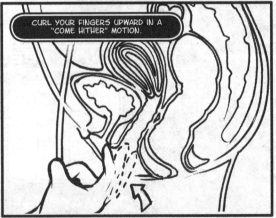

YOU MIGHT FEEL AN AREA THAT IS SWOLLEN OR TEXTURED DIFFERENTLY FROM THE REST OF HER VAGINA. IF YOU DO, YOU ARE PROBABLY ON THE RIGHT SPOT.

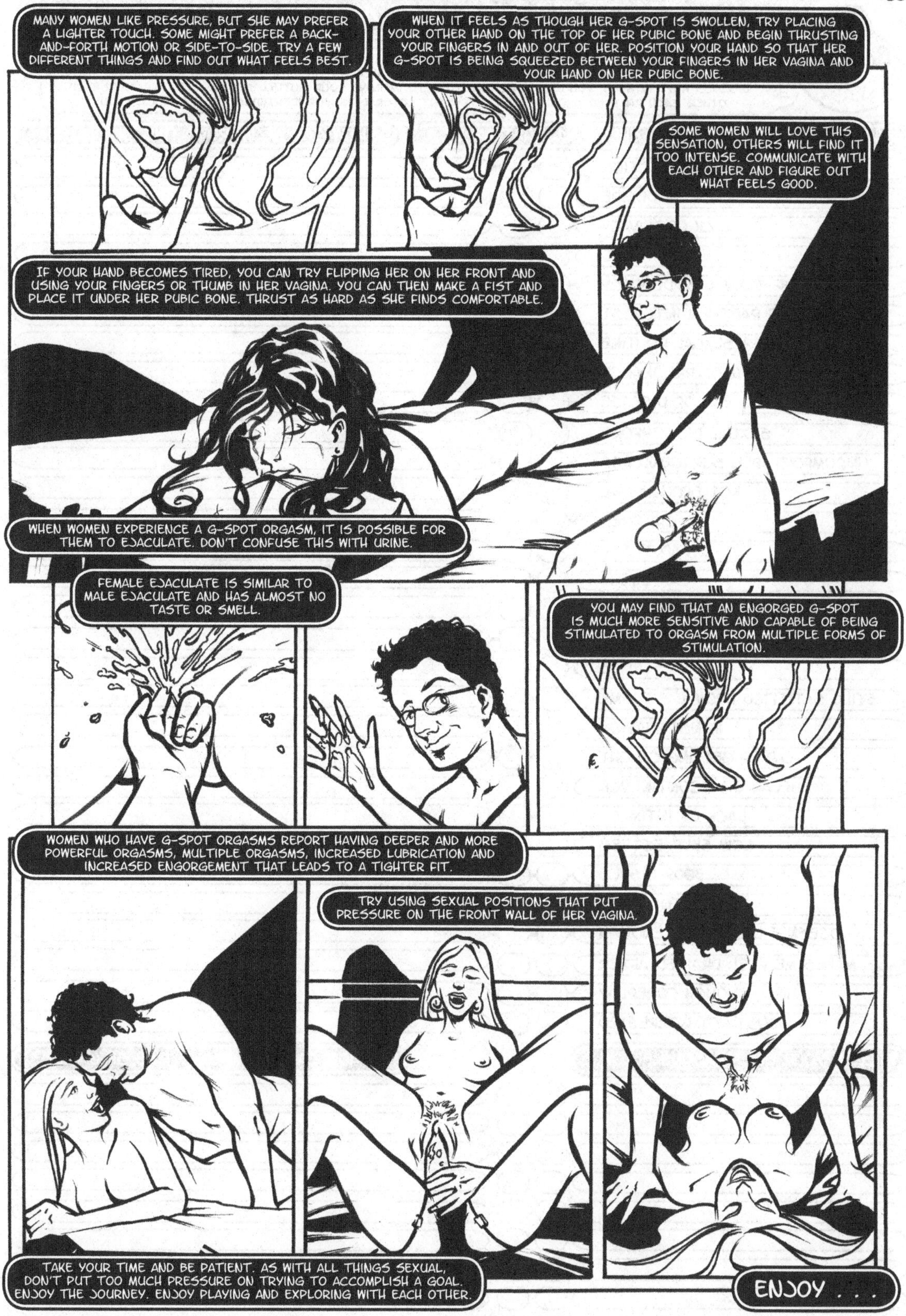
MANY WOMEN LIKE PRESSURE, BUT SHE MAY PREFER A LIGHTER TOUCH. SOME MIGHT PREFER A BACK-AND-FORTH MOTION OR SIDE-TO-SIDE. TRY A FEW DIFFERENT THINGS AND FIND OUT WHAT FEELS BEST.
WHEN IT FEELS AS THOUGH HER G-SPOT IS SWOLLEN, TRY PLACING YOUR OTHER HAND ON THE TOP OF HER PUBIC BONE AND BEGIN THRUSTING YOUR FINGERS IN AND OUT OF HER. POSITION YOUR HAND SO THAT HER G-SPOT IS BEING SQUEEZED BETWEEN YOUR FINGERS IN HER VAGINA AND YOUR HAND ON HER PUBIC BONE.
SOME WOMEN WILL LOVE THIS SENSATION, OTHERS WILL FIND IT TOO INTENSE. COMMUNICATE WITH EACH OTHER AND FIGURE OUT WHAT FEELS GOOD.
IF YOUR HAND BECOMES TIRED, YOU CAN TRY FLIPPING HER ON HER FRONT AND USING YOUR FINGERS OR THUMB IN HER VAGINA. YOU CAN THEN MAKE A FIST AND PLACE IT UNDER HER PUBIC BONE. THRUST AS HARD AS SHE FINDS COMFORTABLE.
WHEN WOMEN EXPERIENCE A G-SPOT ORGASM, IT IS POSSIBLE FOR THEM TO EJACULATE. DON'T CONFUSE THIS WITH URINE.
FEMALE EJACULATE IS SIMILAR TO MALE EJACULATE AND HAS ALMOST NO TASTE OR SMELL.
YOU MAY FIND THAT AN ENGORGED G-SPOT IS MUCH MORE SENSITIVE AND CAPABLE OF BEING STIMULATED TO ORGASM FROM MULTIPLE FORMS OF STIMULATION.
WOMEN WHO HAVE G-SPOT ORGASMS REPORT HAVING DEEPER AND MORE POWERFUL ORGASMS, MULTIPLE ORGASMS, INCREASED LUBRICATION AND INCREASED ENGORGEMENT THAT LEADS TO A TIGHTER FIT.
TRY USING SEXUAL POSITIONS THAT PUT PRESSURE ON THE FRONT WALL OF HER VAGINA.
TAKE YOUR TIME AND BE PATIENT. AS WITH ALL THINGS SEXUAL, DON'T PUT TOO MUCH PRESSURE ON TRYING TO ACCOMPLISH A GOAL. ENJOY THE JOURNEY. ENJOY PLAYING AND EXPLORING WITH EACH OTHER.
ENJOY . . .

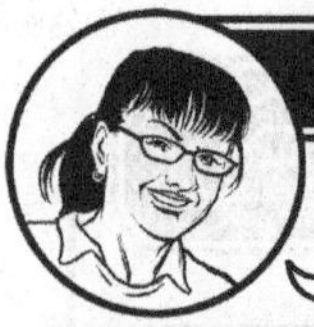

WHY DON'T WE HAVE MORE SEX?

INITIATING SEX CAN BE DIFFICULT FOR MANY PEOPLE. IT IS IMPORTANT TO IDENTIFY THE REASONS THAT KEEP YOU AND YOUR PARTNER(S) FROM INITIATING SEX WITH EACH OTHER. FILL IN THE FORM BELOW AND THEN DISCUSS WAYS IN WHICH YOU CAN WORK TOGETHER TO IMPROVE YOUR MUTUAL SEXUAL INITIATION WITH EACH OTHER. EACH PARTNER SHOULD USE A DIFFERENT COLORED INK FOR IDENTIFICATION AND DISCUSSION.

WHY DO I AVOID HAVING SEX? CHECK ALL THAT APPLY:			HOW CAN WE IMPROVE THIS SITUATION?
FEAR OF REJECTION			
LACK OF DESIRE			
LACK OF PRIVACY			
TOO TIRED			
FEAR OF SEXUAL INADEQUACY			
LACK OF PARTNER INTEREST			
BORING SEXUAL ROUTINE			
FEAR OF PREGNANCY			
FEAR OF DISEASE			
SEXUAL DISCOMFORT			
UNCOMFORTABLE SURROUNDINGS			
NOT ENOUGH TIME			
CHILDREN			
BAD TASTE			
BAD SMELL			
UNRESOLVED RESENTMENT			
TOO BUSY DOING OTHER THINGS			
STRESS			
STILL SATISFIED FROM LAST TIME			
MENSTRUATION			
FEAR OF GETTING CAUGHT			
FEAR OF INCONTINENCE			
LACK OF INTIMACY			
LOW SELF-ESTEEM			
BODY ISSUES			
TAKES TOO LONG			
DOESN'T LAST LONG ENOUGH			
MAKES ME FEEL DRAINED AFTER			
NOT ENOUGH FOREPLAY			
JUST NOT INTERESTED			

FILL IN YOUR OWN REASONS BELOW.			HOW CAN WE IMPROVE THIS SITUATION?

CHAPTER 13

HOW TO FIND AND STIMULATE HIS PROSTATE GLAND

BURIED JUST BEHIND HIS PENIS IS A MAGICAL WALNUT-SHAPED GLAND CALLED THE PROSTATE. IF YOU WANT TO AND, MORE IMPORTANT, IF HE WANTS YOU TO, YOU CAN HELP HIM HAVE LONGER AND MORE POWERFUL ORGASMS BY STIMULATING HIS PROSTATE GLAND FOR HIM.

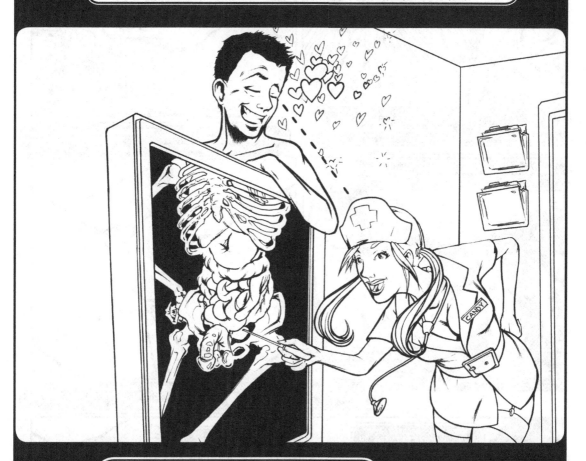

WHAT YOU'LL NEED . . .

LUBRICATION

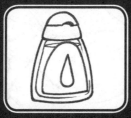

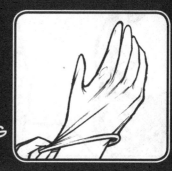

EXAM GLOVES

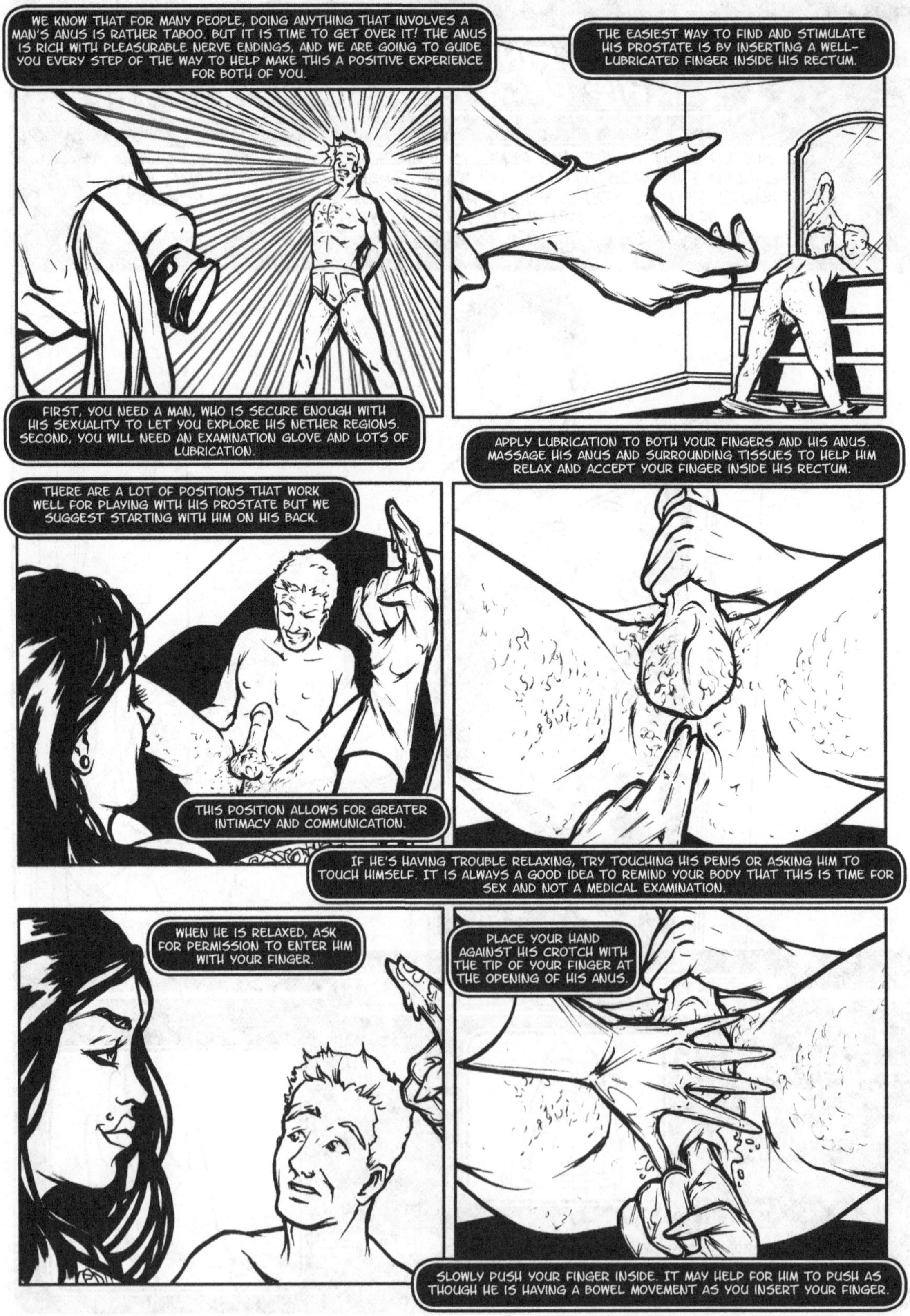
WE KNOW THAT FOR MANY PEOPLE, DOING ANYTHING THAT INVOLVES A MAN'S ANUS IS RATHER TABOO. BUT IT IS TIME TO GET OVER IT! THE ANUS IS RICH WITH PLEASURABLE NERVE ENDINGS, AND WE ARE GOING TO GUIDE YOU EVERY STEP OF THE WAY TO HELP MAKE THIS A POSITIVE EXPERIENCE FOR BOTH OF YOU.
FIRST, YOU NEED A MAN, WHO IS SECURE ENOUGH WITH HIS SEXUALITY TO LET YOU EXPLORE HIS NETHER REGIONS. SECOND, YOU WILL NEED AN EXAMINATION GLOVE AND LOTS OF LUBRICATION.
THE EASIEST WAY TO FIND AND STIMULATE HIS PROSTATE IS BY INSERTING A WELL-LUBRICATED FINGER INSIDE HIS RECTUM.
THERE ARE A LOT OF POSITIONS THAT WORK WELL FOR PLAYING WITH HIS PROSTATE BUT WE SUGGEST STARTING WITH HIM ON HIS BACK.
THIS POSITION ALLOWS FOR GREATER INTIMACY AND COMMUNICATION.
APPLY LUBRICATION TO BOTH YOUR FINGERS AND HIS ANUS. MASSAGE HIS ANUS AND SURROUNDING TISSUES TO HELP HIM RELAX AND ACCEPT YOUR FINGER INSIDE HIS RECTUM.
IF HE'S HAVING TROUBLE RELAXING, TRY TOUCHING HIS PENIS OR ASKING HIM TO TOUCH HIMSELF. IT IS ALWAYS A GOOD IDEA TO REMIND YOUR BODY THAT THIS IS TIME FOR SEX AND NOT A MEDICAL EXAMINATION.
WHEN HE IS RELAXED, ASK FOR PERMISSION TO ENTER HIM WITH YOUR FINGER.
PLACE YOUR HAND AGAINST HIS CROTCH WITH THE TIP OF YOUR FINGER AT THE OPENING OF HIS ANUS.
SLOWLY PUSH YOUR FINGER INSIDE. IT MAY HELP FOR HIM TO PUSH AS THOUGH HE IS HAVING A BOWEL MOVEMENT AS YOU INSERT YOUR FINGER.

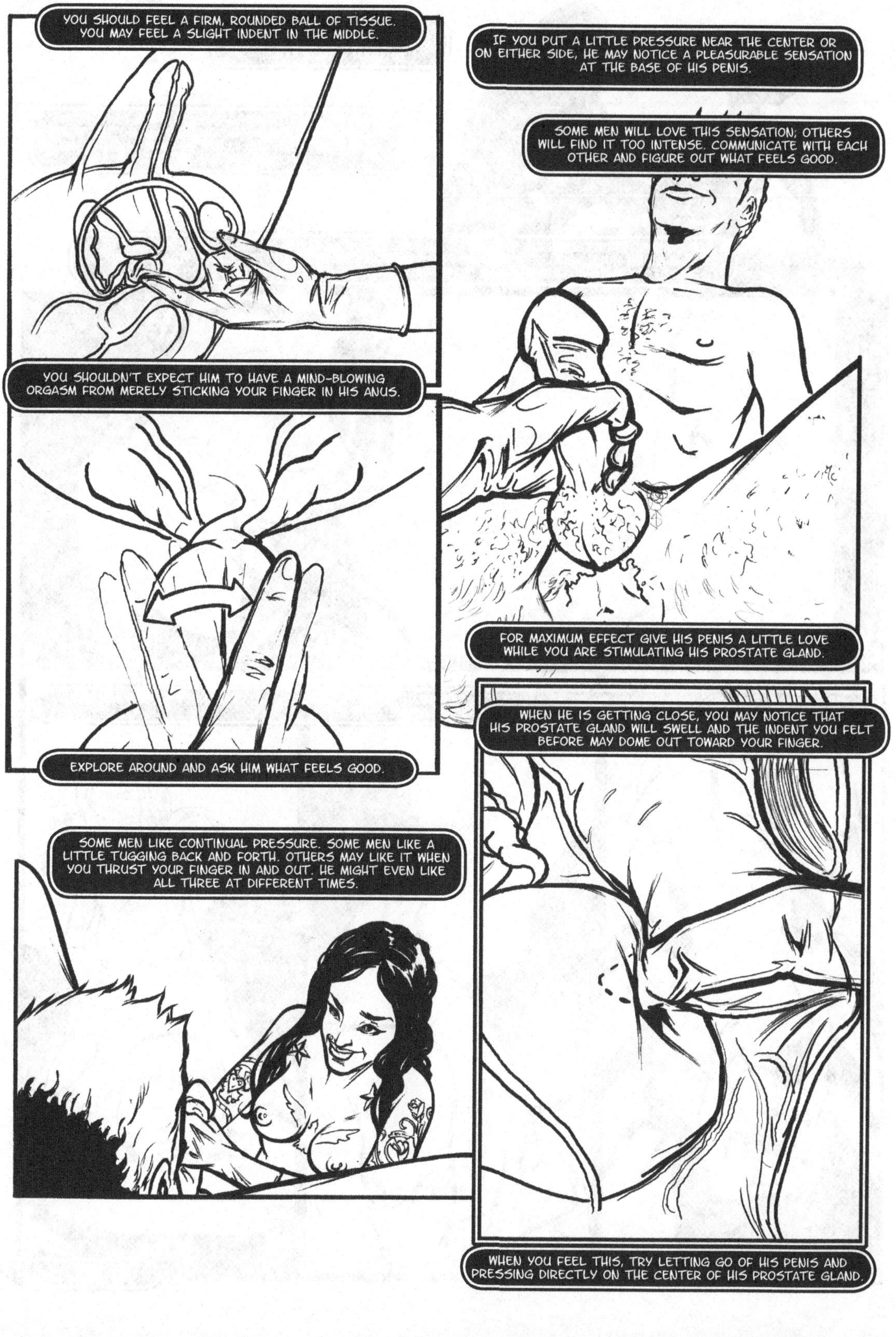
YOU SHOULD FEEL A FIRM, ROUNDED BALL OF TISSUE. YOU MAY FEEL A SLIGHT INDENT IN THE MIDDLE.
IF YOU PUT A LITTLE PRESSURE NEAR THE CENTER OR ON EITHER SIDE, HE MAY NOTICE A PLEASURABLE SENSATION AT THE BASE OF HIS PENIS.
SOME MEN WILL LOVE THIS SENSATION; OTHERS WILL FIND IT TOO INTENSE. COMMUNICATE WITH EACH OTHER AND FIGURE OUT WHAT FEELS GOOD.
YOU SHOULDN'T EXPECT HIM TO HAVE A MIND-BLOWING ORGASM FROM MERELY STICKING YOUR FINGER IN HIS ANUS.
EXPLORE AROUND AND ASK HIM WHAT FEELS GOOD.
FOR MAXIMUM EFFECT GIVE HIS PENIS A LITTLE LOVE WHILE YOU ARE STIMULATING HIS PROSTATE GLAND.
SOME MEN LIKE CONTINUAL PRESSURE. SOME MEN LIKE A LITTLE TUGGING BACK AND FORTH. OTHERS MAY LIKE IT WHEN YOU THRUST YOUR FINGER IN AND OUT. HE MIGHT EVEN LIKE ALL THREE AT DIFFERENT TIMES.
WHEN HE IS GETTING CLOSE, YOU MAY NOTICE THAT HIS PROSTATE GLAND WILL SWELL AND THE INDENT YOU FELT BEFORE MAY DOME OUT TOWARD YOUR FINGER.
WHEN YOU FEEL THIS, TRY LETTING GO OF HIS PENIS AND PRESSING DIRECTLY ON THE CENTER OF HIS PROSTATE GLAND.

WITH SOME PRACTICE, HE MAY BE CAPABLE OF HAVING AN ORGASM WITHOUT EJACULATING.

A NONEJACULATORY ORGASM WILL FEEL AS GOOD AS OR BETTER THAN HAVING AN ORGASM, BUT HE WILL REMAIN AROUSED AND READY TO HAVE ANOTHER AND POSSIBLY EVEN ANOTHER.

OF COURSE, THIS TECHNIQUE IS MORE OF AN ART THAN A SCIENCE, AND HE MIGHT EVEN FIND IT QUITE JARRING WHEN YOU LET GO OF HIS PENIS RIGHT AS HE IS ABOUT TO CLIMAX. YOU ARE IN NEW TERRITORY AND YOU'LL BOTH HAVE TO FIGURE OUT WHAT WORKS BEST WHILE YOU ARE HERE.

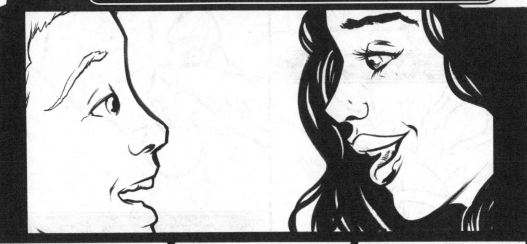

TRY SOME DIFFERENT POSITIONS AND DISCOVER ALL OF THE DIFFERENT WAYS THE TWO OF YOU CAN ENJOY THIS WONDERFUL SOURCE OF PLEASURE.

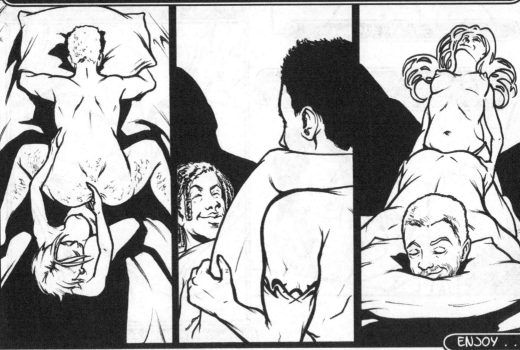

ENJOY . . .

CHAPTER 14

GETTING CAUGHT

MASTURBATION IS OFTEN THOUGHT OF AS AN ACT THAT
YOU PERFORM WITH NINJALIKE STEALTH SO THAT YOU
WON'T FACE THE EMBARRASSMENT OF GETTING CAUGHT.
BUT HAVE YOU EVER CONSIDERED HOW MUCH FUN IT WOULD
BE FOR YOUR PARTNER TO DISCOVER YOU?

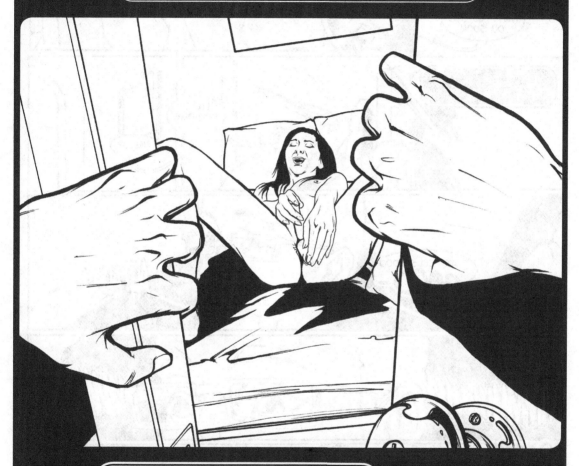

WHAT YOU'LL NEED . . .

LUBRICATION

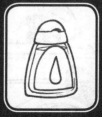

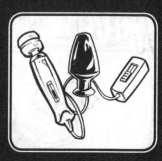

FAVORITE SEX TOY

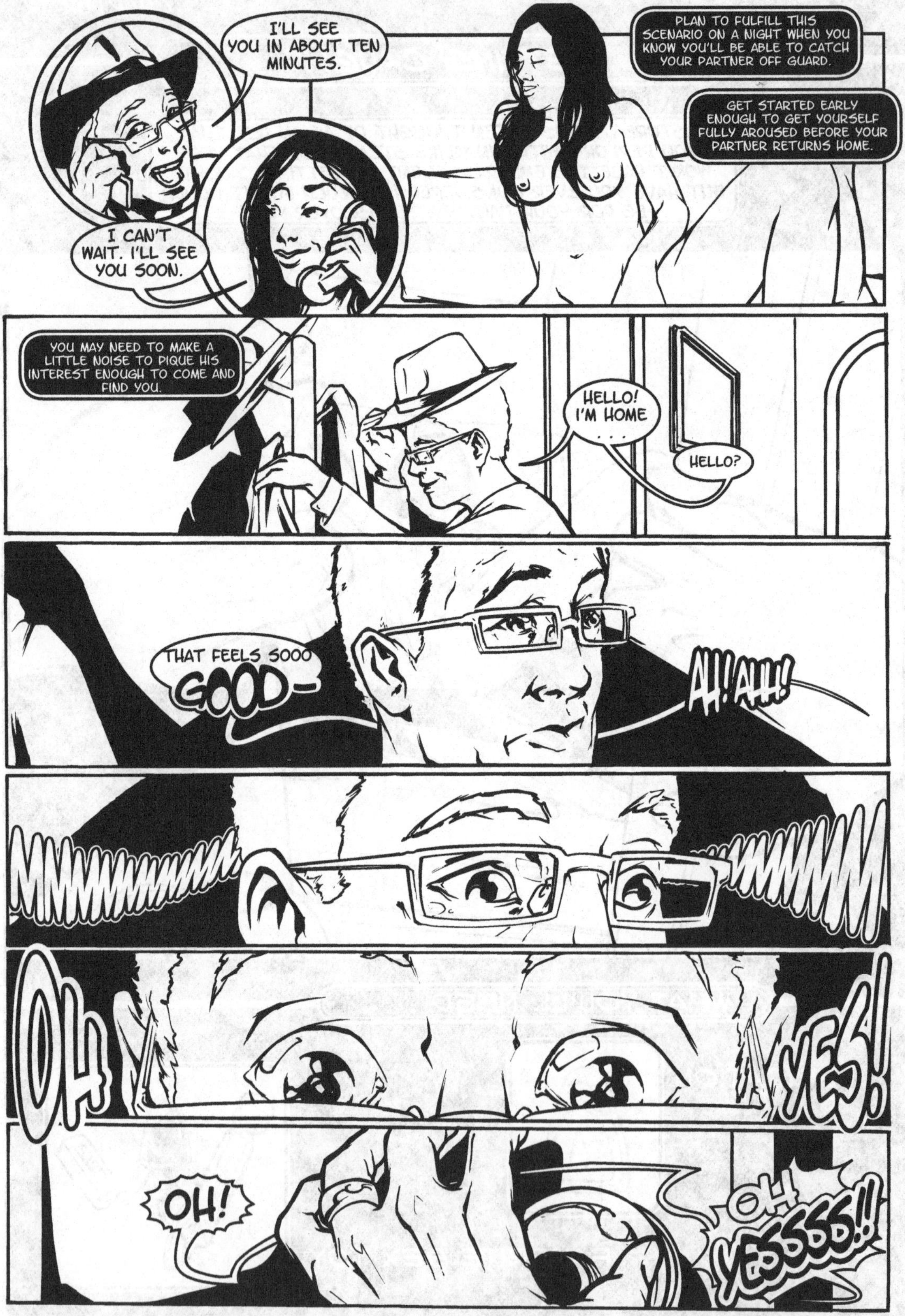
I'LL SEE YOU IN ABOUT TEN MINUTES.
I CAN'T WAIT. I'LL SEE YOU SOON.
PLAN TO FULFILL THIS SCENARIO ON A NIGHT WHEN YOU KNOW YOU'LL BE ABLE TO CATCH YOUR PARTNER OFF GUARD.
GET STARTED EARLY ENOUGH TO GET YOURSELF FULLY AROUSED BEFORE YOUR PARTNER RETURNS HOME.
YOU MAY NEED TO MAKE A LITTLE NOISE TO PIQUE HIS INTEREST ENOUGH TO COME AND FIND YOU.
HELLO! I'M HOME . . .
HELLO?
THAT FEELS SOOO GOOD-
AH! AHH!
MMMMMMMMMMM
MMMMMMMMMMM
OH
YES!
OH!
OH YESSSS!!

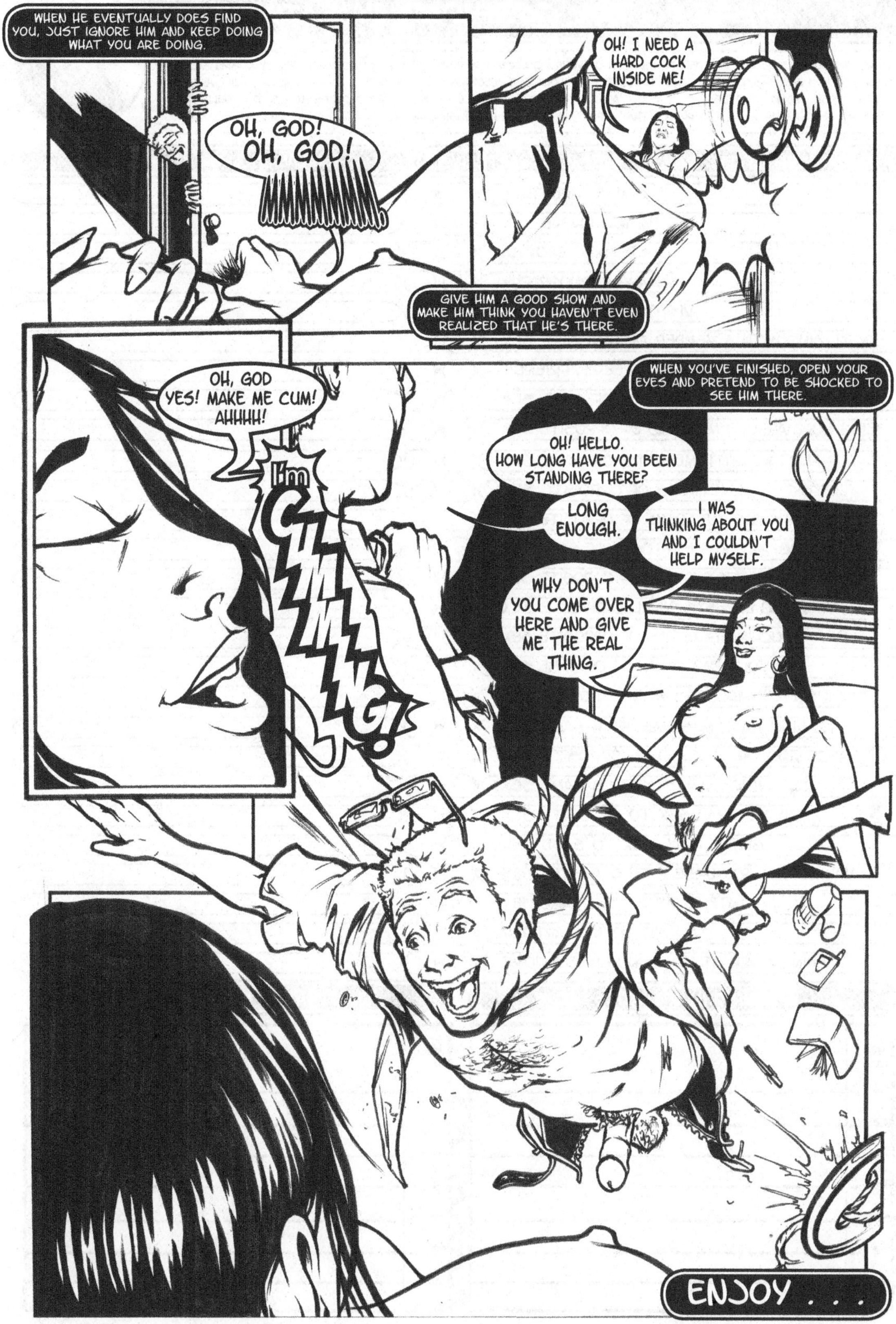
WHEN HE EVENTUALLY DOES FIND YOU, JUST IGNORE HIM AND KEEP DOING WHAT YOU ARE DOING.
OH, GOD! OH, GOD!
MMMMMM
OH! I NEED A HARD COCK INSIDE ME!
GIVE HIM A GOOD SHOW AND MAKE HIM THINK YOU HAVEN'T EVEN REALIZED THAT HE'S THERE.
OH, GOD YES! MAKE ME CUM! AHHHH!
I'm CUMMING!
WHEN YOU'VE FINISHED, OPEN YOUR EYES AND PRETEND TO BE SHOCKED TO SEE HIM THERE.
OH! HELLO. HOW LONG HAVE YOU BEEN STANDING THERE?
LONG ENOUGH.
I WAS THINKING ABOUT YOU AND I COULDN'T HELP MYSELF.
WHY DON'T YOU COME OVER HERE AND GIVE ME THE REAL THING.
ENJOY . . .

WHAT DO YOU CONSIDER CHEATING?

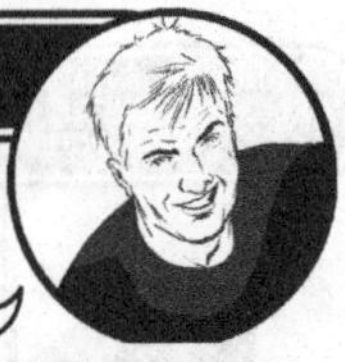

USE THIS FORM TO HELP DEFINE THE BOUNDARIES OF YOUR RELATIONSHIP. MARK THE FOLLOWING ACTIVITIES BY NUMBERING THEM 1 TO 10. 1 DENOTES THAT YOU ARE COMPLETELY COMFORTABLE ALLOWING YOUR PARTNERS TO DO SOMETHING WHENEVER THEY WISH, AND 10 DENOTES THAT IT WOULD ABSOLUTELY MAKE YOU FEEL BETRAYED, AND PERHAPS MEANS YOU WOULD PREFER THAT A PARTNER ASK FOR PERMISSION FIRST.

TO HOW COMFORTABLE ARE YOU WITH YOUR PARTNER'S			EXPLANATION OR HELPFUL TIPS
MASTURBATING			
HAVING PHONE SEX			
READING EROTICA			
VIEWING PORNOGRAPHY			
VISITING A STRIP CLUB			
SOCIALIZING WITH A MEMBER OF OPPOSITE SEX			
DISCUSSING SEX LIFE WITH PEERS/FRIENDS			
BEING NUDE AROUND MEMBERS OF SAME SEX			
BEING NUDE AROUND MEMBERS OF OPPOSITE SEX			
FLIRTING WITH MEMBERS OF SAME SEX			
FLIRTING WITH MEMBERS OF OPPOSITE SEX			
GRABBING/PINCHING BUTTOCKS OF OPPOSITE SEX			
GRABBING/PINCHING BUTTOCKS OF SAME SEX			
TOUCHING BREASTS/NIPPLES OF OPPOSITE SEX			
TOUCHING BREASTS/NIPPLES OF SAME SEX			
TOUCHING GENITALS OF OPPOSITE SEX			
TOUCHING GENITALS OF SAME SEX			
TRADING BACK MASSAGE WITH OPPOSITE SEX			
TRADING BACK MASSAGE WITH SAME SEX			
RECEIVING ORAL SEX FROM OPPOSITE SEX			
RECEIVING ORAL SEX FROM SAME SEX			
GIVING ORAL SEX TO OPPOSITE SEX			
GIVING ORAL SEX TO SAME SEX			
HAVING INTERCOURSE WITH OPPOSITE SEX			
HAVING INTERCOURSE WITH SAME SEX			
TALKING TO EX-PARTNER			
SLEEPING OVER AT SOMEONE ELSE'S HOME			

FILL IN YOUR OWN ACTIVITIES BELOW.	EXPLANATION OR HELPFUL TIPS

CHAPTER 15

RUB RACERS

THIS IS A GREAT GAME WHEN YOU BOTH NEED SEXUAL SATISFACTION AND DON'T HAVE THE TIME OR ENERGY FOR INTERCOURSE. MASTURBATE TOGETHER WITH THE GOAL OF GIVING YOURSELF AN ORGASM BEFORE YOUR PARTNER REACHES HIS OR HER ORGASM.

I'M REALLY HORNY!!
SO AM I, BUT I HAVE WAY TOO MUCH TO DO TO HAVE SEX TONIGHT.
WHATEVER WILL WE DO?

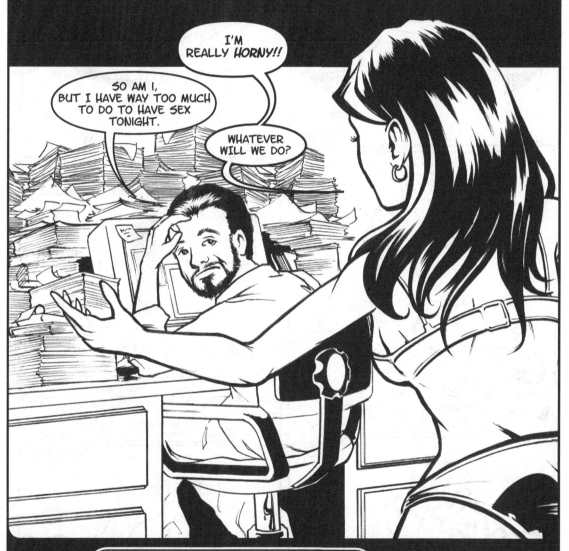

WHAT YOU'LL NEED . . .

LUBRICATION

FAVORITE SEX TOY

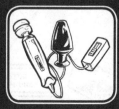

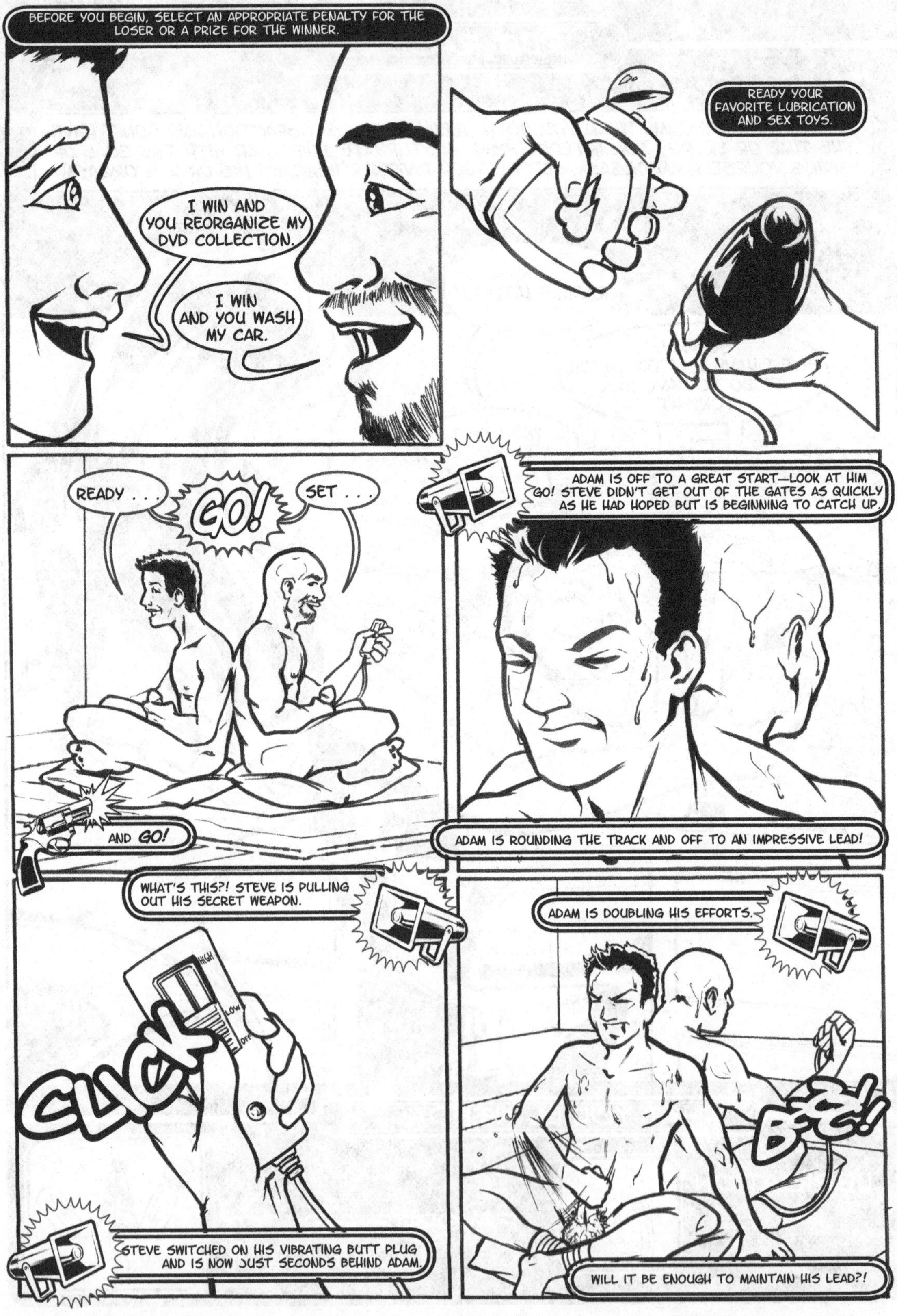
BEFORE YOU BEGIN, SELECT AN APPROPRIATE PENALTY FOR THE LOSER OR A PRIZE FOR THE WINNER.
I WIN AND YOU REORGANIZE MY DVD COLLECTION.
I WIN AND YOU WASH MY CAR.
READY YOUR FAVORITE LUBRICATION AND SEX TOYS.
READY . . .
SET . . .
GO!
AND GO!
ADAM IS OFF TO A GREAT START—LOOK AT HIM GO! STEVE DIDN'T GET OUT OF THE GATES AS QUICKLY AS HE HAD HOPED BUT IS BEGINNING TO CATCH UP.
ADAM IS ROUNDING THE TRACK AND OFF TO AN IMPRESSIVE LEAD!
WHAT'S THIS?! STEVE IS PULLING OUT HIS SECRET WEAPON.
HIGH
LOW
OFF
CLICK
STEVE SWITCHED ON HIS VIBRATING BUTT PLUG AND IS NOW JUST SECONDS BEHIND ADAM.
ADAM IS DOUBLING HIS EFFORTS.
BZZ!
WILL IT BE ENOUGH TO MAINTAIN HIS LEAD?!

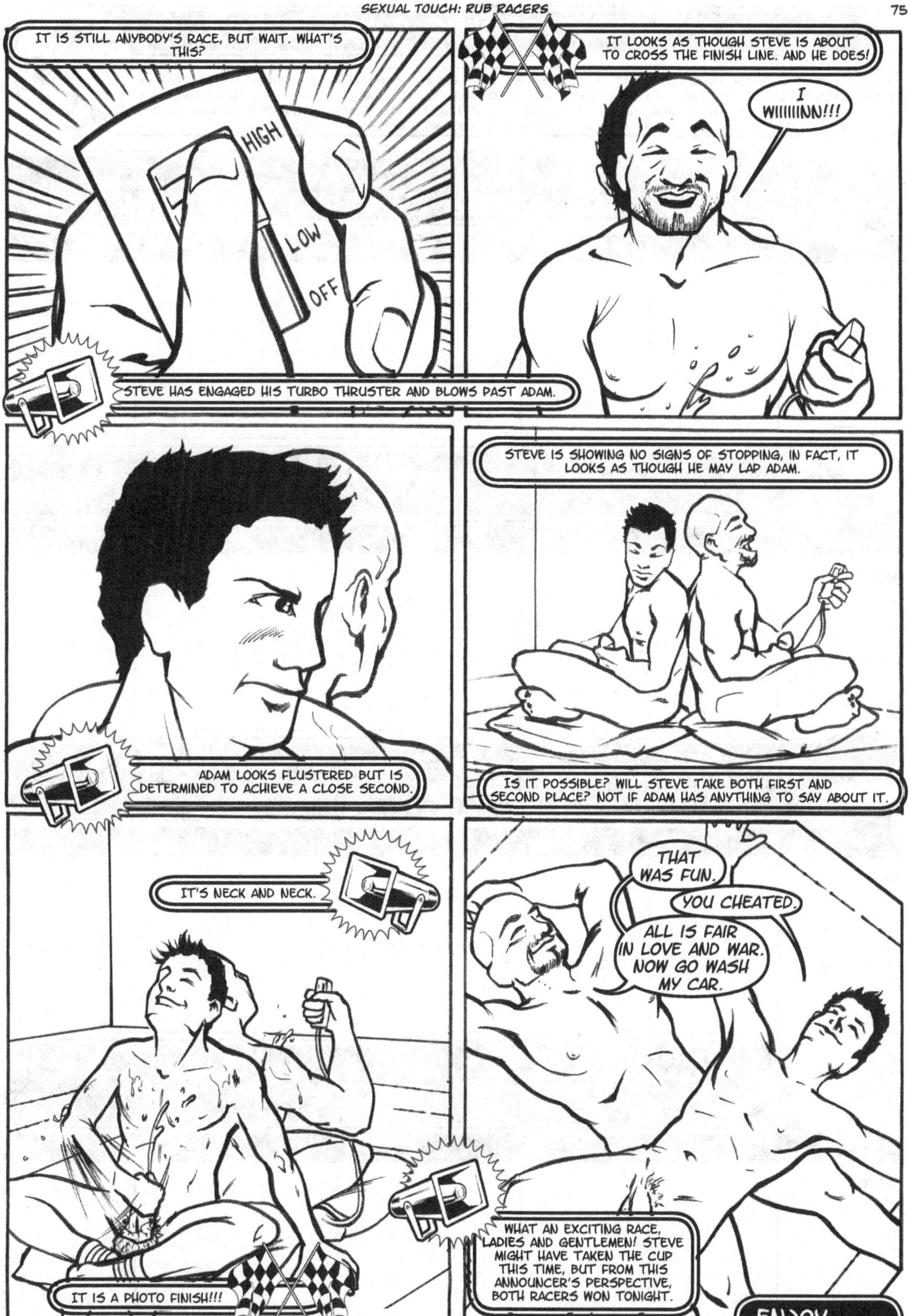
IT IS STILL ANYBODY'S RACE, BUT WAIT. WHAT'S THIS?
HIGH
LOW
OFF
STEVE HAS ENGAGED HIS TURBO THRUSTER AND BLOWS PAST ADAM.
IT LOOKS AS THOUGH STEVE IS ABOUT TO CROSS THE FINISH LINE. AND HE DOES!
I WIIIIINN!!!
ADAM LOOKS FLUSTERED BUT IS DETERMINED TO ACHIEVE A CLOSE SECOND.
STEVE IS SHOWING NO SIGNS OF STOPPING, IN FACT, IT LOOKS AS THOUGH HE MAY LAP ADAM.
IS IT POSSIBLE? WILL STEVE TAKE BOTH FIRST AND SECOND PLACE? NOT IF ADAM HAS ANYTHING TO SAY ABOUT IT.
IT'S NECK AND NECK.
IT IS A PHOTO FINISH!!!
THAT WAS FUN.
YOU CHEATED.
ALL IS FAIR IN LOVE AND WAR. NOW GO WASH MY CAR.
WHAT AN EXCITING RACE, LADIES AND GENTLEMEN! STEVE MIGHT HAVE TAKEN THE CUP THIS TIME, BUT FROM THIS ANNOUNCER'S PERSPECTIVE, BOTH RACERS WON TONIGHT.
ENJOY . . .

INTIMACY TRAINING EXERCISES

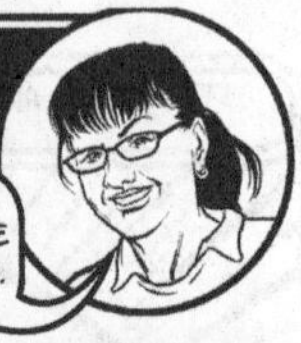

INTIMACY, WHEN IT IS WORKING IN YOUR FAVOR, MAKES YOU FEEL ALL WARM INSIDE WHEN YOU ARE WITH YOUR PARTNER. WHEN INTIMACY FEELS A BIT OFF, IT SOMETIMES SEEMS LIKE THERE IS NOTHING THAT YOU CAN DO TO GET BACK TO A COMFORTABLE PLACE WITH YOUR PARTNER. THESE EXERCISES ARE DESIGNED TO HELP INCREASE AND MAINTAIN INTIMACY WITH YOUR PARTNER. TRY THEM FOR A WEEK AND SEE IF YOU BOTH FEEL A BIT MORE CUDDLY WITH EACH OTHER.

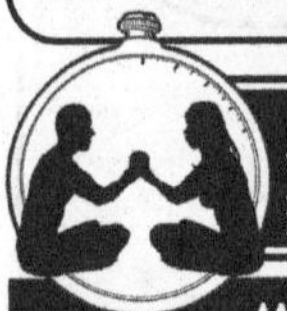

GAZING EXERCISE

SPEND THREE MINUTES EVERY DAY FACING YOUR PARTNER, CLOSE ENOUGH TO COMFORTABLY HOLD HANDS. DON'T TALK—JUST LOOK INTO EACH OTHER'S EYES. IF YOU HAVE TROUBLE COMPLETING THE WHOLE THREE MINUTES, DON'T WORRY; INTIMACY TAKES TIME TO ESTABLISH. WRITE DOWN YOUR TIME IN THE CALENDAR BELOW AND TRY TO GO LONGER TOMORROW.

M	T	W	T	F	S	S
NOTES:						

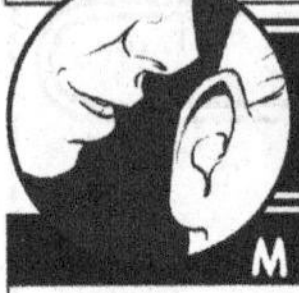

SWEET NOTHINGS

GIVE YOUR PARTNER A COMPLIMENT EVERY DAY. BE HONEST BUT TRY TO COMPLIMENT YOUR PARTNER ON SOMETHING THAT HE OR SHE TAKES PRIDE IN. PUT A LITTLE MARK EACH DAY IN THE CALENDAR BELOW TO MAKE SURE YOU'VE MADE GOOD ON THE EXERCISE.

M	T	W	T	F	S	S
NOTES:						

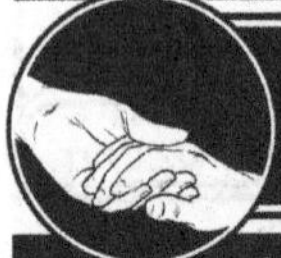

HELPING HAND

FIND ONE WAY TO HELP YOUR PARTNER EACH DAY. PERHAPS YOU CAN PERFORM AN ERRAND FOR YOUR PARTNER, OR YOU CAN DELIVER LUNCH, OR YOU CAN CLEAN THE CAR, OR YOU CAN MAKE A FAVORITE BEVERAGE. DO YOUR BEST TO FIND A WAY TO MAKE HER FEEL LIKE YOU ARE WILLING TO PUT A LITTLE EFFORT INTO MAKING HER HAPPY. MAKE A NOTE AS TO WHAT YOU DID EACH DAY.

M	T	W	T	F	S	S
NOTES:						

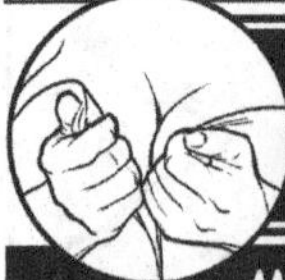

SEXY FLIRTATION

FIND A SIMPLE WAY EACH DAY TO REMIND YOUR PARTNER THAT YOU ARE A SEXUAL BEING AND THAT YOU SEE YOUR PARTNER AS A SEXUAL BEING. FLASH HIM ON YOUR WAY OUT OF THE SHOWER. TEASE HIM A BIT AS YOU GET DRESSED. WHISPER SOMETHING NAUGHTY IN HIS EAR BEFORE YOU LEAVE FOR WORK. CALL HIM AND LET HIM KNOW YOU ARE AROUSED SIMPLY BY THE THOUGHT OF HIM. MARK THE CALENDAR BELOW.

M	T	W	T	F	S	S
NOTES:						

Heading: A DAY AT THE SPA

CHAPTER 16

A DAY AT THE SPA

WHEN YOU REALLY WANT TO DO SOMETHING NICE FOR YOUR LOVER, TRY GIVING YOUR PARTNER A FULL-SERVICE SPA TREATMENT.

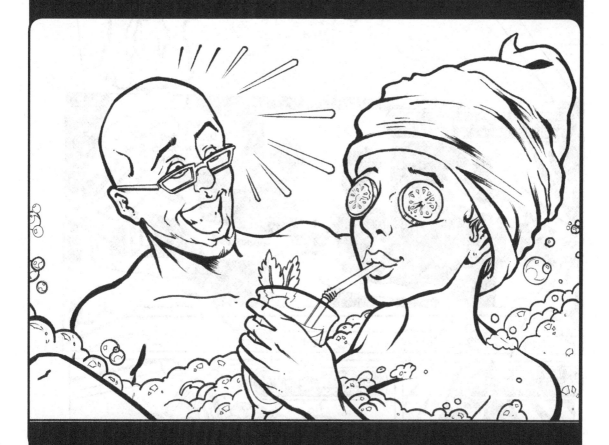

WHAT YOU'LL NEED . . .

TOWELS & ROBE

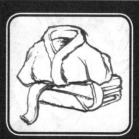

TOILETRIES

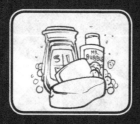

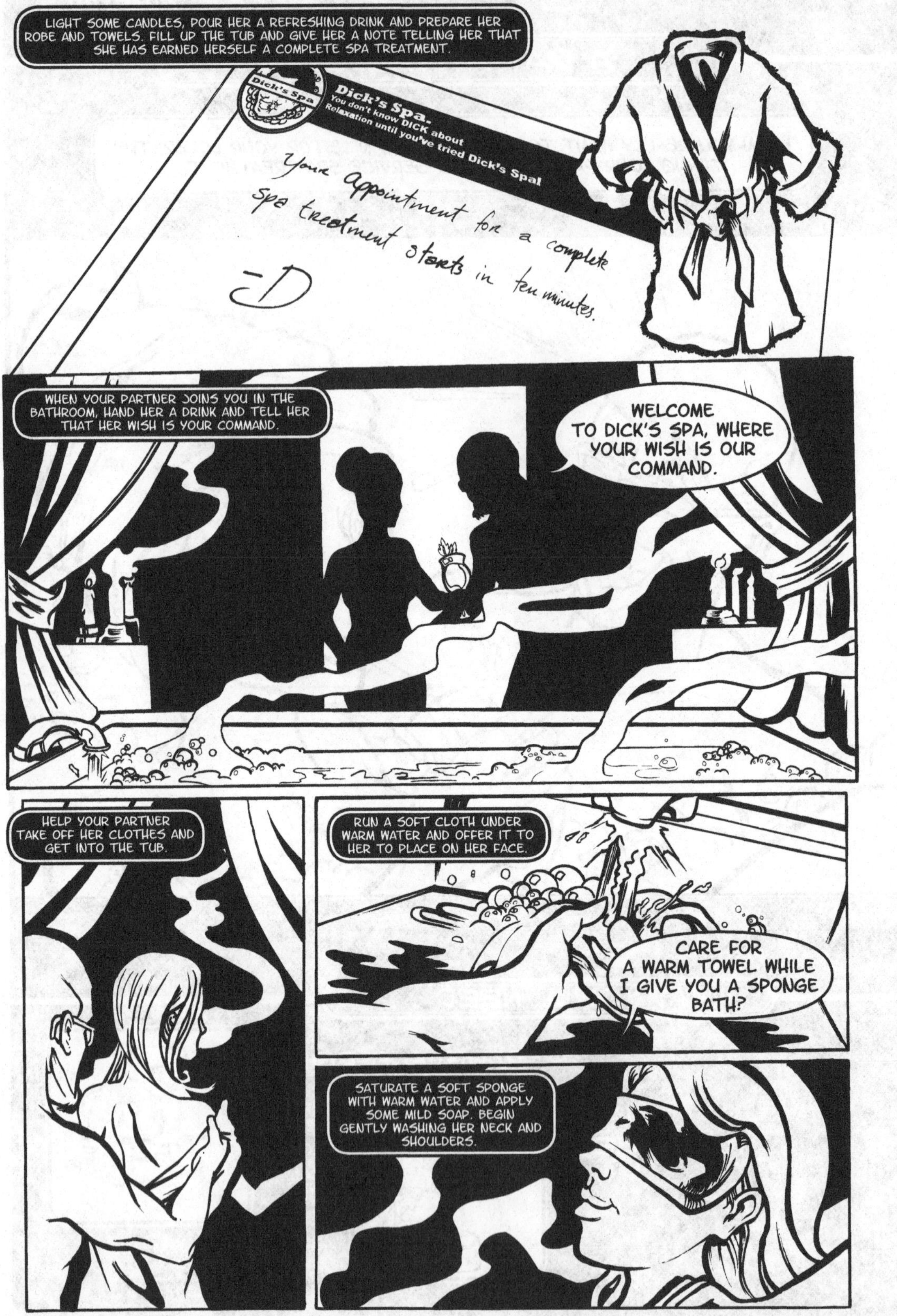
LIGHT SOME CANDLES, POUR HER A REFRESHING DRINK AND PREPARE HER ROBE AND TOWELS. FILL UP THE TUB AND GIVE HER A NOTE TELLING HER THAT SHE HAS EARNED HERSELF A COMPLETE SPA TREATMENT.
Dick's Spa
Dick's Spa.
You don't know DICK about Relaxation until you've tried Dick's Spa!
Your appointment for a complete spa treatment starts in ten minutes.
-D
WHEN YOUR PARTNER JOINS YOU IN THE BATHROOM, HAND HER A DRINK AND TELL HER THAT HER WISH IS YOUR COMMAND.
WELCOME TO DICK'S SPA, WHERE YOUR WISH IS OUR COMMAND.
HELP YOUR PARTNER TAKE OFF HER CLOTHES AND GET INTO THE TUB.
RUN A SOFT CLOTH UNDER WARM WATER AND OFFER IT TO HER TO PLACE ON HER FACE.
CARE FOR A WARM TOWEL WHILE I GIVE YOU A SPONGE BATH?
SATURATE A SOFT SPONGE WITH WARM WATER AND APPLY SOME MILD SOAP. BEGIN GENTLY WASHING HER NECK AND SHOULDERS.

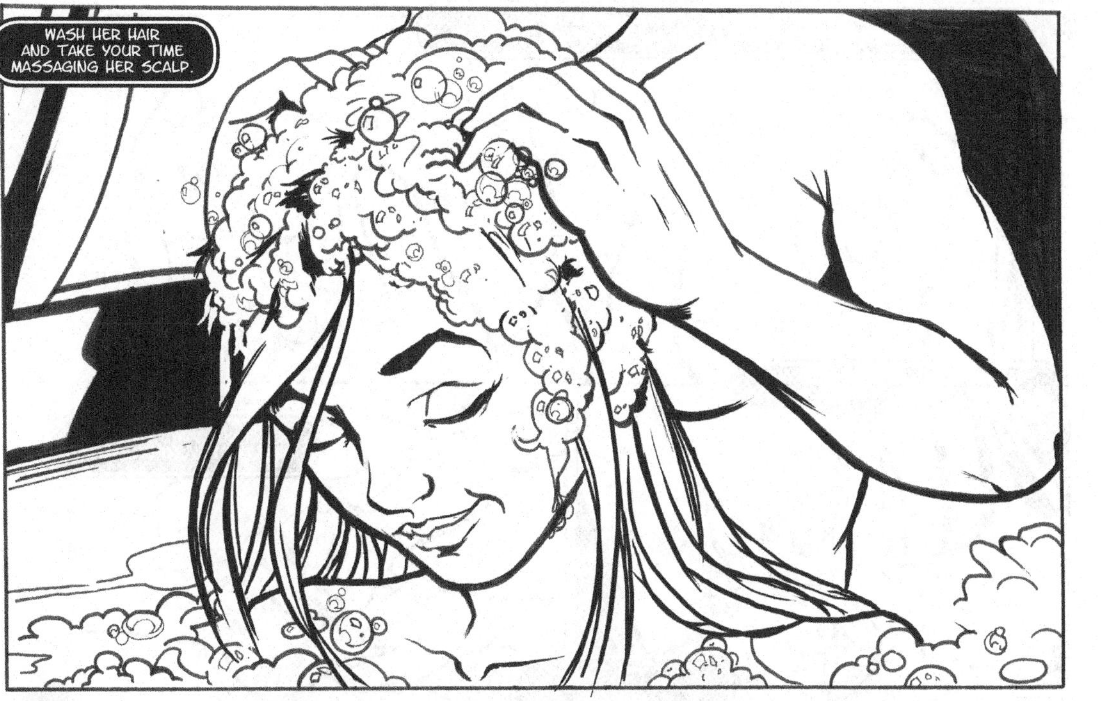
WASH HER HAIR AND TAKE YOUR TIME MASSAGING HER SCALP.

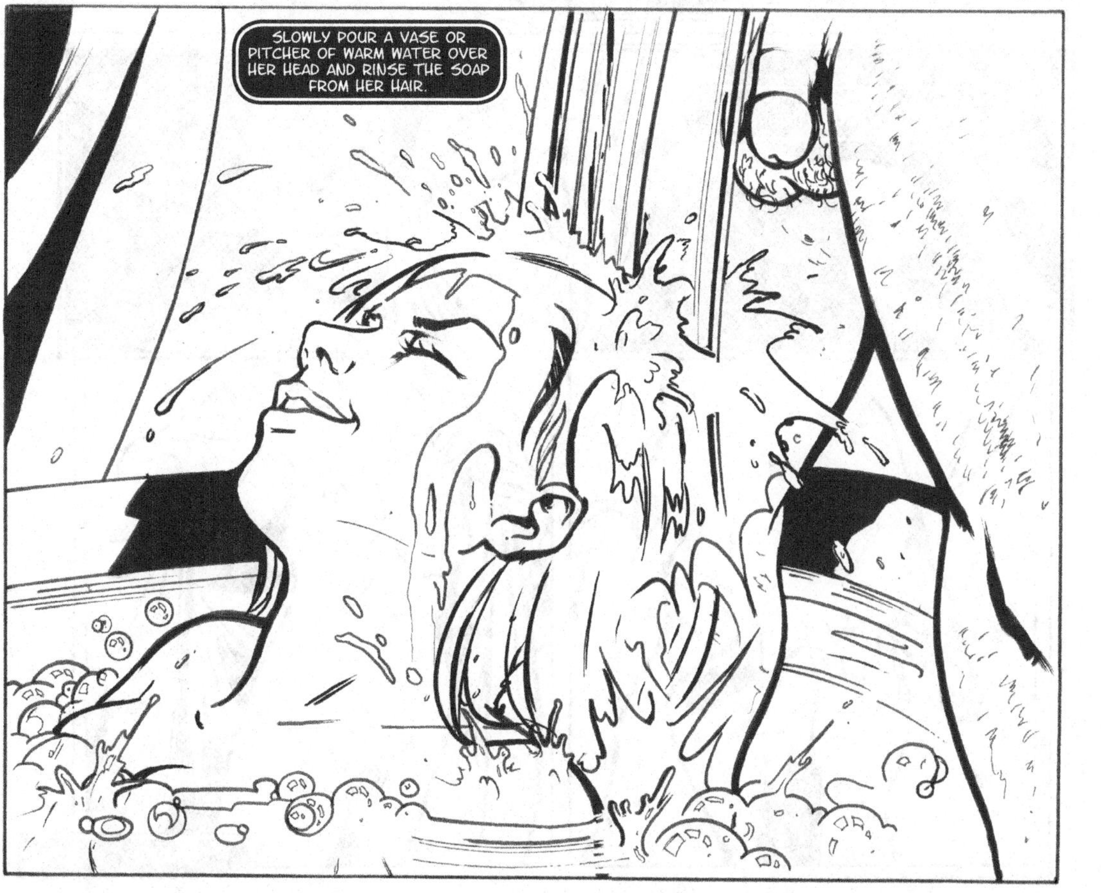
SLOWLY POUR A VASE OR PITCHER OF WARM WATER OVER HER HEAD AND RINSE THE SOAP FROM HER HAIR.

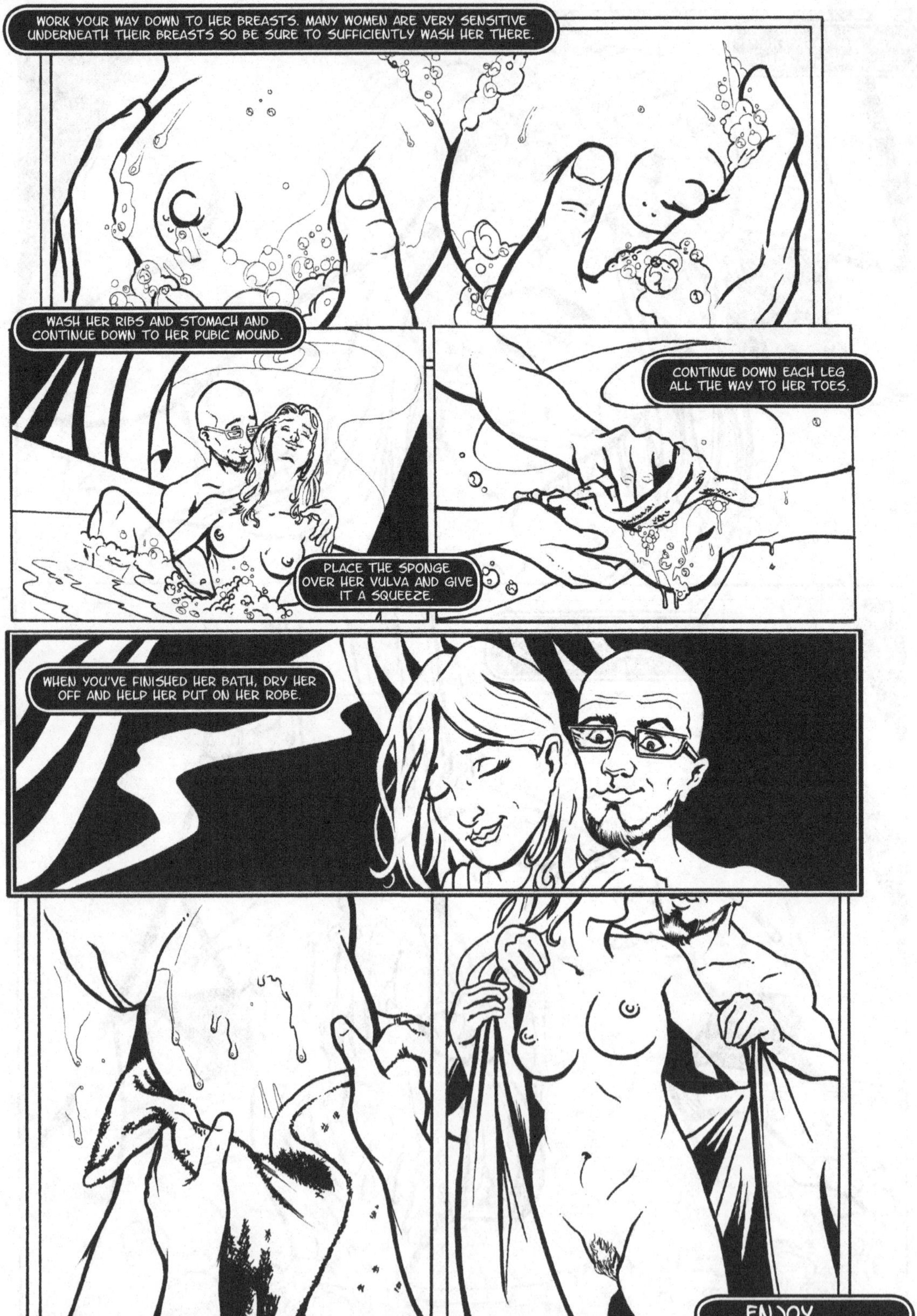
WORK YOUR WAY DOWN TO HER BREASTS. MANY WOMEN ARE VERY SENSITIVE UNDERNEATH THEIR BREASTS SO BE SURE TO SUFFICIENTLY WASH HER THERE.
WASH HER RIBS AND STOMACH AND CONTINUE DOWN TO HER PUBIC MOUND.
PLACE THE SPONGE OVER HER VULVA AND GIVE IT A SQUEEZE.
CONTINUE DOWN EACH LEG ALL THE WAY TO HER TOES.
WHEN YOU'VE FINISHED HER BATH, DRY HER OFF AND HELP HER PUT ON HER ROBE.
ENJOY . . .

CHAPTER 17

FUN WITH BLINDFOLDS

IN THIS GAME OF SENSUAL TOUCH, YOU'LL DISCOVER THAT A BLINDFOLD CAN TURN COMMON OBJECTS INTO DIVINE DEVICES OF SEXY STIMULATION.

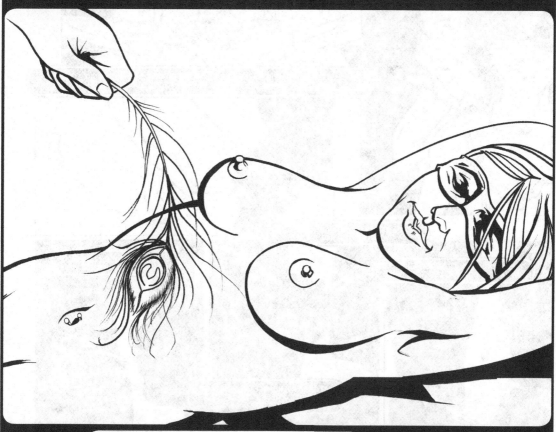

WHAT YOU'LL NEED . . .

 BLINDFOLD

 FEATHER

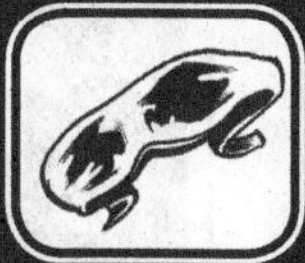

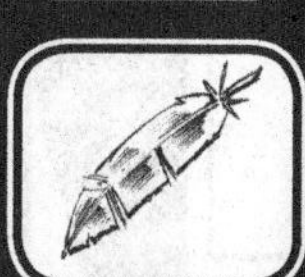

HAIRBRUSH

HANDHELD VIBRATOR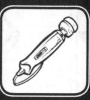

CHAMOIS CLOTH OR ANIMAL FUR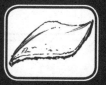

DRINKING STRAW

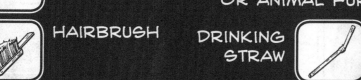

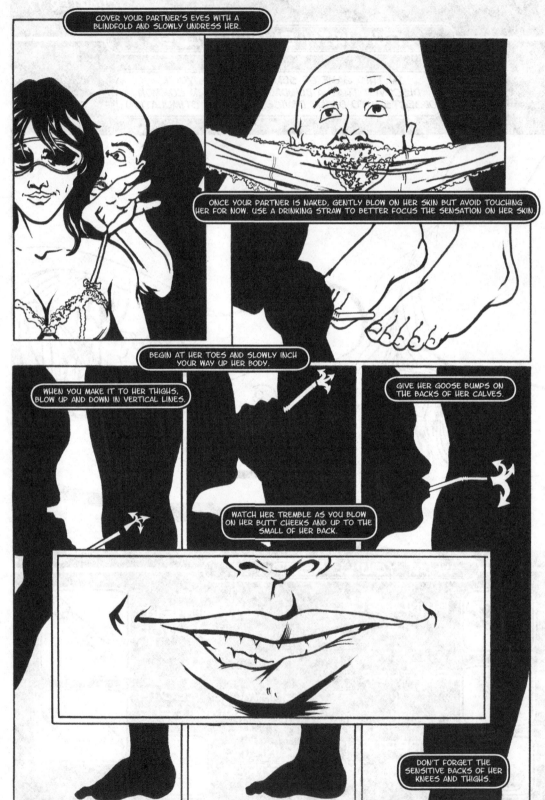

COVER YOUR PARTNER'S EYES WITH A BLINDFOLD AND SLOWLY UNDRESS HER.

ONCE YOUR PARTNER IS NAKED, GENTLY BLOW ON HER SKIN BUT AVOID TOUCHING HER FOR NOW. USE A DRINKING STRAW TO BETTER FOCUS THE SENSATION ON HER SKIN.

BEGIN AT HER TOES AND SLOWLY INCH YOUR WAY UP HER BODY.

WHEN YOU MAKE IT TO HER THIGHS, BLOW UP AND DOWN IN VERTICAL LINES.

GIVE HER GOOSE BUMPS ON THE BACKS OF HER CALVES.

WATCH HER TREMBLE AS YOU BLOW ON HER BUTT CHEEKS AND UP TO THE SMALL OF HER BACK.

DON'T FORGET THE SENSITIVE BACKS OF HER KNEES AND THIGHS.

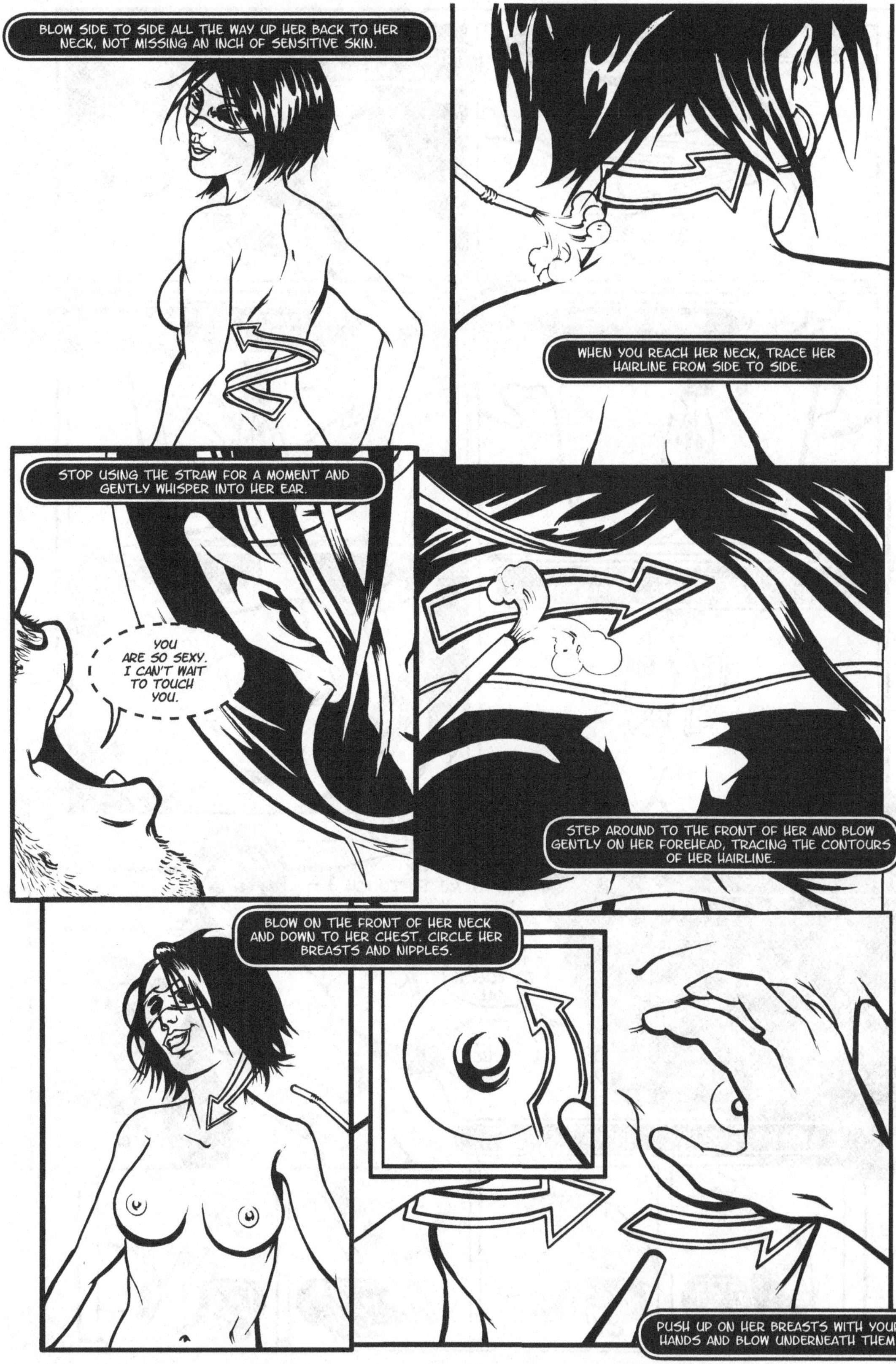
BLOW SIDE TO SIDE ALL THE WAY UP HER BACK TO HER NECK, NOT MISSING AN INCH OF SENSITIVE SKIN.
WHEN YOU REACH HER NECK, TRACE HER HAIRLINE FROM SIDE TO SIDE.
STOP USING THE STRAW FOR A MOMENT AND GENTLY WHISPER INTO HER EAR.
YOU ARE SO SEXY. I CAN'T WAIT TO TOUCH YOU.
STEP AROUND TO THE FRONT OF HER AND BLOW GENTLY ON HER FOREHEAD, TRACING THE CONTOURS OF HER HAIRLINE.
BLOW ON THE FRONT OF HER NECK AND DOWN TO HER CHEST. CIRCLE HER BREASTS AND NIPPLES.
PUSH UP ON HER BREASTS WITH YOUR HANDS AND BLOW UNDERNEATH THEM.

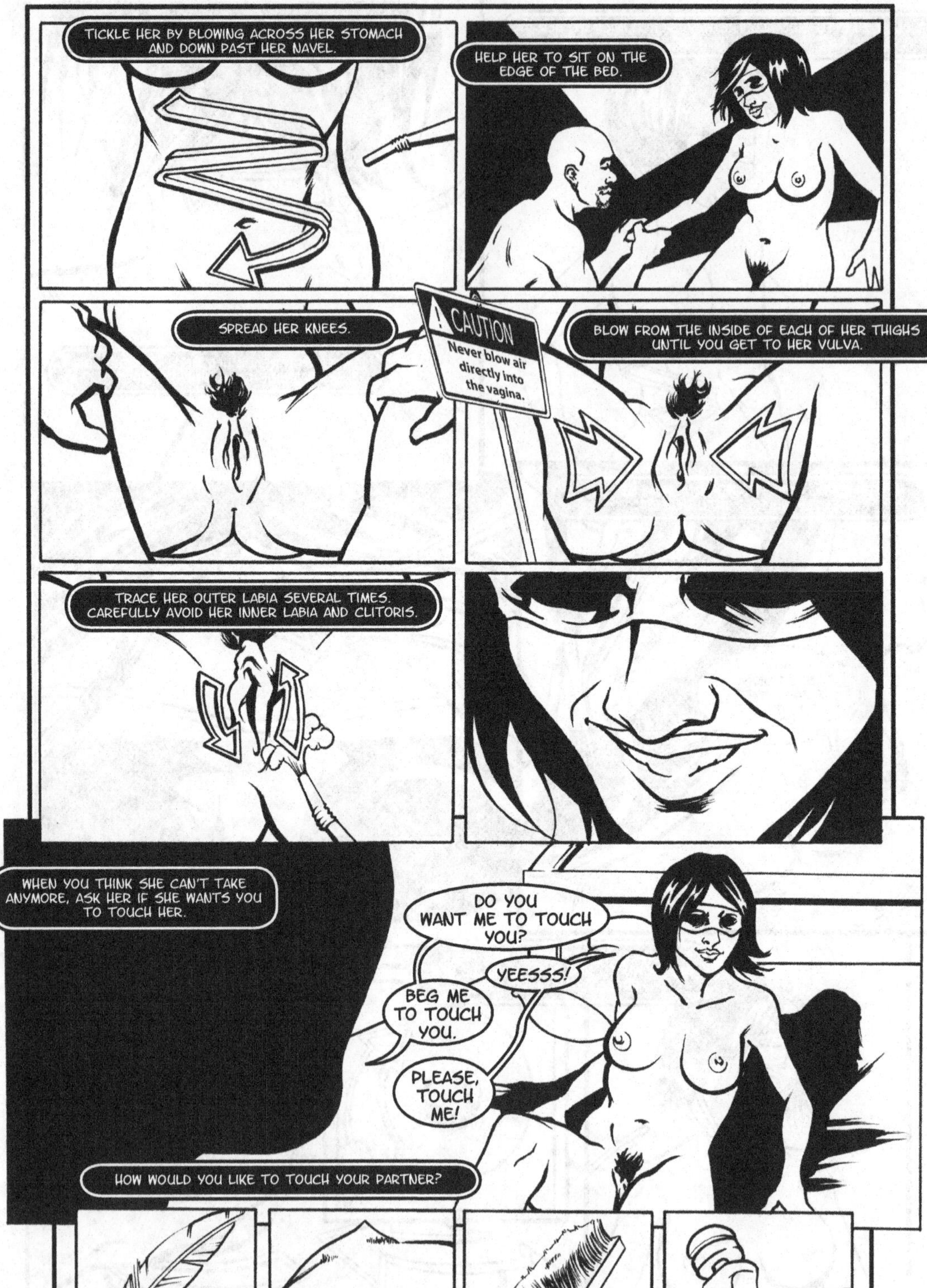
TICKLE HER BY BLOWING ACROSS HER STOMACH AND DOWN PAST HER NAVEL.
HELP HER TO SIT ON THE EDGE OF THE BED.
SPREAD HER KNEES.
CAUTION
Never blow air directly into the vagina.
BLOW FROM THE INSIDE OF EACH OF HER THIGHS UNTIL YOU GET TO HER VULVA.
TRACE HER OUTER LABIA SEVERAL TIMES. CAREFULLY AVOID HER INNER LABIA AND CLITORIS.
WHEN YOU THINK SHE CAN'T TAKE ANYMORE, ASK HER IF SHE WANTS YOU TO TOUCH HER.
DO YOU WANT ME TO TOUCH YOU?
YEESSS!
BEG ME TO TOUCH YOU.
PLEASE, TOUCH ME!
HOW WOULD YOU LIKE TO TOUCH YOUR PARTNER?
PAGE 85!
PAGE 87!
PAGE 88!
PAGE 89!

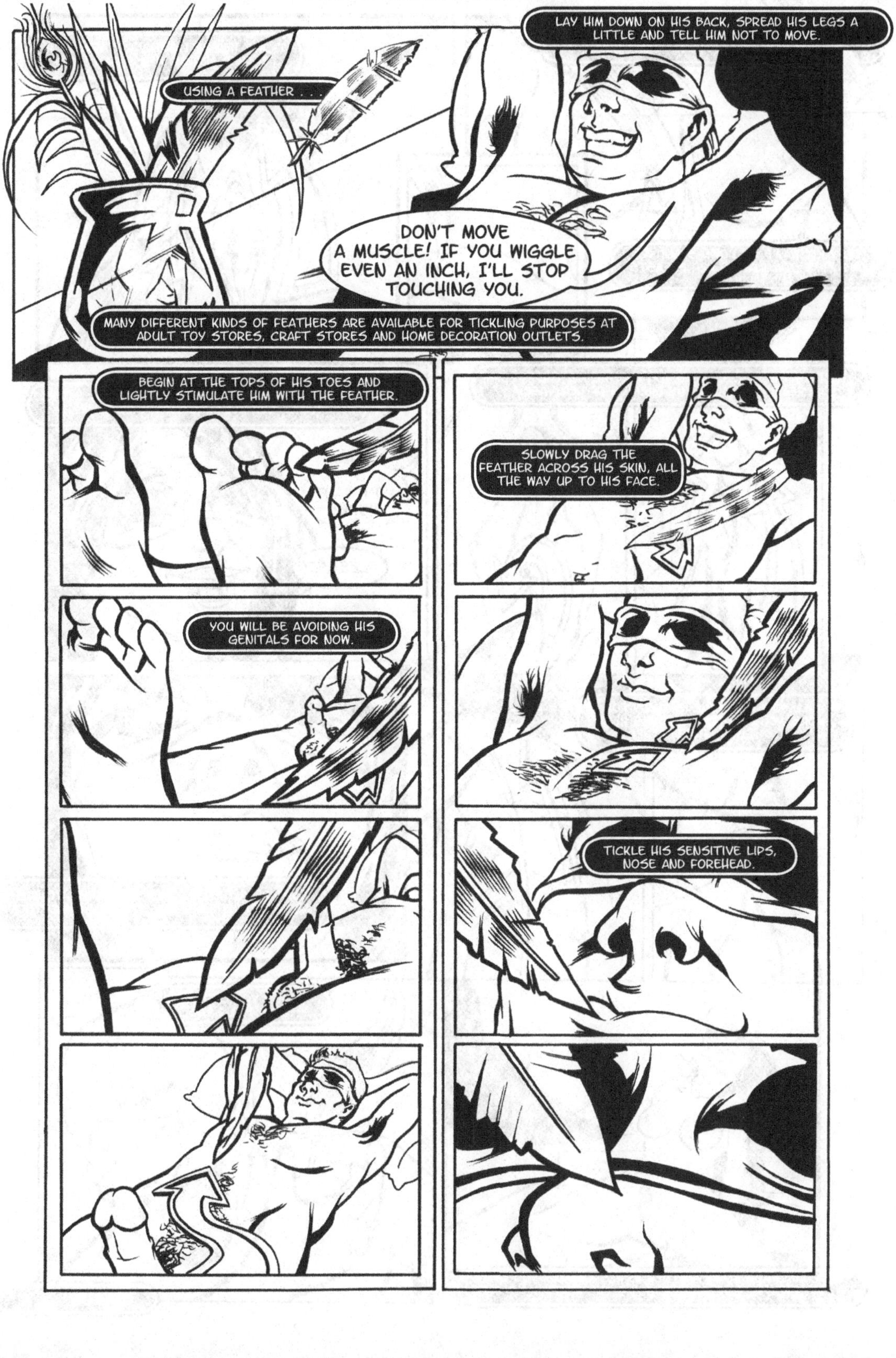
USING A FEATHER . . .
LAY HIM DOWN ON HIS BACK, SPREAD HIS LEGS A LITTLE AND TELL HIM NOT TO MOVE.
DON'T MOVE A MUSCLE! IF YOU WIGGLE EVEN AN INCH, I'LL STOP TOUCHING YOU.
MANY DIFFERENT KINDS OF FEATHERS ARE AVAILABLE FOR TICKLING PURPOSES AT ADULT TOY STORES, CRAFT STORES AND HOME DECORATION OUTLETS.
BEGIN AT THE TOPS OF HIS TOES AND LIGHTLY STIMULATE HIM WITH THE FEATHER.
SLOWLY DRAG THE FEATHER ACROSS HIS SKIN, ALL THE WAY UP TO HIS FACE.
YOU WILL BE AVOIDING HIS GENITALS FOR NOW.
TICKLE HIS SENSITIVE LIPS, NOSE AND FOREHEAD.

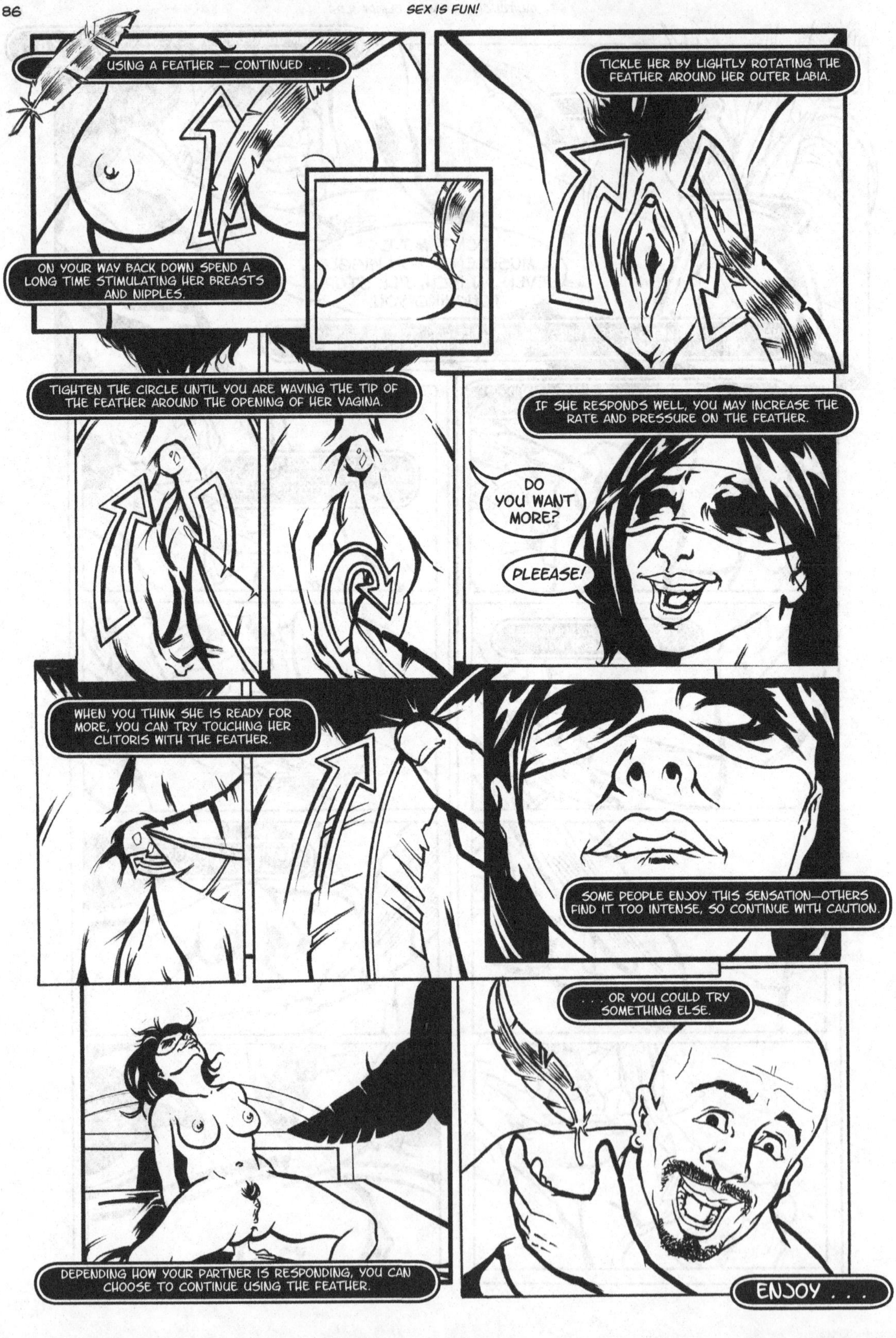
USING A FEATHER — CONTINUED . . .
ON YOUR WAY BACK DOWN SPEND A LONG TIME STIMULATING HER BREASTS AND NIPPLES.
TICKLE HER BY LIGHTLY ROTATING THE FEATHER AROUND HER OUTER LABIA.
TIGHTEN THE CIRCLE UNTIL YOU ARE WAVING THE TIP OF THE FEATHER AROUND THE OPENING OF HER VAGINA.
IF SHE RESPONDS WELL, YOU MAY INCREASE THE RATE AND PRESSURE ON THE FEATHER.
DO YOU WANT MORE?
PLEEASE!
WHEN YOU THINK SHE IS READY FOR MORE, YOU CAN TRY TOUCHING HER CLITORIS WITH THE FEATHER.
SOME PEOPLE ENJOY THIS SENSATION—OTHERS FIND IT TOO INTENSE, SO CONTINUE WITH CAUTION.
DEPENDING HOW YOUR PARTNER IS RESPONDING, YOU CAN CHOOSE TO CONTINUE USING THE FEATHER.
. . . OR YOU COULD TRY SOMETHING ELSE.
ENJOY . . .

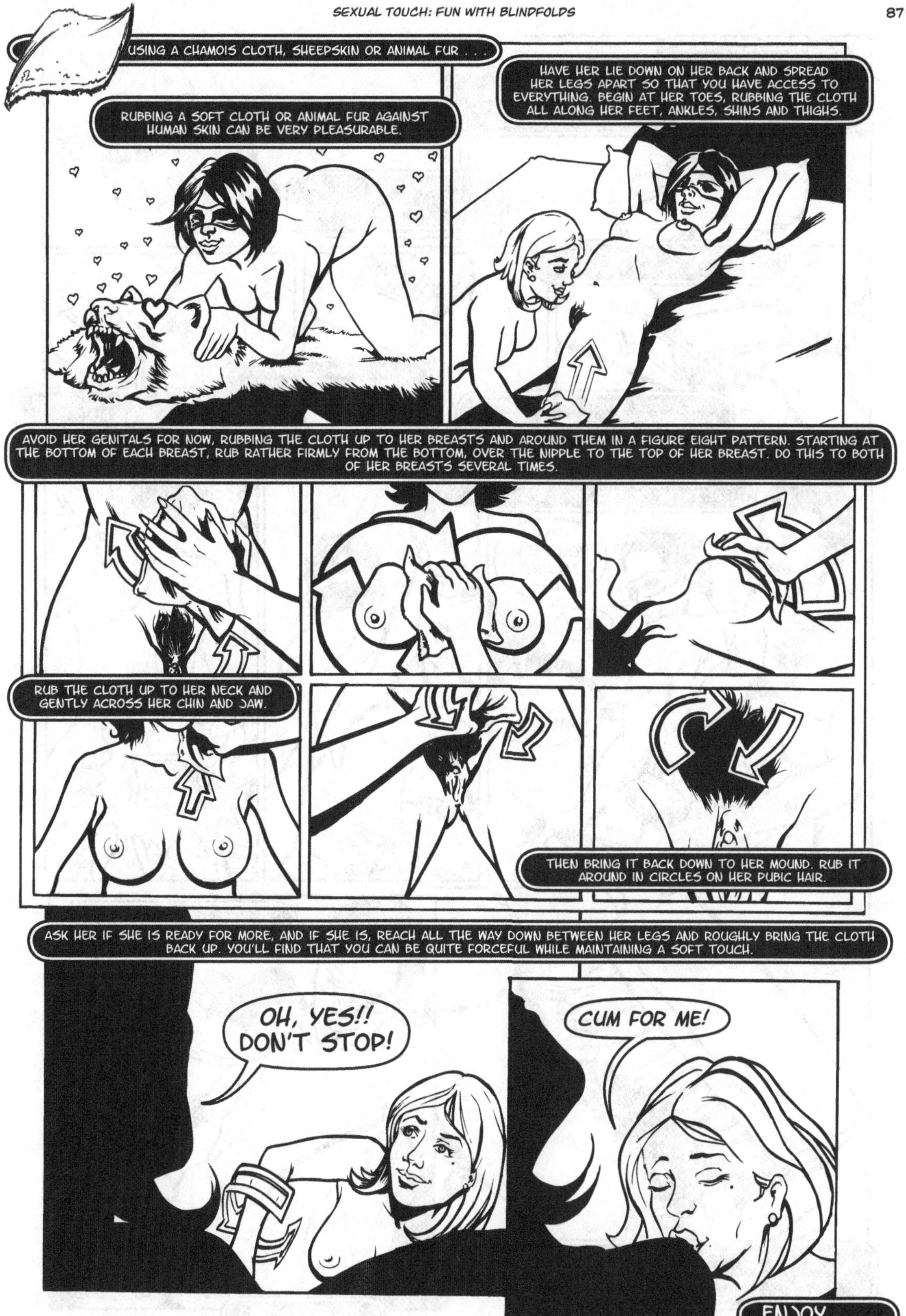
USING A CHAMOIS CLOTH, SHEEPSKIN OR ANIMAL FUR . . .
RUBBING A SOFT CLOTH OR ANIMAL FUR AGAINST HUMAN SKIN CAN BE VERY PLEASURABLE.
HAVE HER LIE DOWN ON HER BACK AND SPREAD HER LEGS APART SO THAT YOU HAVE ACCESS TO EVERYTHING. BEGIN AT HER TOES, RUBBING THE CLOTH ALL ALONG HER FEET, ANKLES, SHINS AND THIGHS.
AVOID HER GENITALS FOR NOW, RUBBING THE CLOTH UP TO HER BREASTS AND AROUND THEM IN A FIGURE EIGHT PATTERN. STARTING AT THE BOTTOM OF EACH BREAST, RUB RATHER FIRMLY FROM THE BOTTOM, OVER THE NIPPLE TO THE TOP OF HER BREAST. DO THIS TO BOTH OF HER BREASTS SEVERAL TIMES.
RUB THE CLOTH UP TO HER NECK AND GENTLY ACROSS HER CHIN AND JAW.
THEN BRING IT BACK DOWN TO HER MOUND. RUB IT AROUND IN CIRCLES ON HER PUBIC HAIR.
ASK HER IF SHE IS READY FOR MORE, AND IF SHE IS, REACH ALL THE WAY DOWN BETWEEN HER LEGS AND ROUGHLY BRING THE CLOTH BACK UP. YOU'LL FIND THAT YOU CAN BE QUITE FORCEFUL WHILE MAINTAINING A SOFT TOUCH.
OH, YES!! DON'T STOP!
CUM FOR ME!
ENJOY . . .

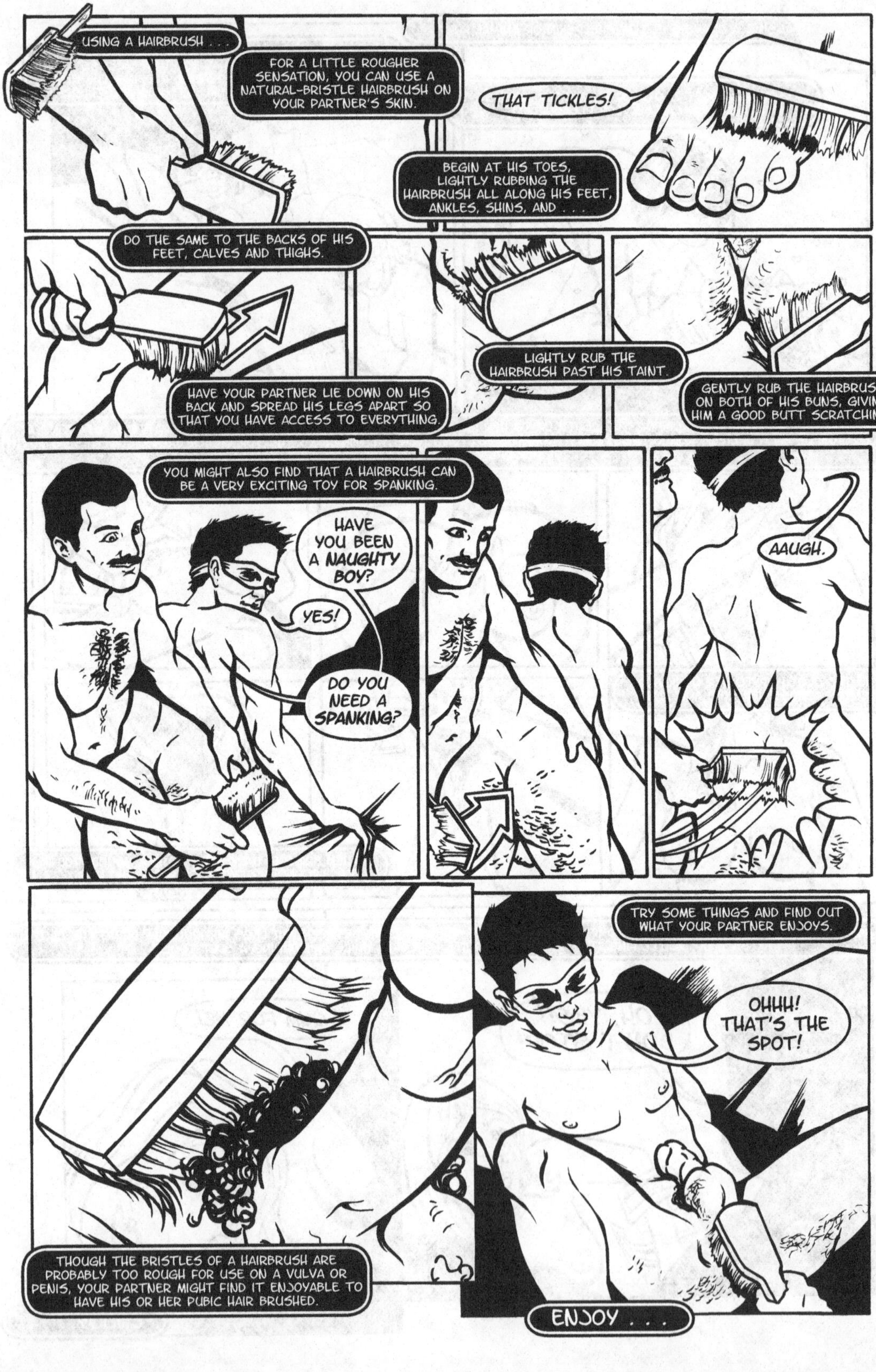
USING A HAIRBRUSH . . .
FOR A LITTLE ROUGHER SENSATION, YOU CAN USE A NATURAL-BRISTLE HAIRBRUSH ON YOUR PARTNER'S SKIN.
THAT TICKLES!
BEGIN AT HIS TOES, LIGHTLY RUBBING THE HAIRBRUSH ALL ALONG HIS FEET, ANKLES, SHINS, AND . . .
DO THE SAME TO THE BACKS OF HIS FEET, CALVES AND THIGHS.
HAVE YOUR PARTNER LIE DOWN ON HIS BACK AND SPREAD HIS LEGS APART SO THAT YOU HAVE ACCESS TO EVERYTHING.
LIGHTLY RUB THE HAIRBRUSH PAST HIS TAINT.
GENTLY RUB THE HAIRBRUSH ON BOTH OF HIS BUNS, GIVING HIM A GOOD BUTT SCRATCHING.
YOU MIGHT ALSO FIND THAT A HAIRBRUSH CAN BE A VERY EXCITING TOY FOR SPANKING.
HAVE YOU BEEN A NAUGHTY BOY?
YES!
DO YOU NEED A SPANKING?
AAUGH.
THOUGH THE BRISTLES OF A HAIRBRUSH ARE PROBABLY TOO ROUGH FOR USE ON A VULVA OR PENIS, YOUR PARTNER MIGHT FIND IT ENJOYABLE TO HAVE HIS OR HER PUBIC HAIR BRUSHED.
TRY SOME THINGS AND FIND OUT WHAT YOUR PARTNER ENJOYS.
OHHH! THAT'S THE SPOT!
ENJOY . . .

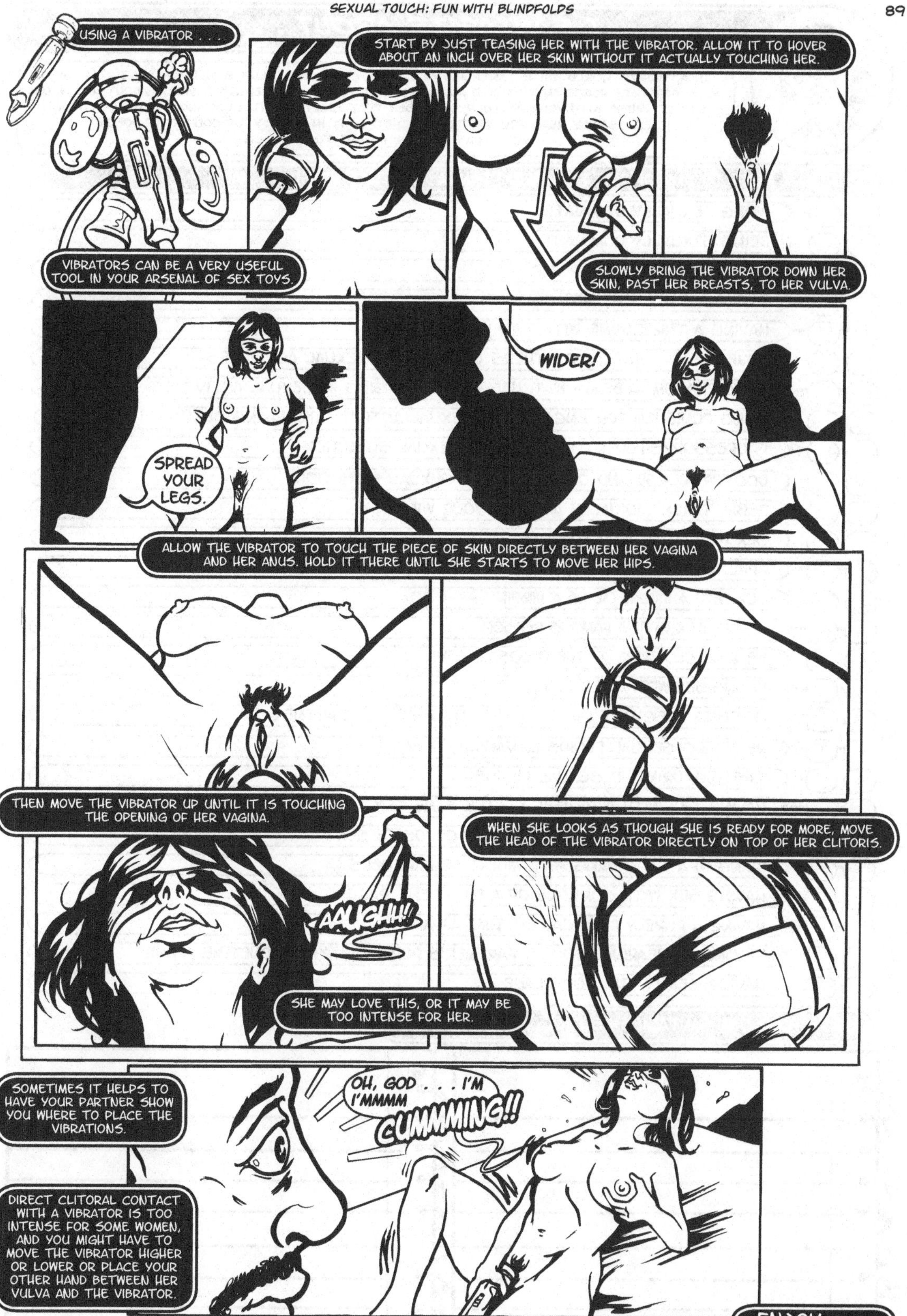
USING A VIBRATOR . . .
VIBRATORS CAN BE A VERY USEFUL TOOL IN YOUR ARSENAL OF SEX TOYS.
START BY JUST TEASING HER WITH THE VIBRATOR. ALLOW IT TO HOVER ABOUT AN INCH OVER HER SKIN WITHOUT IT ACTUALLY TOUCHING HER.
SLOWLY BRING THE VIBRATOR DOWN HER SKIN, PAST HER BREASTS, TO HER VULVA.
SPREAD YOUR LEGS.
WIDER!
ALLOW THE VIBRATOR TO TOUCH THE PIECE OF SKIN DIRECTLY BETWEEN HER VAGINA AND HER ANUS. HOLD IT THERE UNTIL SHE STARTS TO MOVE HER HIPS.
THEN MOVE THE VIBRATOR UP UNTIL IT IS TOUCHING THE OPENING OF HER VAGINA.
AAUGHH!
SHE MAY LOVE THIS, OR IT MAY BE TOO INTENSE FOR HER.
WHEN SHE LOOKS AS THOUGH SHE IS READY FOR MORE, MOVE THE HEAD OF THE VIBRATOR DIRECTLY ON TOP OF HER CLITORIS.
SOMETIMES IT HELPS TO HAVE YOUR PARTNER SHOW YOU WHERE TO PLACE THE VIBRATIONS.
DIRECT CLITORAL CONTACT WITH A VIBRATOR IS TOO INTENSE FOR SOME WOMEN, AND YOU MIGHT HAVE TO MOVE THE VIBRATOR HIGHER OR LOWER OR PLACE YOUR OTHER HAND BETWEEN HER VULVA AND THE VIBRATOR.
OH, GOD . . . I'M I'MMMM CUMMMING!!
ENJOY . . .

I FANTASIZE ABOUT . . .

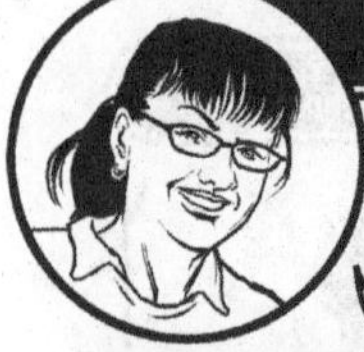

IN A PERFECT WORLD WHERE FANTASIES COULD ALL COME TRUE, WHAT WOULD YOU LOVE TO DO WITH YOUR PARTNER? PLACE AN "X" AFTER ANYTHING THAT YOU'VE ENJOYED FANTASIZING ABOUT AND WOULD LIKE TO SHARE WITH YOUR PARTNER. REMEMBER THAT ADMITTING TO ENJOYING A FANTASY DOESN'T NECESSARILY MEAN YOU WANT OR NEED TO DO IT IN REALITY. OF COURSE, IT DOESN'T MEAN THAT YOU DON'T WANT TO DO IT, EITHER.

PUT AN X NEXT TO ANY OF THE FOLLOWING FANTASIES THAT YOU HAVE HAD.

- BEING SEXUALLY DOMINATED
- BEING SEXUALLY DOMINANT
- HAVING SEX WITH A STRANGER
- HAVING A THREESOME WITH TWO MEN
- HAVING A THREESOME WITH TWO WOMEN
- VOYEURISM — WATCHING OTHERS ENGAGING IN SEXUAL ACTIVITIES
- EXHIBITIONISM — BEING WATCHED WHILE ENGAGING IN SEXUAL ACTIVITIES
- BEING PUNISHED FOR ENGAGING IN SEXUAL ACTIVITY OR HAVING SEXUAL THOUGHTS
- PROFESSOR/STUDENT ENGAGING IN SEXUAL SITUATION
- DOCTOR/NURSE AND OTHER MEDICAL SEXUAL SITUATION
- BEING TAKEN SEXUALLY AGAINST YOUR WILL
- SEX WITH OR AS A PROSTITUTE
- APPEARING IN A SEXUALLY EXPLICIT MOVIE OR PHOTOGRAPH
- SEX WITH A VIRGIN OR AS A VIRGIN
- HAVING SEX WITH A FAMOUS PERSON
- WEARING CLOTHING OF THE OPPOSITE SEX
- HAVING SEX WITH AN EX-LOVER
- GETTING PREGNANT OR IMPREGNATING A SEXUAL PARTNER
- RECEIVING SEXUAL FLUIDS IN VAGINA OR ANUS
- TASTING/DRINKING SEXUAL FLUIDS
- HAVING SEX WITH A MEMBER OF THE SAME SEX
- HAVING SEX WITH A MEMBER OF THE OPPOSITE SEX
- BEING IN A GANG BANG WITH MULTIPLE PARTNERS
- HAVING SEX WITH SOMEONE OF A DIFFERENT RACE
- HAVING A PURELY PHYSICAL ONETIME AFFAIR
- VIEWING OR HEARING ABOUT A PARTNER'S PURELY PHYSICAL ONETIME AFFAIR
- HAVING SEX IN THE WORKPLACE

WRITE YOUR OWN FANTASIES BELOW.

CHAPTER 18

SEXY SUDS

NOTHING QUITE COMPARES TO THE SENSATION OF SOAPING UP AND SLIPPING AND SLIDING YOUR BODY AGAINST YOUR PARTNER'S. WE'LL SHOW YOU HOW IN THIS SCENARIO OF GOOD CLEAN FUN.

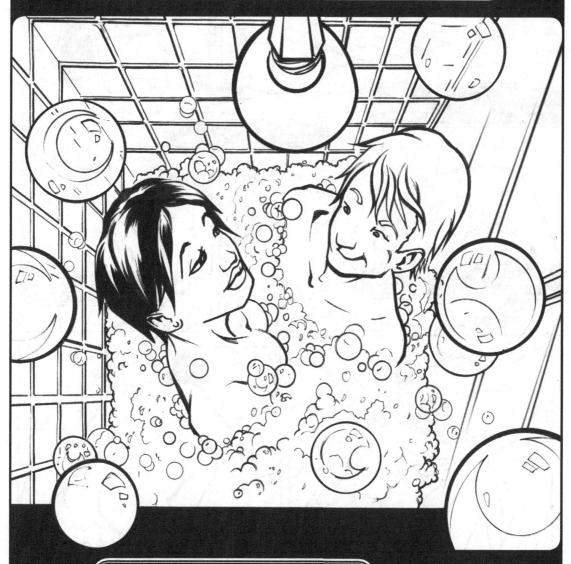

WHAT YOU'LL NEED . . .

pH-BALANCED SOAP OR SILICONE-BASED LUBRICATION

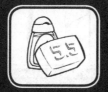

A SOFT YET WATER-RESISTANT SURFACE

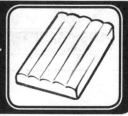

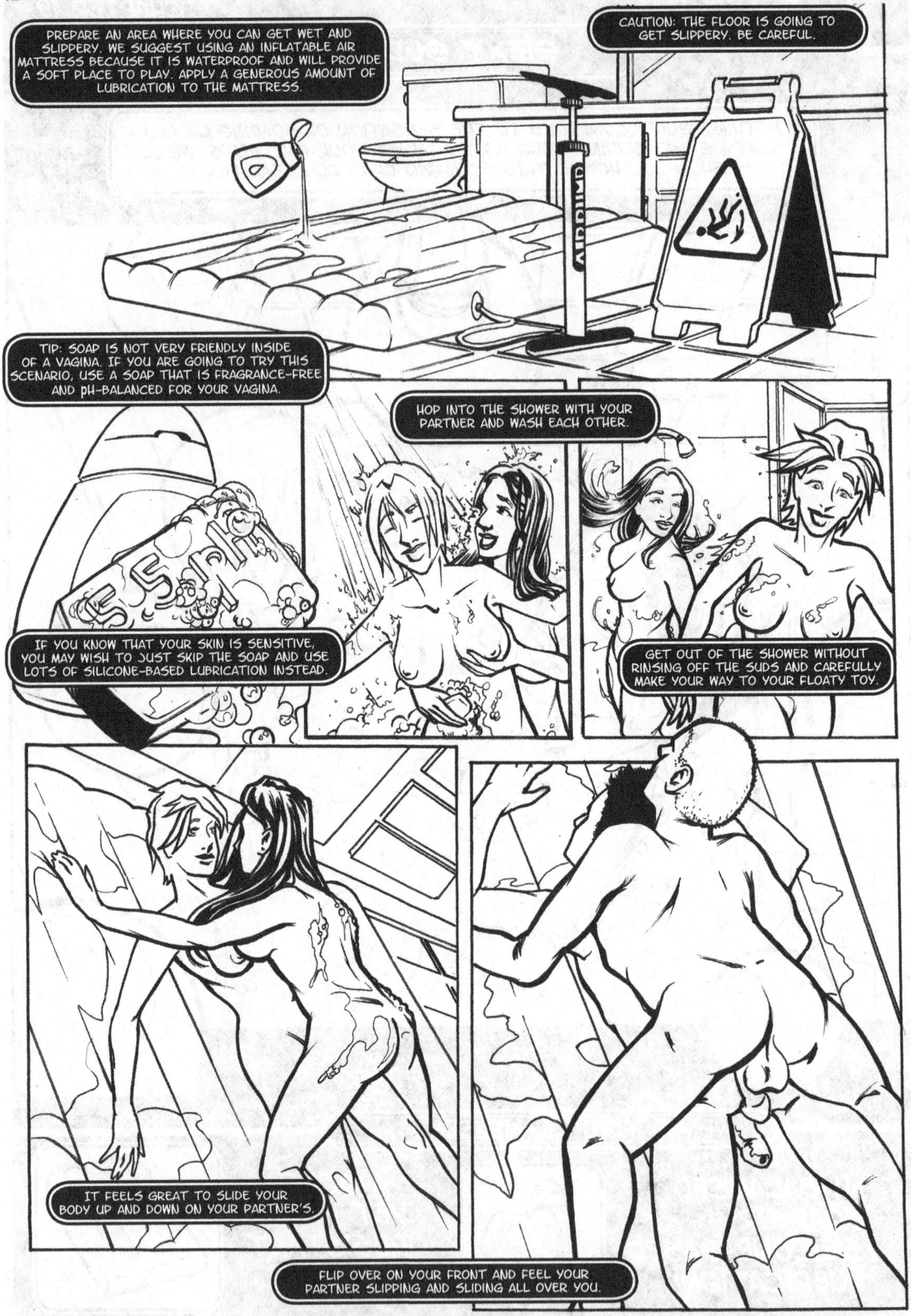
PREPARE AN AREA WHERE YOU CAN GET WET AND SLIPPERY. WE SUGGEST USING AN INFLATABLE AIR MATTRESS BECAUSE IT IS WATERPROOF AND WILL PROVIDE A SOFT PLACE TO PLAY. APPLY A GENEROUS AMOUNT OF LUBRICATION TO THE MATTRESS.
CAUTION: THE FLOOR IS GOING TO GET SLIPPERY. BE CAREFUL.
TIP: SOAP IS NOT VERY FRIENDLY INSIDE OF A VAGINA. IF YOU ARE GOING TO TRY THIS SCENARIO, USE A SOAP THAT IS FRAGRANCE-FREE AND pH-BALANCED FOR YOUR VAGINA.
IF YOU KNOW THAT YOUR SKIN IS SENSITIVE, YOU MAY WISH TO JUST SKIP THE SOAP AND USE LOTS OF SILICONE-BASED LUBRICATION INSTEAD.
HOP INTO THE SHOWER WITH YOUR PARTNER AND WASH EACH OTHER.
GET OUT OF THE SHOWER WITHOUT RINSING OFF THE SUDS AND CAREFULLY MAKE YOUR WAY TO YOUR FLOATY TOY.
IT FEELS GREAT TO SLIDE YOUR BODY UP AND DOWN ON YOUR PARTNER'S.
FLIP OVER ON YOUR FRONT AND FEEL YOUR PARTNER SLIPPING AND SLIDING ALL OVER YOU.

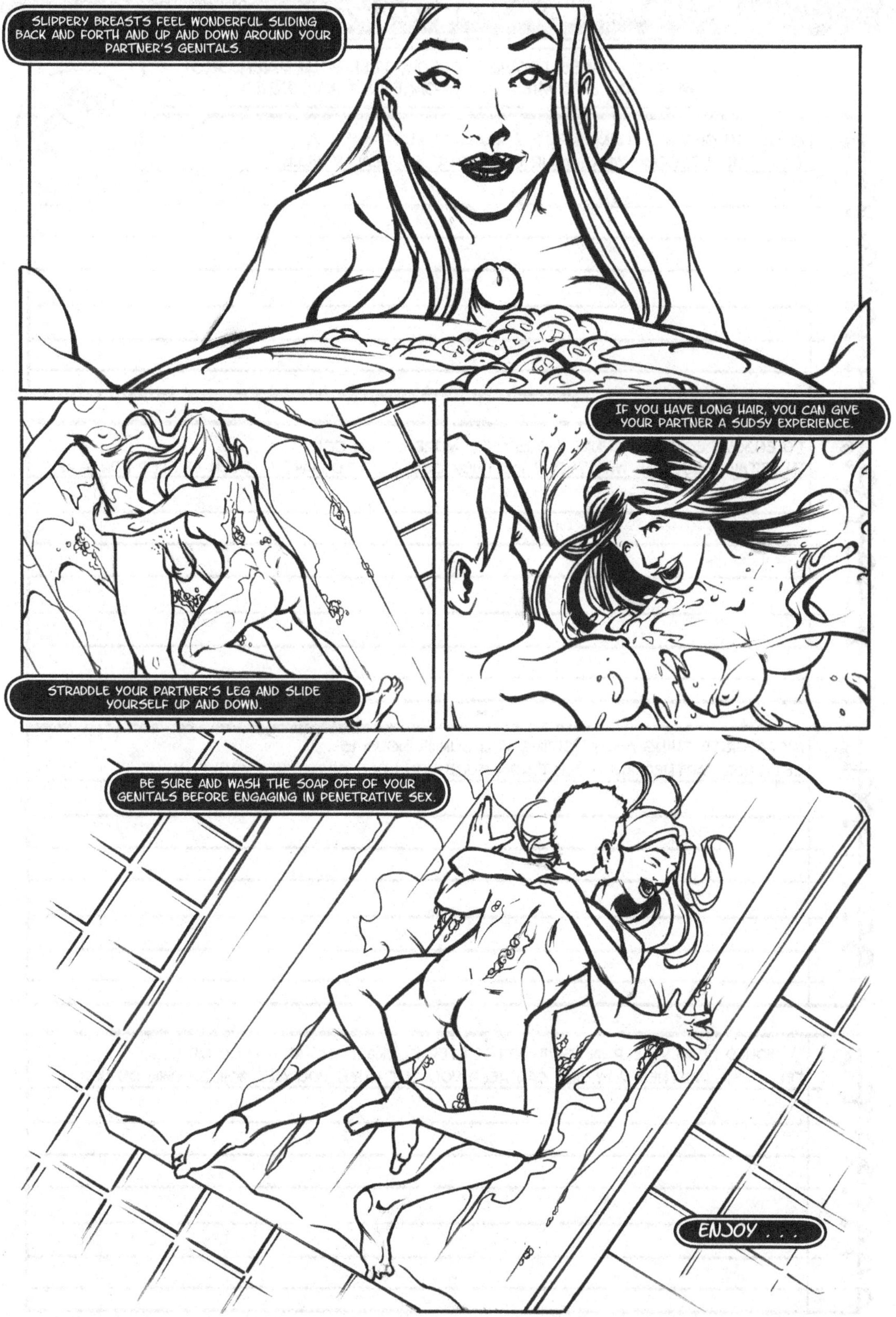
SLIPPERY BREASTS FEEL WONDERFUL SLIDING BACK AND FORTH AND UP AND DOWN AROUND YOUR PARTNER'S GENITALS.
STRADDLE YOUR PARTNER'S LEG AND SLIDE YOURSELF UP AND DOWN.
IF YOU HAVE LONG HAIR, YOU CAN GIVE YOUR PARTNER A SUDSY EXPERIENCE.
BE SURE AND WASH THE SOAP OFF OF YOUR GENITALS BEFORE ENGAGING IN PENETRATIVE SEX.
ENJOY . . .

CUNNILINGUS: IT IS ALL ABOUT PERSONAL TASTES.

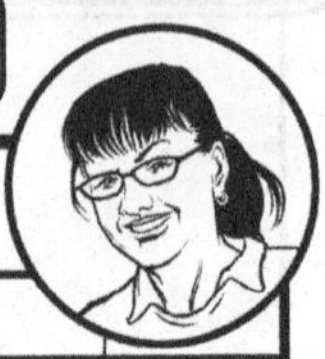
IN THE SPACES PROVIDED BELOW, TELL YOUR PARTNER(S) WHAT YOU LIKE WHEN YOU ENGAGE IN CUNNILINGUS.

WHEN YOU GIVE ME CUNNILINGUS, I REALLY LIKE IT WHEN YOU . . .
IN DETAIL, DESCRIBE WHAT YOUR PARTNER DOES REALLY WELL.

I'D ENJOY RECEIVING CUNNILINGUS EVEN MORE IF YOU COULD . . .
IN DETAIL, DESCRIBE WHAT YOUR PARTNER COULD DO TO MAKE IT EVEN BETTER FOR YOU.

MY FAVORITE THING ABOUT GIVING YOU CUNNILINGUS IS . . .
LET YOUR PARTNER KNOW JUST HOW MUCH YOU LOVE GIVING HER CUNNILINGUS.

IT WOULD REALLY HELP ME GIVE YOU BETTER CUNNILINGUS IF YOU COULD . . .
TELL YOUR PARTNER HOW SHE CAN HELP YOU OUT WHEN YOU ARE GOING DOWN ON HER.

CHAPTER 19

HOW TO GIVE GREAT CUNNILINGUS

WHEN YOU REALLY WANT TO GIVE HER SELFLESS PLEASURE, IT IS HARD TO BEAT CUNNILINGUS. IN THIS SCENARIO, WE WILL SHOW YOU SOME TECHNIQUES TO MAKE IT MORE COMFORTABLE FOR YOU AND EVEN MORE PLEASURABLE FOR HER.

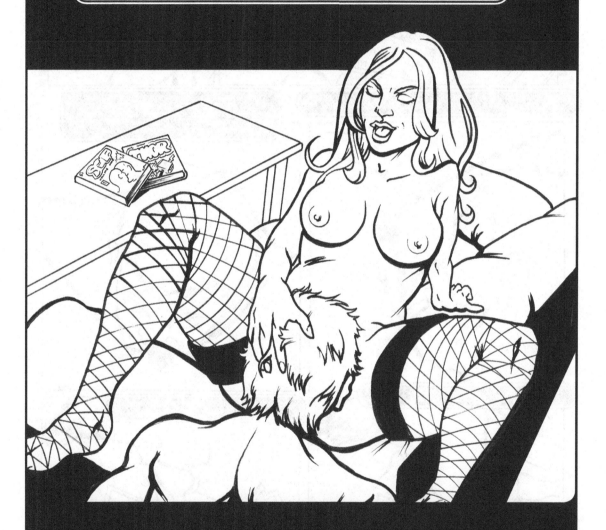

WE'LL SHOW YOU HOW . . .

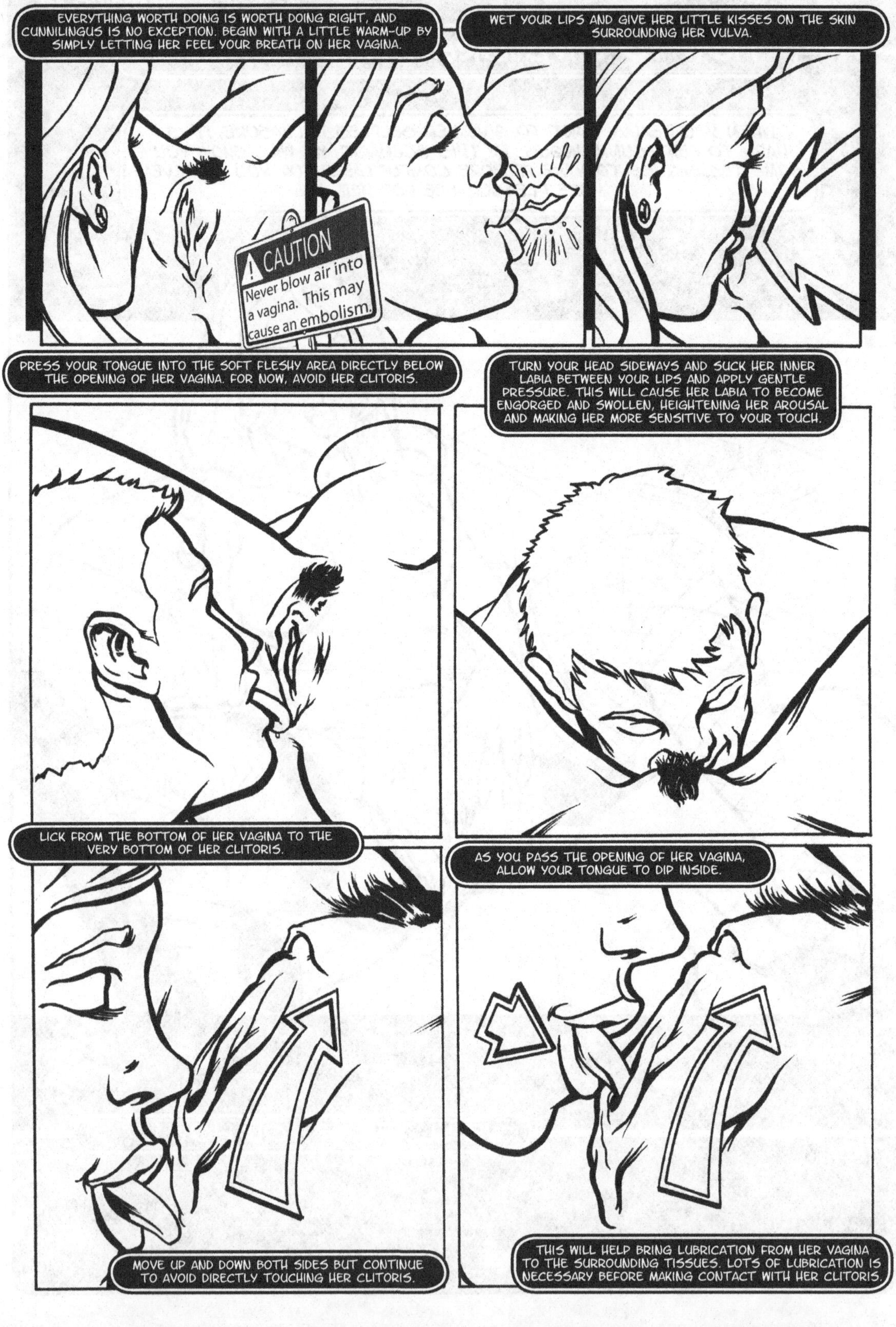
EVERYTHING WORTH DOING IS WORTH DOING RIGHT, AND CUNNILINGUS IS NO EXCEPTION. BEGIN WITH A LITTLE WARM-UP BY SIMPLY LETTING HER FEEL YOUR BREATH ON HER VAGINA.
CAUTION
Never blow air into a vagina. This may cause an embolism.
WET YOUR LIPS AND GIVE HER LITTLE KISSES ON THE SKIN SURROUNDING HER VULVA.
PRESS YOUR TONGUE INTO THE SOFT FLESHY AREA DIRECTLY BELOW THE OPENING OF HER VAGINA. FOR NOW, AVOID HER CLITORIS.
TURN YOUR HEAD SIDEWAYS AND SUCK HER INNER LABIA BETWEEN YOUR LIPS AND APPLY GENTLE PRESSURE. THIS WILL CAUSE HER LABIA TO BECOME ENGORGED AND SWOLLEN, HEIGHTENING HER AROUSAL AND MAKING HER MORE SENSITIVE TO YOUR TOUCH.
LICK FROM THE BOTTOM OF HER VAGINA TO THE VERY BOTTOM OF HER CLITORIS.
MOVE UP AND DOWN BOTH SIDES BUT CONTINUE TO AVOID DIRECTLY TOUCHING HER CLITORIS.
AS YOU PASS THE OPENING OF HER VAGINA, ALLOW YOUR TONGUE TO DIP INSIDE.
THIS WILL HELP BRING LUBRICATION FROM HER VAGINA TO THE SURROUNDING TISSUES. LOTS OF LUBRICATION IS NECESSARY BEFORE MAKING CONTACT WITH HER CLITORIS.

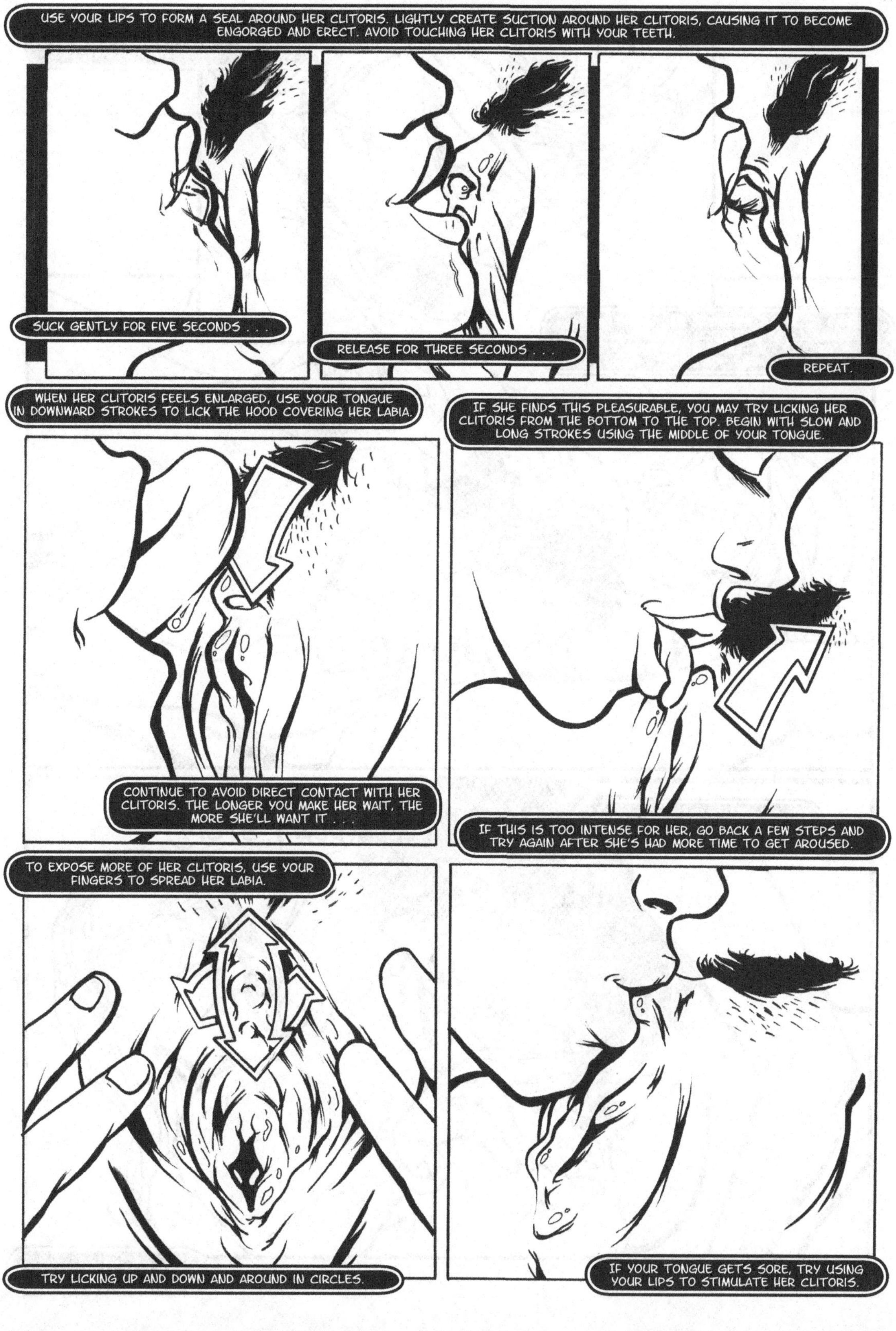
USE YOUR LIPS TO FORM A SEAL AROUND HER CLITORIS. LIGHTLY CREATE SUCTION AROUND HER CLITORIS, CAUSING IT TO BECOME ENGORGED AND ERECT. AVOID TOUCHING HER CLITORIS WITH YOUR TEETH.
SUCK GENTLY FOR FIVE SECONDS . . .
RELEASE FOR THREE SECONDS . . .
REPEAT.
WHEN HER CLITORIS FEELS ENLARGED, USE YOUR TONGUE IN DOWNWARD STROKES TO LICK THE HOOD COVERING HER LABIA.
CONTINUE TO AVOID DIRECT CONTACT WITH HER CLITORIS. THE LONGER YOU MAKE HER WAIT, THE MORE SHE'LL WANT IT . . .
IF SHE FINDS THIS PLEASURABLE, YOU MAY TRY LICKING HER CLITORIS FROM THE BOTTOM TO THE TOP. BEGIN WITH SLOW AND LONG STROKES USING THE MIDDLE OF YOUR TONGUE.
IF THIS IS TOO INTENSE FOR HER, GO BACK A FEW STEPS AND TRY AGAIN AFTER SHE'S HAD MORE TIME TO GET AROUSED.
TO EXPOSE MORE OF HER CLITORIS, USE YOUR FINGERS TO SPREAD HER LABIA.
TRY LICKING UP AND DOWN AND AROUND IN CIRCLES.
IF YOUR TONGUE GETS SORE, TRY USING YOUR LIPS TO STIMULATE HER CLITORIS.

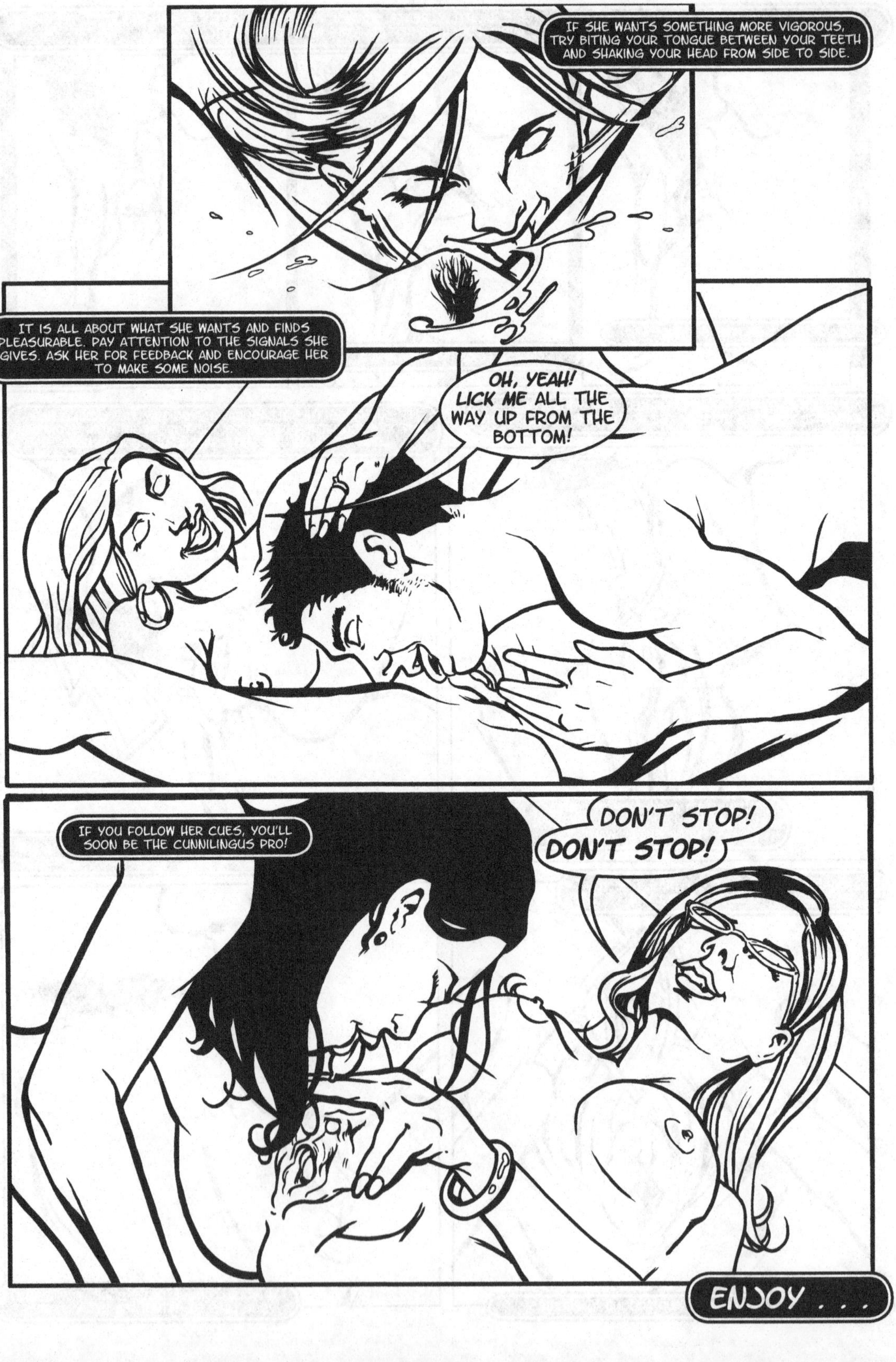
IF SHE WANTS SOMETHING MORE VIGOROUS, TRY BITING YOUR TONGUE BETWEEN YOUR TEETH AND SHAKING YOUR HEAD FROM SIDE TO SIDE.
IT IS ALL ABOUT WHAT SHE WANTS AND FINDS PLEASURABLE. PAY ATTENTION TO THE SIGNALS SHE GIVES. ASK HER FOR FEEDBACK AND ENCOURAGE HER TO MAKE SOME NOISE.
OH, YEAH! LICK ME ALL THE WAY UP FROM THE BOTTOM!
IF YOU FOLLOW HER CUES, YOU'LL SOON BE THE CUNNILINGUS PRO!
DON'T STOP! DON'T STOP!
ENJOY . . .

CHAPTER 20

HOW TO GIVE GREAT FELLATIO

FOR MANY MEN, FELLATIO IS A SPECIAL FAVORITE. IT GIVES YOUR PARTNER AN OPPORTUNITY TO RELAX AND RECEIVE PLEASURE WITHOUT THE PRESSURE TO PERFORM SEXUALLY. IN THIS SCENARIO, WE WILL SHOW YOU HOW TO USE YOUR LIPS, TONGUE AND MOUTH TO MAXIMIZE THE PLEASURE FOR BOTH OF YOU.

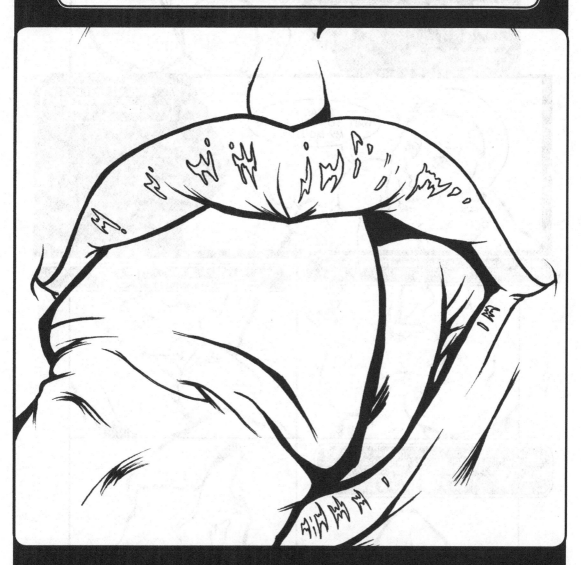

WE'LL SHOW YOU HOW . . .

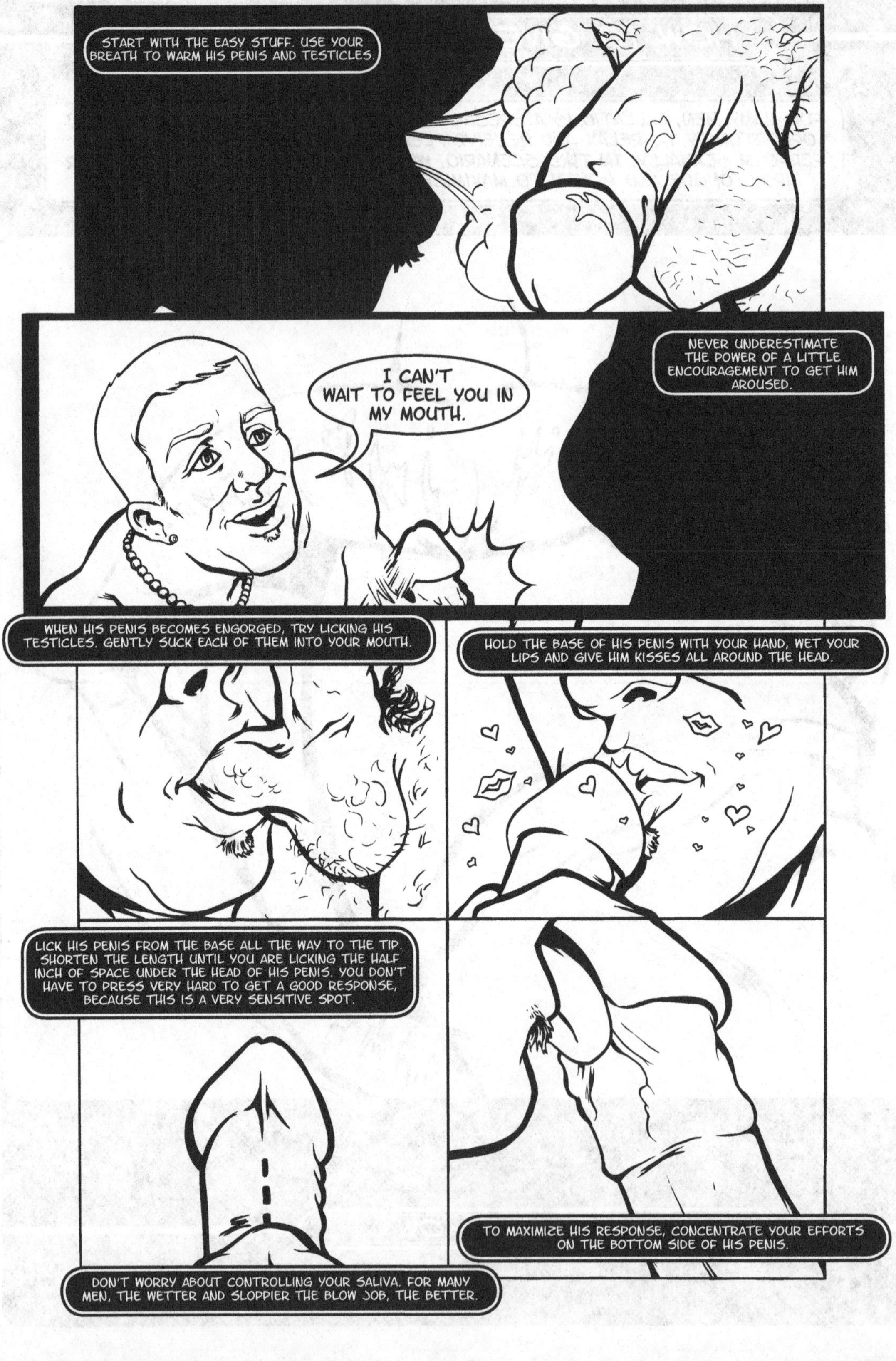
START WITH THE EASY STUFF. USE YOUR BREATH TO WARM HIS PENIS AND TESTICLES.
I CAN'T WAIT TO FEEL YOU IN MY MOUTH.
NEVER UNDERESTIMATE THE POWER OF A LITTLE ENCOURAGEMENT TO GET HIM AROUSED.
WHEN HIS PENIS BECOMES ENGORGED, TRY LICKING HIS TESTICLES. GENTLY SUCK EACH OF THEM INTO YOUR MOUTH.
HOLD THE BASE OF HIS PENIS WITH YOUR HAND, WET YOUR LIPS AND GIVE HIM KISSES ALL AROUND THE HEAD.
LICK HIS PENIS FROM THE BASE ALL THE WAY TO THE TIP. SHORTEN THE LENGTH UNTIL YOU ARE LICKING THE HALF INCH OF SPACE UNDER THE HEAD OF HIS PENIS. YOU DON'T HAVE TO PRESS VERY HARD TO GET A GOOD RESPONSE, BECAUSE THIS IS A VERY SENSITIVE SPOT.
DON'T WORRY ABOUT CONTROLLING YOUR SALIVA. FOR MANY MEN, THE WETTER AND SLOPPIER THE BLOW JOB, THE BETTER.
TO MAXIMIZE HIS RESPONSE, CONCENTRATE YOUR EFFORTS ON THE BOTTOM SIDE OF HIS PENIS.

WHEN YOU ARE READY TO ALLOW HIS PENIS TO ENTER YOUR MOUTH, BE SURE TO GRAB THE BASE OF HIS PENIS WITH YOUR HAND. THIS WILL ENABLE YOU TO SIMULATE A DEEP-THROAT TECHNIQUE WITHOUT ACTUALLY HAVING TO GAG ON THE FULL LENGTH OF HIS PENIS.

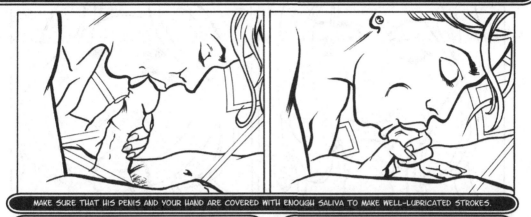

MAKE SURE THAT HIS PENIS AND YOUR HAND ARE COVERED WITH ENOUGH SALIVA TO MAKE WELL-LUBRICATED STROKES.

WITH YOUR HAND IN PLACE YOU ONLY NEED TO TAKE THE VERY TIP OF HIS PENIS INTO YOUR MOUTH TO MAKE HIM FEEL AS THOUGH HE'S GETTING THE REAL DEAL. COVER YOUR TEETH WITH YOUR LIPS AND STICK OUT YOUR TONGUE SO THAT IT IS RUBBING ON THE BOTTOM OF HIS PENIS.

UNLESS YOU ARE BOTH EXPERIENCED WITH ROUGH ORAL SEX, DON'T GRAB YOUR PARTNER'S HEAD AND DO NOT THRUST YOUR HIPS. JUST LIE BACK AND ENJOY IT.

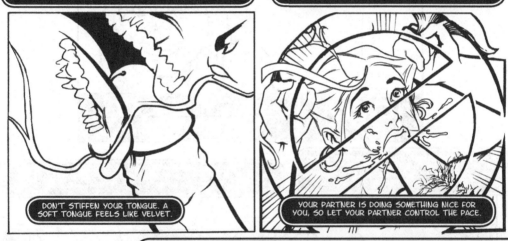

DON'T STIFFEN YOUR TONGUE. A SOFT TONGUE FEELS LIKE VELVET.

YOUR PARTNER IS DOING SOMETHING NICE FOR YOU, SO LET YOUR PARTNER CONTROL THE PACE.

MANY MEN FIND IT DIFFICULT TO ACHIEVE ORGASM FROM ORAL SEX ALONE. SHOWING HIM THAT YOU ARE REALLY ENJOYING THE ACT WILL ALLOW HIM TO LET GO AND REALLY ENJOY THE EXPERIENCE. IF HE'S WORRIED ABOUT YOUR COMFORT, HE WON'T EVER BE ABLE TO ENJOY HIMSELF.

IF YOUR MOUTH AND TONGUE GET SORE, TAKE A BREAK BUT CONTINUE STROKING HIM WITH YOUR HAND.

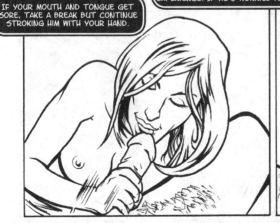

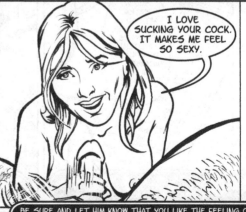

I LOVE SUCKING YOUR COCK. IT MAKES ME FEEL SO SEXY.

BE SURE AND LET HIM KNOW THAT YOU LIKE THE FEELING OF HIS PENIS IN YOUR MOUTH AS MUCH AS HE DOES.

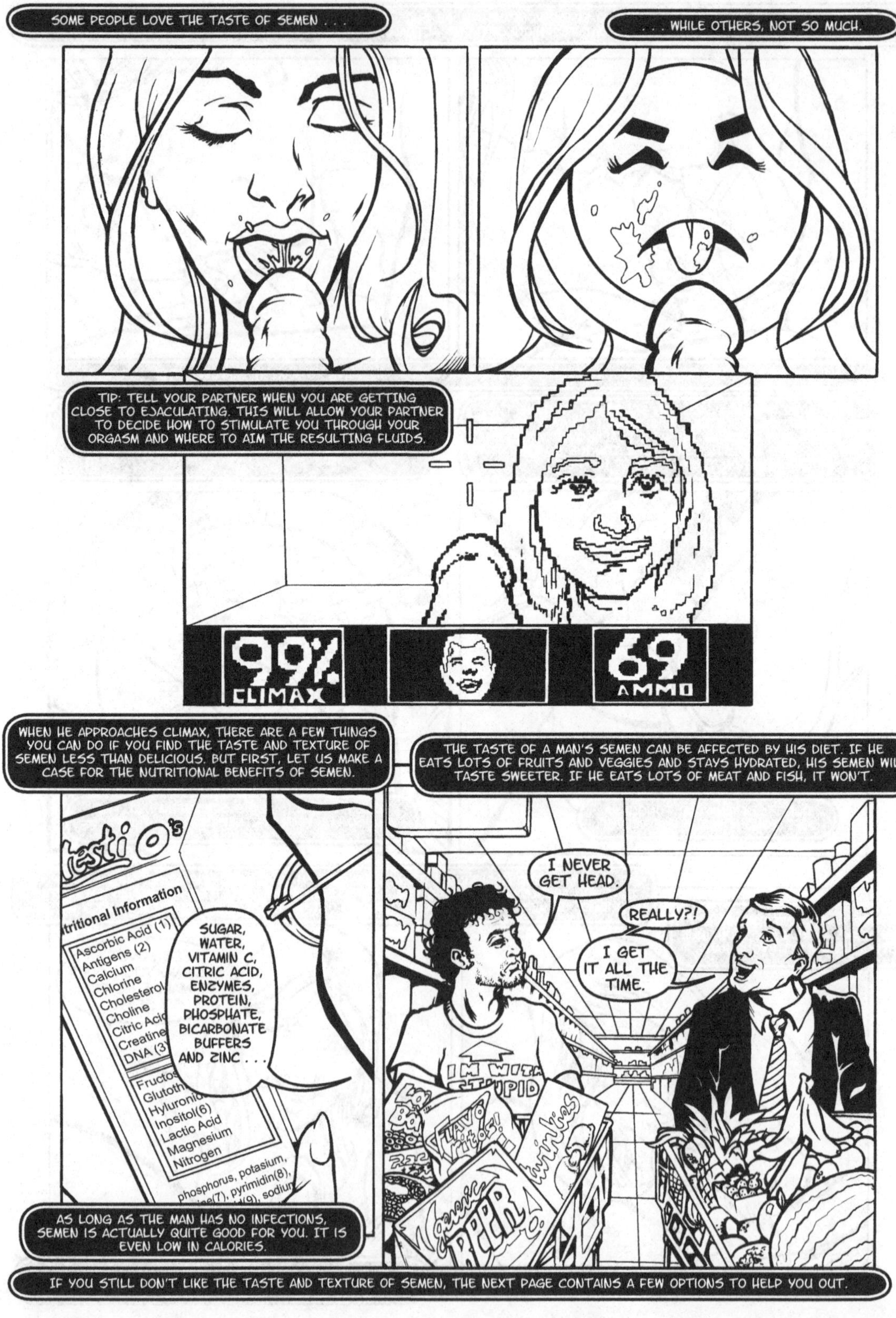
SOME PEOPLE LOVE THE TASTE OF SEMEN . . .
. . . WHILE OTHERS, NOT SO MUCH.
TIP: TELL YOUR PARTNER WHEN YOU ARE GETTING CLOSE TO EJACULATING. THIS WILL ALLOW YOUR PARTNER TO DECIDE HOW TO STIMULATE YOU THROUGH YOUR ORGASM AND WHERE TO AIM THE RESULTING FLUIDS.
99%
CLIMAX
69
AMMO
WHEN HE APPROACHES CLIMAX, THERE ARE A FEW THINGS YOU CAN DO IF YOU FIND THE TASTE AND TEXTURE OF SEMEN LESS THAN DELICIOUS. BUT FIRST, LET US MAKE A CASE FOR THE NUTRITIONAL BENEFITS OF SEMEN.
Ascorbic Acid (1)
Antigens (2)
Calcium
Chlorine
Choline
Inositol(6)
Lactic Acid
Magnesium
Nitrogen
SUGAR, WATER, VITAMIN C, CITRIC ACID, ENZYMES, PROTEIN, PHOSPHATE, BICARBONATE BUFFERS AND ZINC . . .
AS LONG AS THE MAN HAS NO INFECTIONS, SEMEN IS ACTUALLY QUITE GOOD FOR YOU. IT IS EVEN LOW IN CALORIES.
THE TASTE OF A MAN'S SEMEN CAN BE AFFECTED BY HIS DIET. IF HE EATS LOTS OF FRUITS AND VEGGIES AND STAYS HYDRATED, HIS SEMEN WILL TASTE SWEETER. IF HE EATS LOTS OF MEAT AND FISH, IT WON'T.
I NEVER GET HEAD.
REALLY?!
I GET IT ALL THE TIME.
IF YOU STILL DON'T LIKE THE TASTE AND TEXTURE OF SEMEN, THE NEXT PAGE CONTAINS A FEW OPTIONS TO HELP YOU OUT.

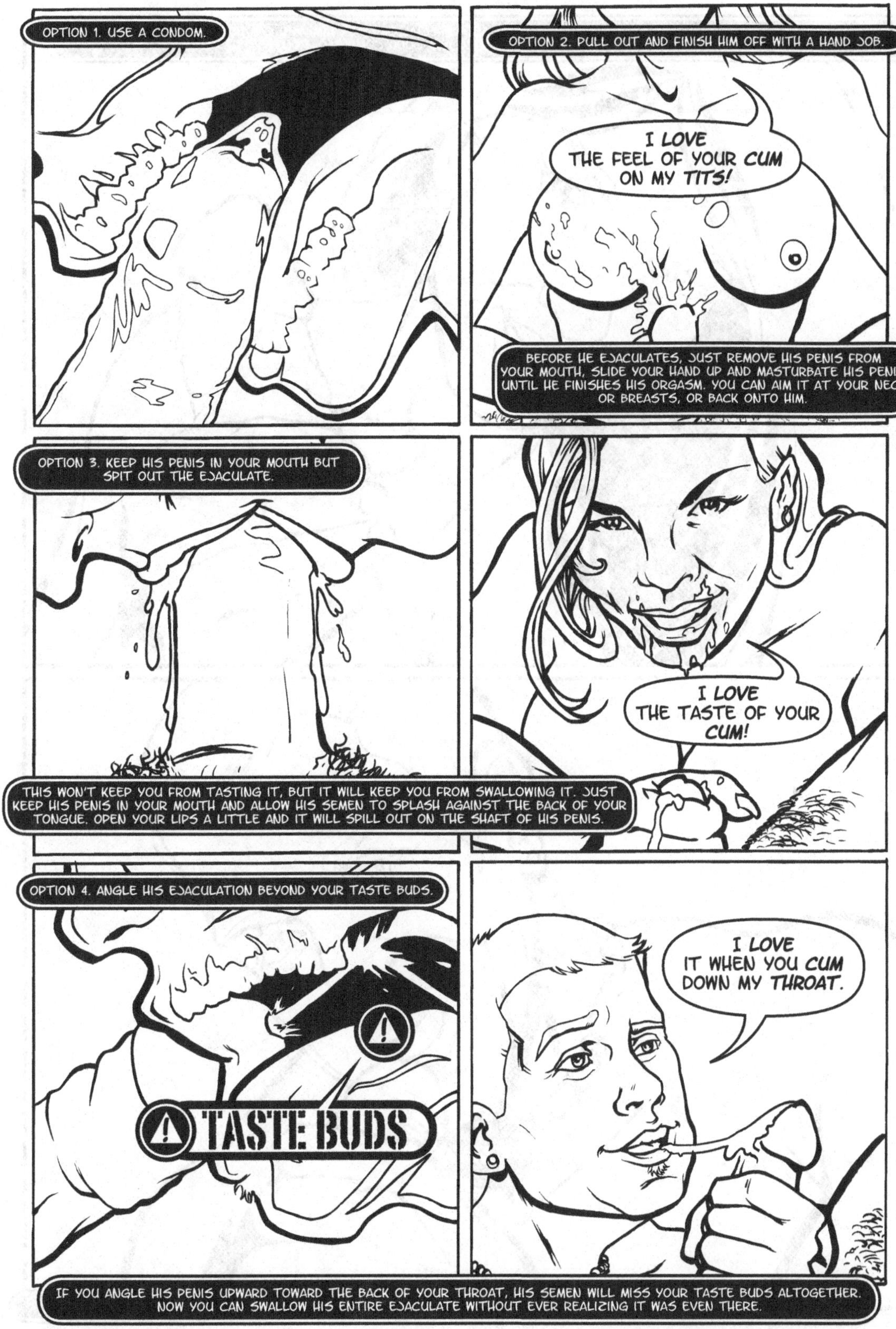
OPTION 1. USE A CONDOM.
OPTION 2. PULL OUT AND FINISH HIM OFF WITH A HAND JOB.
I LOVE THE FEEL OF YOUR CUM ON MY TITS!
BEFORE HE EJACULATES, JUST REMOVE HIS PENIS FROM YOUR MOUTH, SLIDE YOUR HAND UP AND MASTURBATE HIS PENIS UNTIL HE FINISHES HIS ORGASM. YOU CAN AIM IT AT YOUR NECK OR BREASTS, OR BACK ONTO HIM.
OPTION 3. KEEP HIS PENIS IN YOUR MOUTH BUT SPIT OUT THE EJACULATE.
I LOVE THE TASTE OF YOUR CUM!
THIS WON'T KEEP YOU FROM TASTING IT, BUT IT WILL KEEP YOU FROM SWALLOWING IT. JUST KEEP HIS PENIS IN YOUR MOUTH AND ALLOW HIS SEMEN TO SPLASH AGAINST THE BACK OF YOUR TONGUE. OPEN YOUR LIPS A LITTLE AND IT WILL SPILL OUT ON THE SHAFT OF HIS PENIS.
OPTION 4. ANGLE HIS EJACULATION BEYOND YOUR TASTE BUDS.
TASTE BUDS
I LOVE IT WHEN YOU CUM DOWN MY THROAT.
IF YOU ANGLE HIS PENIS UPWARD TOWARD THE BACK OF YOUR THROAT, HIS SEMEN WILL MISS YOUR TASTE BUDS ALTOGETHER. NOW YOU CAN SWALLOW HIS ENTIRE EJACULATE WITHOUT EVER REALIZING IT WAS EVEN THERE.

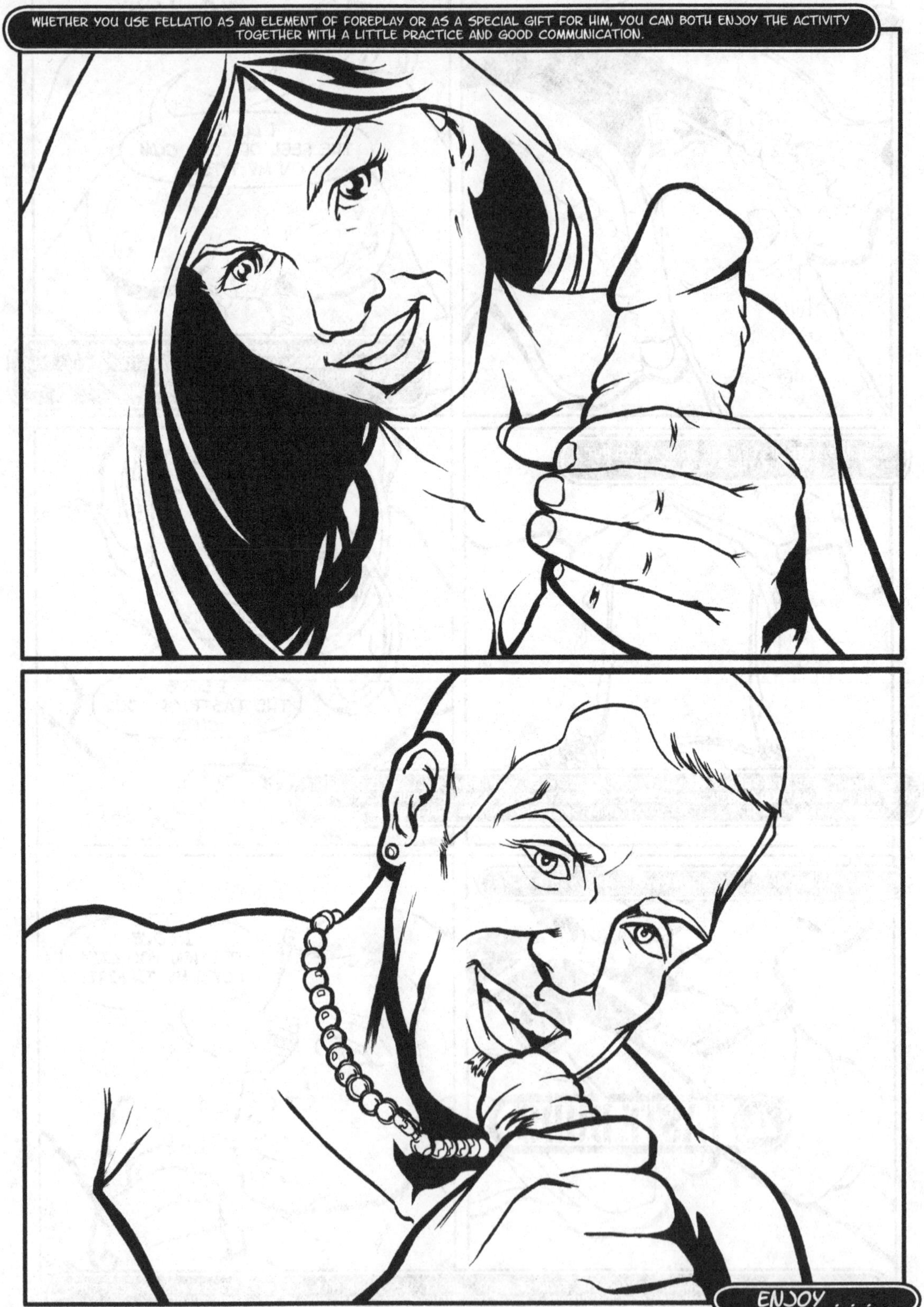
WHETHER YOU USE FELLATIO AS AN ELEMENT OF FOREPLAY OR AS A SPECIAL GIFT FOR HIM, YOU CAN BOTH ENJOY THE ACTIVITY TOGETHER WITH A LITTLE PRACTICE AND GOOD COMMUNICATION.
ENJOY . . .

CHAPTER 21

THE TWENTY-ONE CUNNILINGUS SHUFFLE

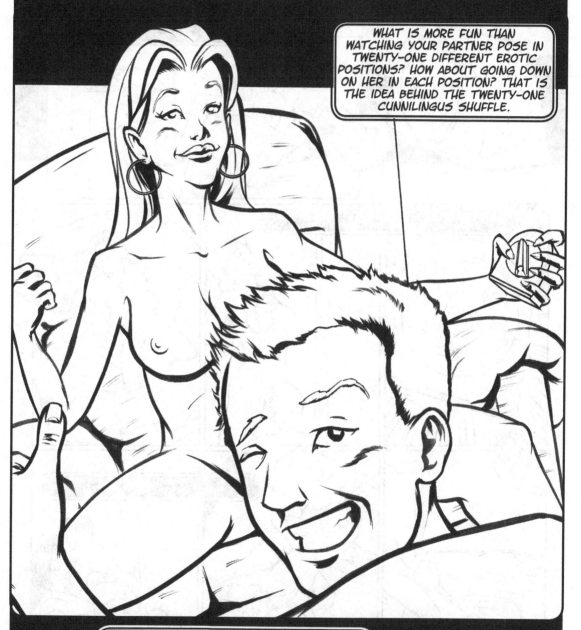

WHAT IS MORE FUN THAN WATCHING YOUR PARTNER POSE IN TWENTY-ONE DIFFERENT EROTIC POSITIONS? HOW ABOUT GOING DOWN ON HER IN EACH POSITION? THAT IS THE IDEA BEHIND THE TWENTY-ONE CUNNILINGUS SHUFFLE.

WHAT YOU'LL NEED . . .

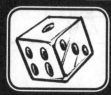

SIX-SIDED DIE

KITCHEN TIMER

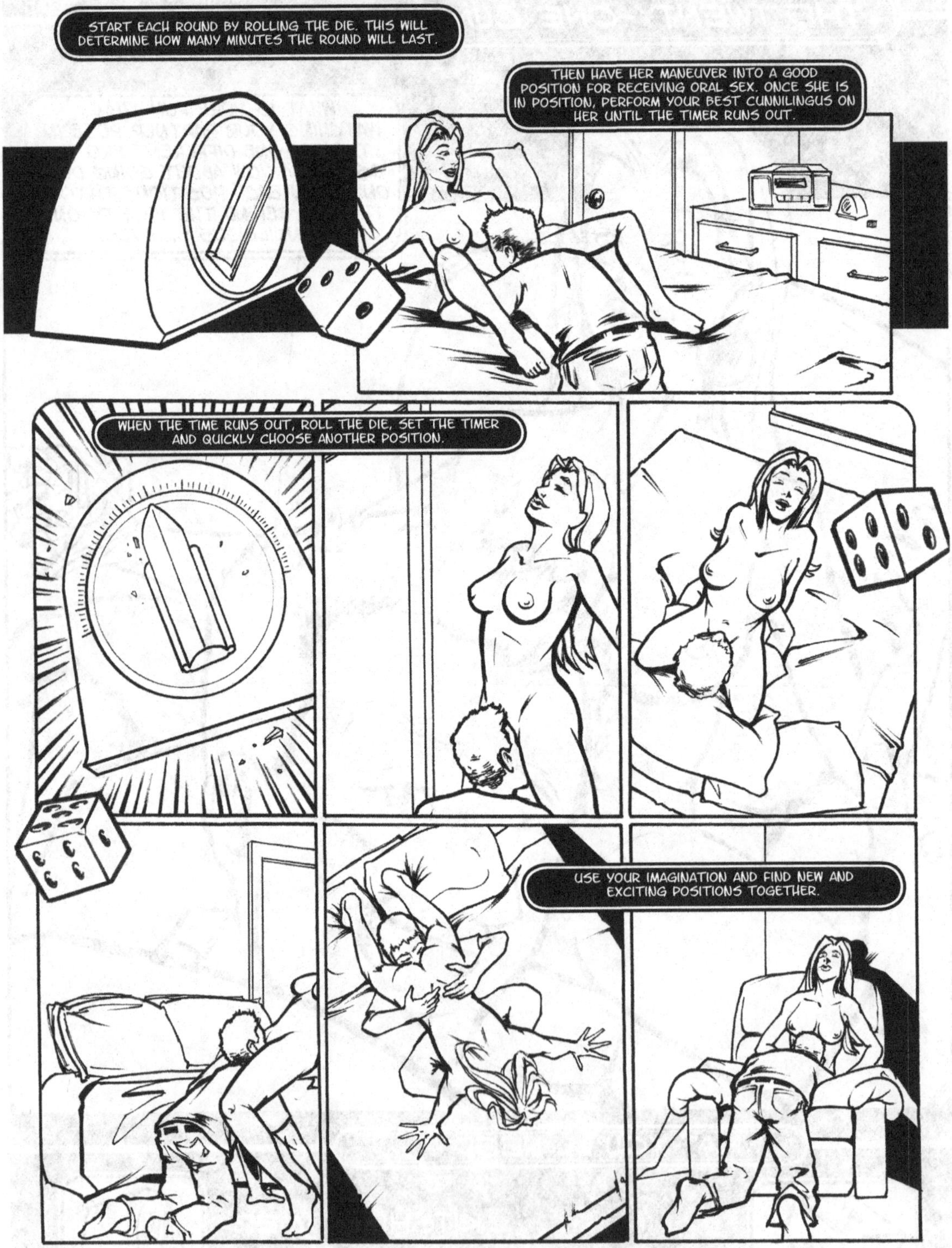
START EACH ROUND BY ROLLING THE DIE. THIS WILL DETERMINE HOW MANY MINUTES THE ROUND WILL LAST.
THEN HAVE HER MANEUVER INTO A GOOD POSITION FOR RECEIVING ORAL SEX. ONCE SHE IS IN POSITION, PERFORM YOUR BEST CUNNILINGUS ON HER UNTIL THE TIMER RUNS OUT.
WHEN THE TIME RUNS OUT, ROLL THE DIE, SET THE TIMER AND QUICKLY CHOOSE ANOTHER POSITION.
USE YOUR IMAGINATION AND FIND NEW AND EXCITING POSITIONS TOGETHER.

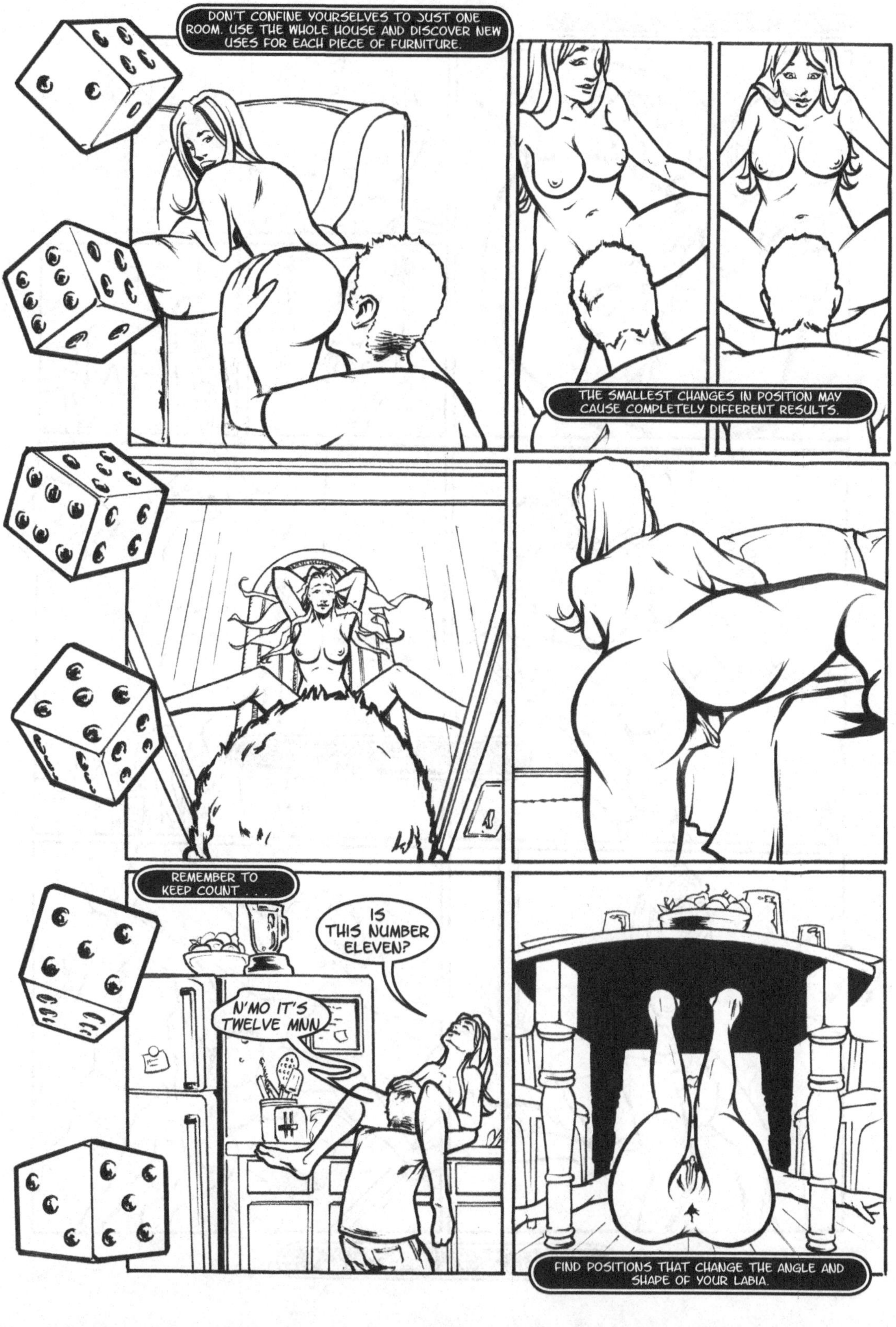
DON'T CONFINE YOURSELVES TO JUST ONE ROOM. USE THE WHOLE HOUSE AND DISCOVER NEW USES FOR EACH PIECE OF FURNITURE.
THE SMALLEST CHANGES IN POSITION MAY CAUSE COMPLETELY DIFFERENT RESULTS.
REMEMBER TO KEEP COUNT . . .
IS THIS NUMBER ELEVEN?
N'MO IT'S TWELVE MNN
FIND POSITIONS THAT CHANGE THE ANGLE AND SHAPE OF YOUR LABIA.

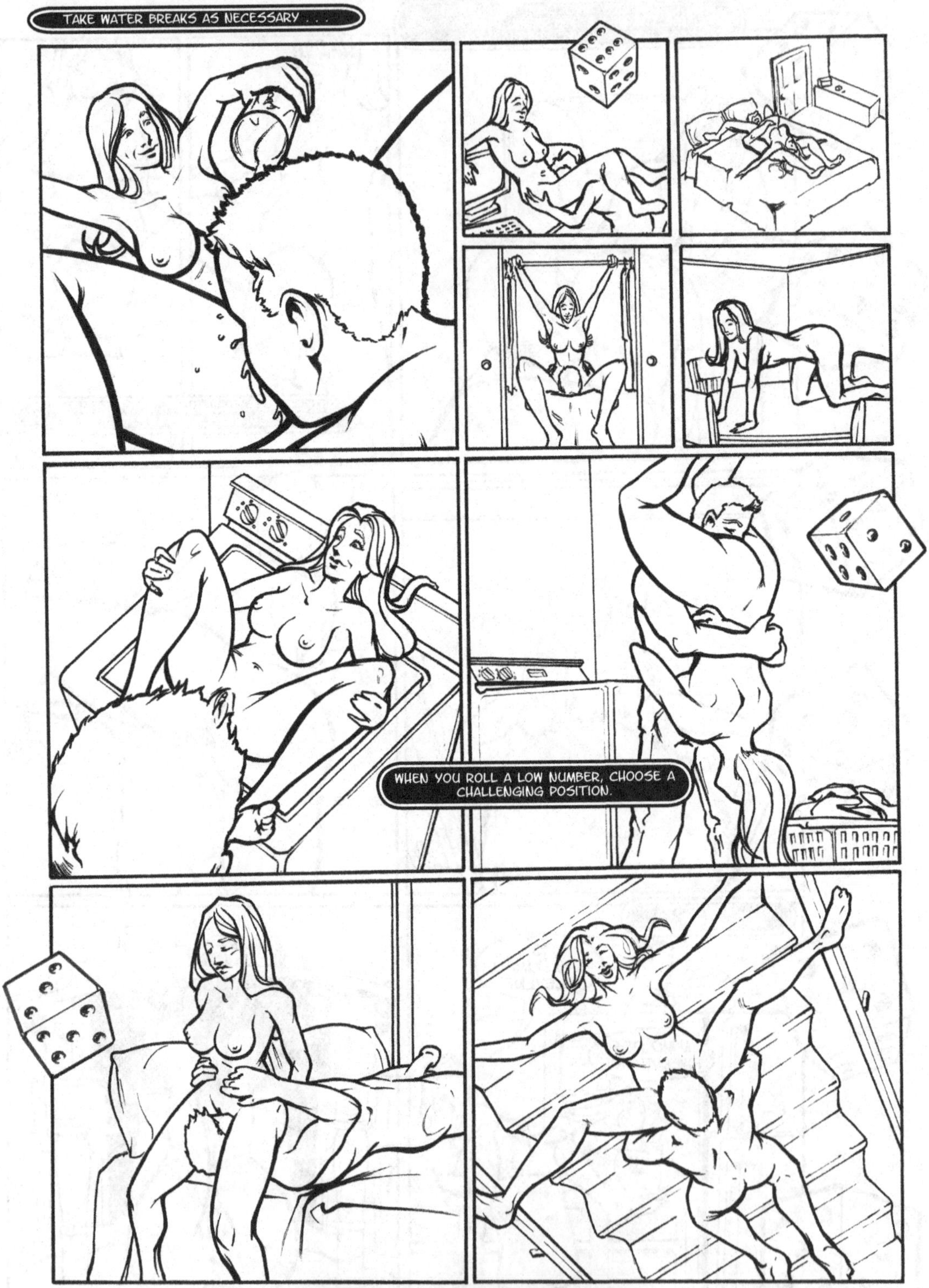
TAKE WATER BREAKS AS NECESSARY . . .
WHEN YOU ROLL A LOW NUMBER, CHOOSE A CHALLENGING POSITION.
THINK OUTSIDE OF THE BOX AND TRY SOMETHING YOU'VE NEVER TRIED BEFORE.

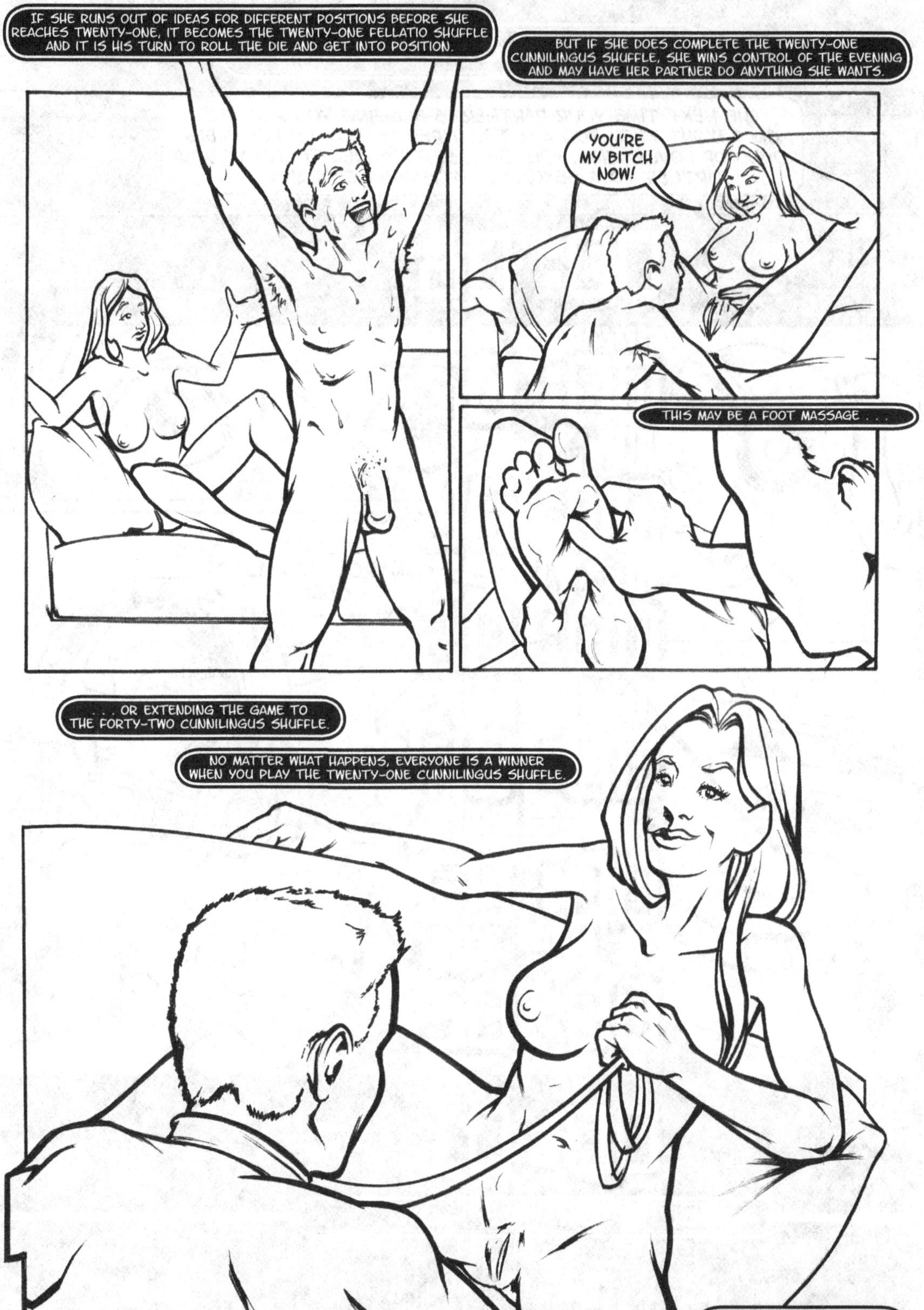
IF SHE RUNS OUT OF IDEAS FOR DIFFERENT POSITIONS BEFORE SHE REACHES TWENTY-ONE, IT BECOMES THE TWENTY-ONE FELLATIO SHUFFLE AND IT IS HIS TURN TO ROLL THE DIE AND GET INTO POSITION.
BUT IF SHE DOES COMPLETE THE TWENTY-ONE CUNNILINGUS SHUFFLE, SHE WINS CONTROL OF THE EVENING AND MAY HAVE HER PARTNER DO ANYTHING SHE WANTS.
YOU'RE MY BITCH NOW!
THIS MAY BE A FOOT MASSAGE . . .
. . . OR EXTENDING THE GAME TO THE FORTY-TWO CUNNILINGUS SHUFFLE.
NO MATTER WHAT HAPPENS, EVERYONE IS A WINNER WHEN YOU PLAY THE TWENTY-ONE CUNNILINGUS SHUFFLE.
ENJOY . . .

CHAPTER 22

GET HIM OFF QUICKLY

THE NEXT TIME YOUR PARTNER IS BEGGING YOU FOR SEX ON A NIGHT WHEN YOU ARE TOO TIRED OR NOT UP FOR A BIG ROUND OF LOVEMAKING, YOU CAN USE THIS IDEA TO TREAT YOUR PARTNER TO A SEXUALLY SATISFYING EXPERIENCE.

00: 08

00: 07
00: 06
GROUND CONTROL TO MAJOR CUM.
00: 05
00: 04
LAUNCH
00: 03
00: 02

00: 01 . . .

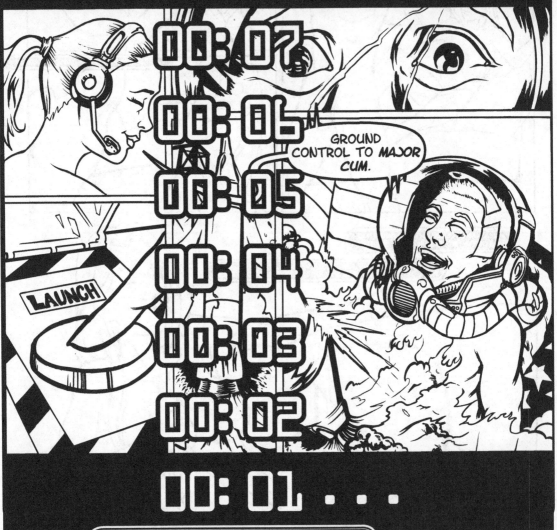

WE'LL SHOW YOU HOW . . .

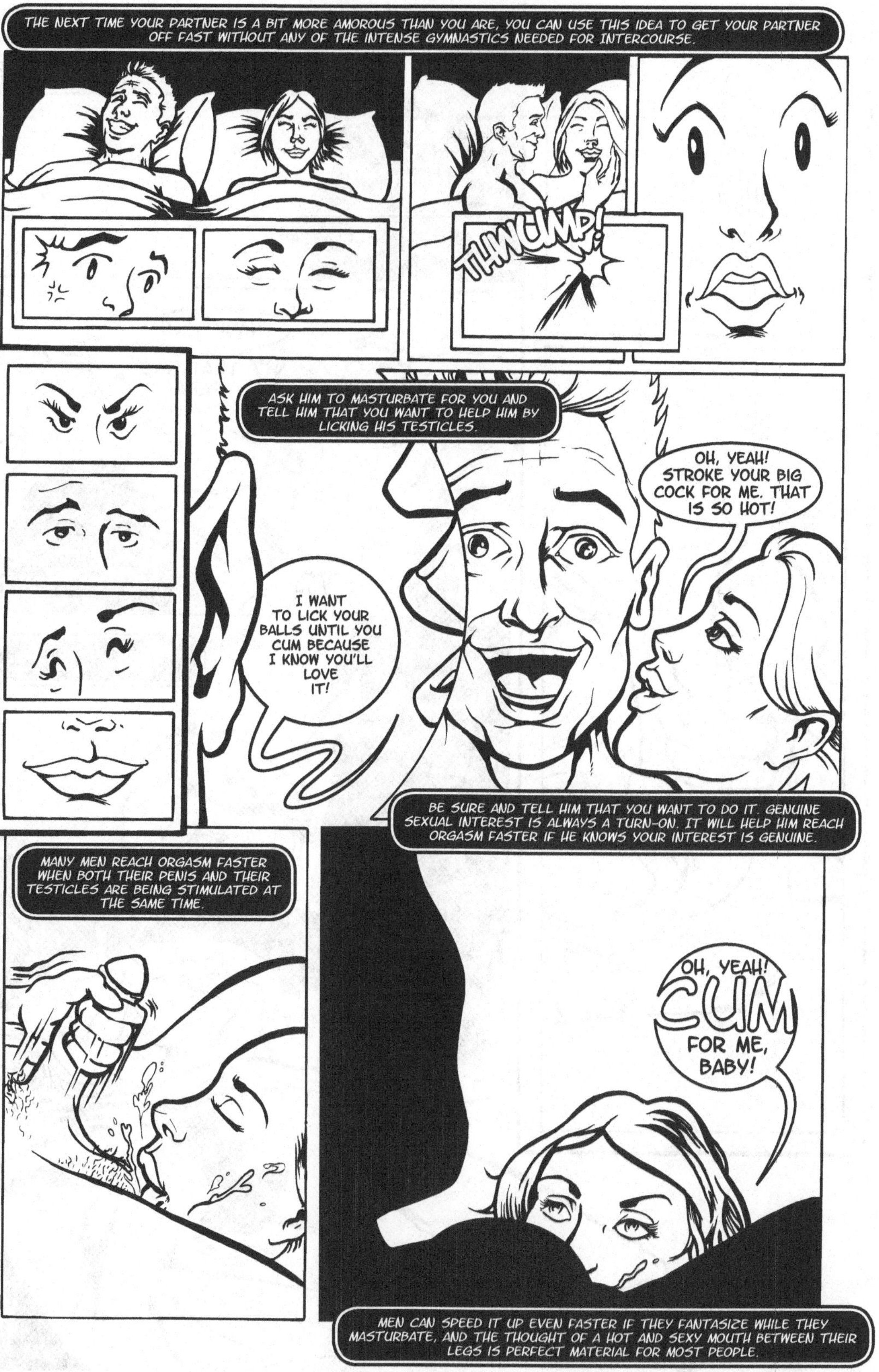
THE NEXT TIME YOUR PARTNER IS A BIT MORE AMOROUS THAN YOU ARE, YOU CAN USE THIS IDEA TO GET YOUR PARTNER OFF FAST WITHOUT ANY OF THE INTENSE GYMNASTICS NEEDED FOR INTERCOURSE.
THWUMP!
ASK HIM TO MASTURBATE FOR YOU AND TELL HIM THAT YOU WANT TO HELP HIM BY LICKING HIS TESTICLES.
I WANT TO LICK YOUR BALLS UNTIL YOU CUM BECAUSE I KNOW YOU'LL LOVE IT!
OH, YEAH! STROKE YOUR BIG COCK FOR ME. THAT IS SO HOT!
BE SURE AND TELL HIM THAT YOU WANT TO DO IT. GENUINE SEXUAL INTEREST IS ALWAYS A TURN-ON. IT WILL HELP HIM REACH ORGASM FASTER IF HE KNOWS YOUR INTEREST IS GENUINE.
MANY MEN REACH ORGASM FASTER WHEN BOTH THEIR PENIS AND THEIR TESTICLES ARE BEING STIMULATED AT THE SAME TIME.
OH, YEAH! CUM FOR ME, BABY!
MEN CAN SPEED IT UP EVEN FASTER IF THEY FANTASIZE WHILE THEY MASTURBATE, AND THE THOUGHT OF A HOT AND SEXY MOUTH BETWEEN THEIR LEGS IS PERFECT MATERIAL FOR MOST PEOPLE.

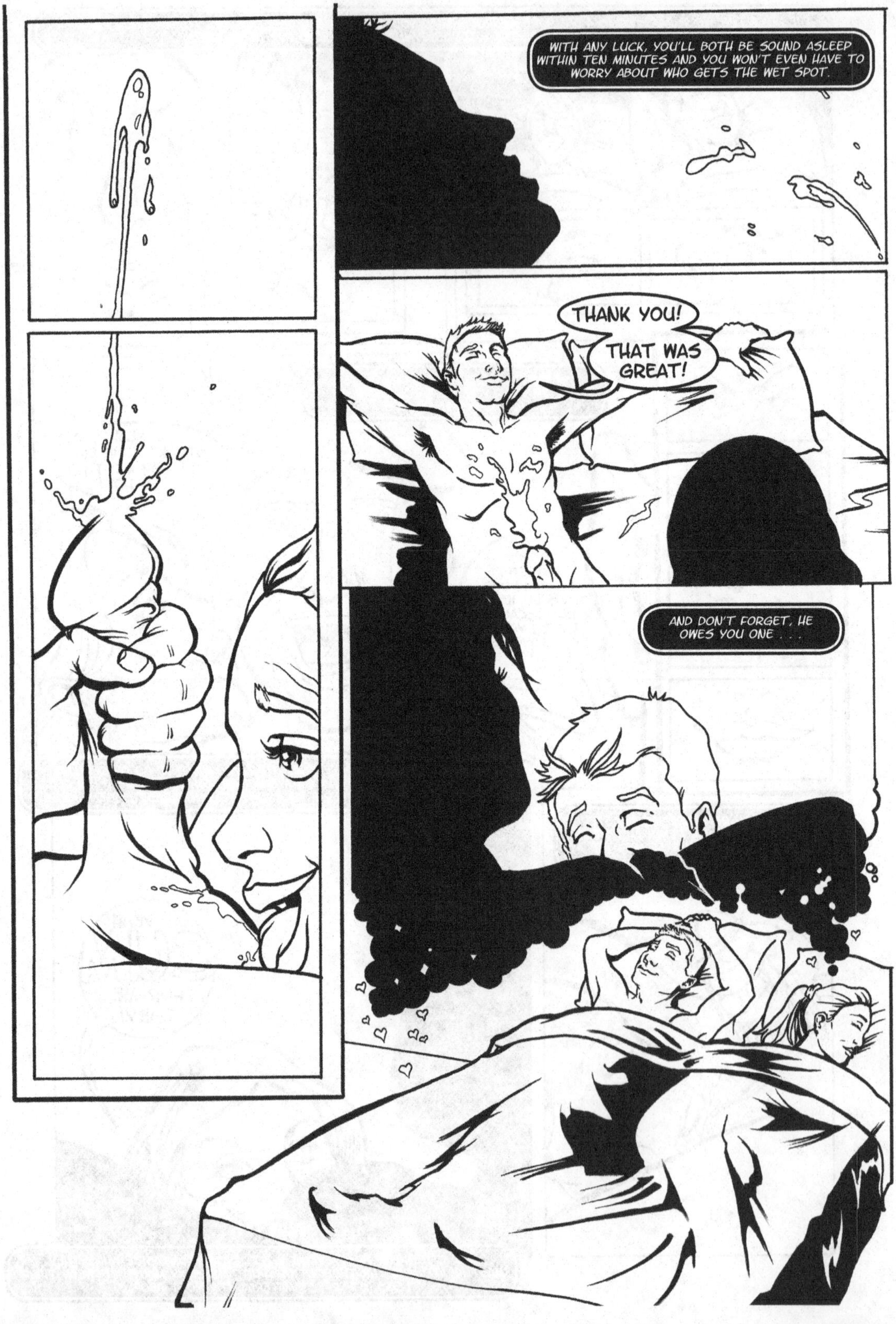
WITH ANY LUCK, YOU'LL BOTH BE SOUND ASLEEP WITHIN TEN MINUTES AND YOU WON'T EVEN HAVE TO WORRY ABOUT WHO GETS THE WET SPOT.
THANK YOU!
THAT WAS GREAT!
AND DON'T FORGET, HE OWES YOU ONE . . .

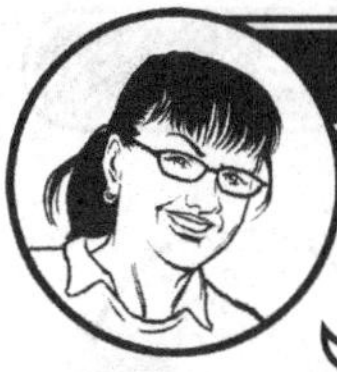

INTIMACY: IT ISN'T JUST FOR SEX ANYMORE

ARE YOU RECEIVING ENOUGH INTIMACY FROM YOUR PARTNER? LET PARTNERS KNOW WHAT INTIMATE ACTIVITIES YOU APPRECIATE FROM THEM.
MARK THE BOXES WITH NUMBERS FROM 1 TO 10, WITH 10 MEANING "YOU ARE DOING GREAT," OR WIITH A 1 TO LET YOUR PARTNER KNOW THAT YOU'D LOVE TO HAVE SOME MORE OF THAT.

- RANDOM HUGS FOR NO REASON AT ALL
- RANDOM KISSES AT ANY TIME OF DAY OR NIGHT
- HOT OPEN-MOUTH KISSES WHEN APPROPRIATE
- OFFERING TO HELP ME OUT WHEN I'VE GOT A LOT ON MY PLATE
- FLIRTING WITH ME WHEN APPROPRIATE
- COPPING A PRIVATE FEEL UNDER THE TABLE OR IN PASSING WHEN NOBODY'S LOOKING
- CALLING/WRITING AND LETTING ME KNOW YOU APPRECIATE ME
- MAKING TIME FOR THE TWO OF US TO TALK
- TAKING A GENUINE INTEREST IN MY SEXUALITY
- TELLING ME ABOUT YOUR SEXUAL FANTASIES AND INTIMATE THOUGHTS
- ALLOWING ME TO SEE YOUR BODY AT APPROPRIATE TIMES
- COOKING FOR ME OR GOING OUT TO DINNER WITH ME
- PROVIDING A ROMANTIC ENVIRONMENT FOR THE TWO OF US
- TOUCHING ME IN WAYS THAT MAKE ME FEEL GOOD, RELAXED AND COMFORTABLE
- SPENDING TIME WITH ME AFTER WE HAVE SEX
- COMPLIMENTING ME ON MY ACHIEVEMENTS OR ON MY VALIANT ATTEMPTS TO DO WELL
- LETTING ME KNOW THAT YOU FIND ME ATTRACTIVE
- MAKING ME FEEL THAT I CAN TRUST YOU WITH MY FANTASIES
- REMEMBERING IMPORTANT DATES AND MILESTONES IN OUR RELATIONSHIP
- BEING GENEROUS WITH ME AND SHOWING ME THAT YOU APPRECIATE MY GENEROSITY
- TAKING A GENUINE INTEREST IN MY ENJOYMENT OF OUR SEX
- LISTENING TO ME WHEN I TELL YOU SOMETHING THAT I FIND IMPORTANT
- SURPRISING ME FROM TIME TO TIME WITH UNEXPECTED TOKENS OF YOUR AFFECTION
- DEMONSTRATING A WILLINGNESS TO TRY YOUR BEST TO SATISFY MY SEXUAL NEEDS
- SHOWING INTEREST WHEN I TELL YOU ABOUT MY DAY
- RANDOM ACTS OF ROMANTIC KINDNESS
- LETTING ME KNOW THAT YOU MISS ME WHEN I AM AWAY

IN THE SPACES BELOW, WRITE A COUPLE OF YOUR FONDEST MEMORIES OF YOUR PARTNER DOING HIS OR HER BEST TO BE INTIMATE WITH YOU.

FELLATIO: IT IS ALL ABOUT PERSONAL TASTES

IN THE SPACES PROVIDED BELOW, TELL YOUR PARTNER(S) WHAT YOU LIKE WHEN YOU ENGAGE IN FELLATIO.

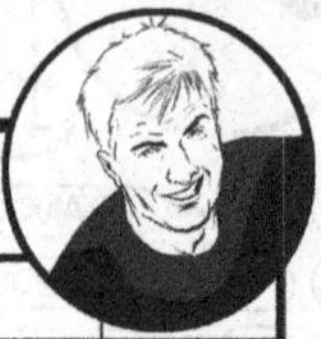

WHEN YOU GIVE ME FELLATIO, I REALLY LIKE IT WHEN YOU . . .
IN DETAIL, DESCRIBE WHAT YOUR PARTNER DOES REALLY WELL.

I'D ENJOY RECEIVING FELLATIO EVEN MORE IF YOU COULD . . .
IN DETAIL, DESCRIBE WHAT YOUR PARTNER COULD DO TO MAKE IT EVEN BETTER FOR YOU.

MY FAVORITE THING ABOUT GIVING YOU FELLATIO IS . . .
LET YOUR PARTNER KNOW JUST HOW MUCH YOU LOVE GIVING HIM FELLATIO.

IT WOULD REALLY HELP ME GIVE YOU BETTER FELLATIO IF YOU COULD . . .
TELL YOUR PARTNER HOW HE CAN HELP YOU OUT WHEN YOU ARE GOING DOWN ON HIM.

CHAPTER 23

ICE CREAM TREATS

HERE IS A TASTY TREAT ON A HOT DAY OR A STEAMY NIGHT. TURN YOUR PARTNER INTO A SEXY ICE CREAM DELICACY.

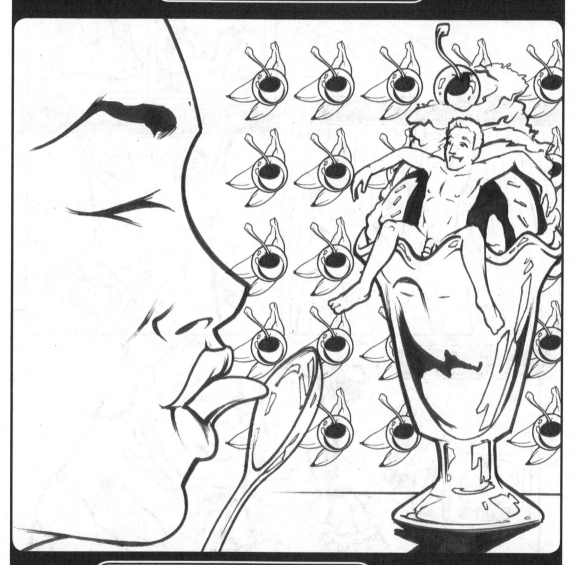

WHAT YOU'LL NEED . . .

SUNDAE-MAKING SUPPLIES

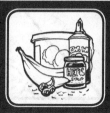

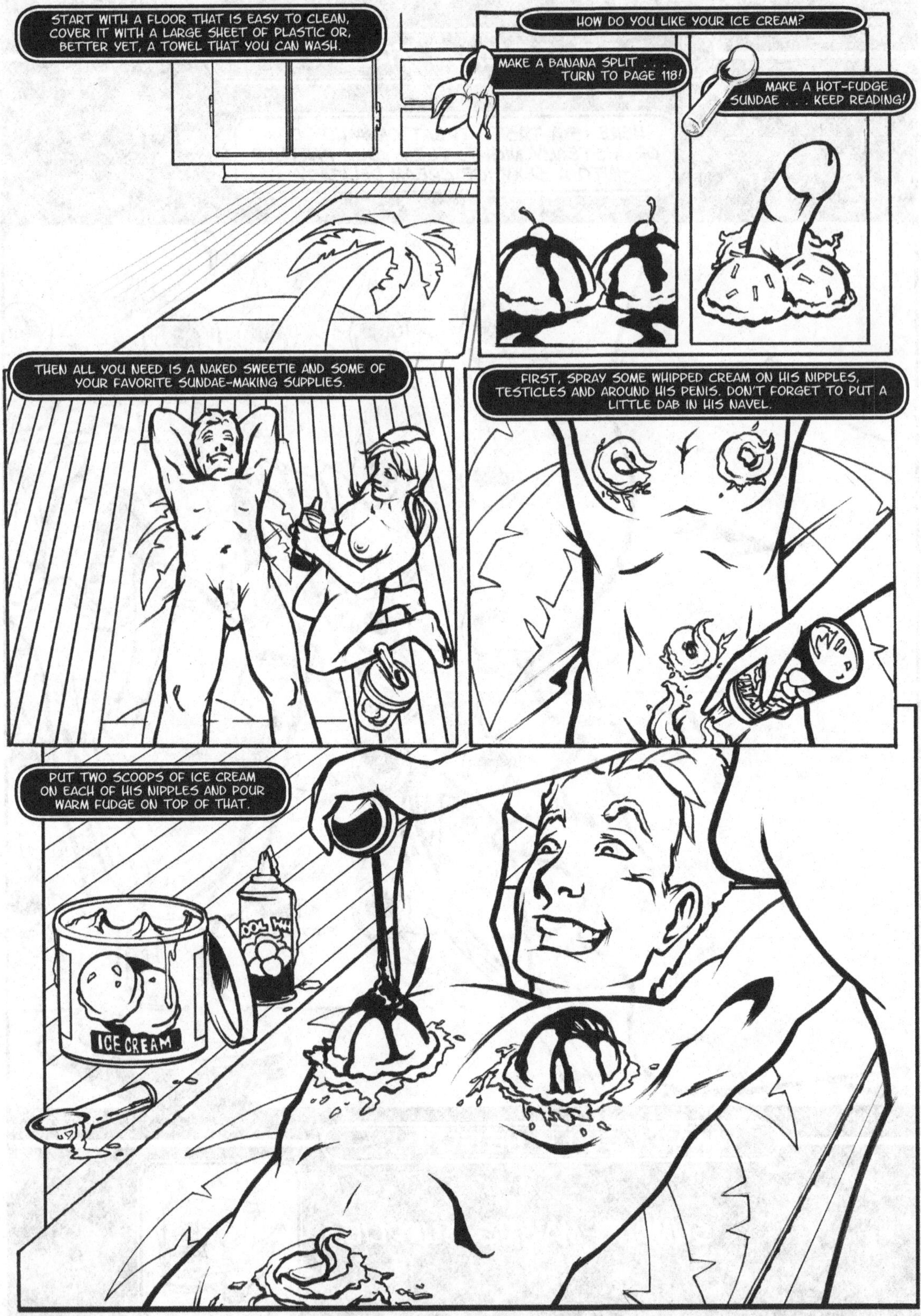
START WITH A FLOOR THAT IS EASY TO CLEAN, COVER IT WITH A LARGE SHEET OF PLASTIC OR, BETTER YET, A TOWEL THAT YOU CAN WASH.
HOW DO YOU LIKE YOUR ICE CREAM?
MAKE A BANANA SPLIT . . . TURN TO PAGE 118!
MAKE A HOT-FUDGE SUNDAE . . . KEEP READING!
THEN ALL YOU NEED IS A NAKED SWEETIE AND SOME OF YOUR FAVORITE SUNDAE-MAKING SUPPLIES.
FIRST, SPRAY SOME WHIPPED CREAM ON HIS NIPPLES, TESTICLES AND AROUND HIS PENIS. DON'T FORGET TO PUT A LITTLE DAB IN HIS NAVEL.
PUT TWO SCOOPS OF ICE CREAM ON EACH OF HIS NIPPLES AND POUR WARM FUDGE ON TOP OF THAT.
ICE CREAM

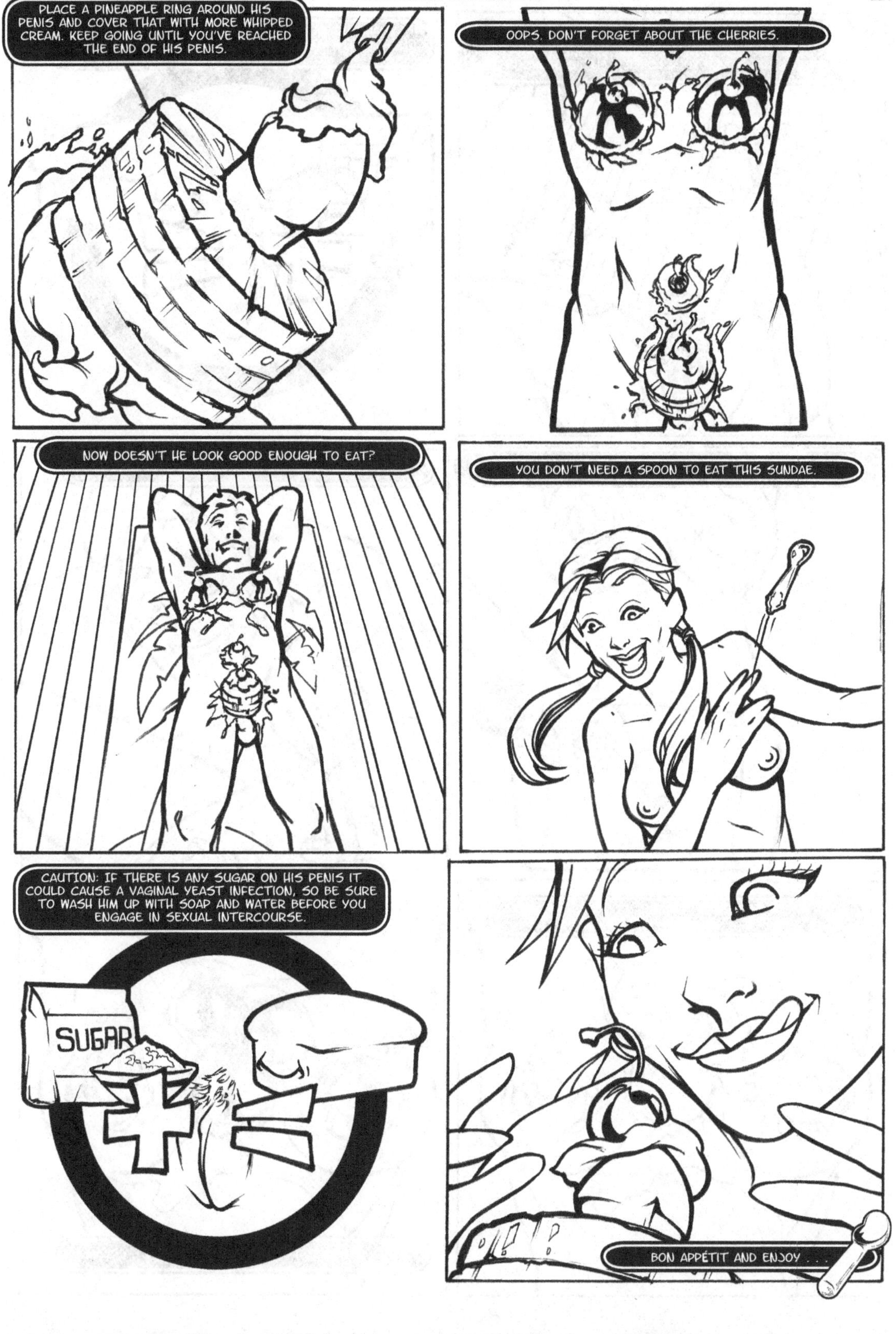
PLACE A PINEAPPLE RING AROUND HIS PENIS AND COVER THAT WITH MORE WHIPPED CREAM. KEEP GOING UNTIL YOU'VE REACHED THE END OF HIS PENIS.
OOPS. DON'T FORGET ABOUT THE CHERRIES.
NOW DOESN'T HE LOOK GOOD ENOUGH TO EAT?
YOU DON'T NEED A SPOON TO EAT THIS SUNDAE.
CAUTION: IF THERE IS ANY SUGAR ON HIS PENIS IT COULD CAUSE A VAGINAL YEAST INFECTION, SO BE SURE TO WASH HIM UP WITH SOAP AND WATER BEFORE YOU ENGAGE IN SEXUAL INTERCOURSE.
SUGAR
BON APPÉTIT AND ENJOY . . .

118

SEX IS FUN!

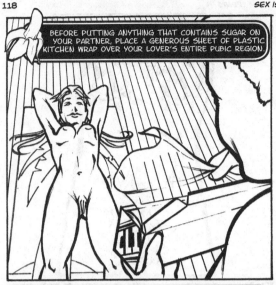

BEFORE PUTTING ANYTHING THAT CONTAINS SUGAR ON YOUR PARTNER, PLACE A GENEROUS SHEET OF PLASTIC KITCHEN WRAP OVER YOUR LOVER'S ENTIRE PUBIC REGION.

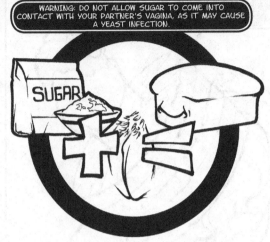

WARNING: DO NOT ALLOW SUGAR TO COME INTO CONTACT WITH YOUR PARTNER'S VAGINA, AS IT MAY CAUSE A YEAST INFECTION.

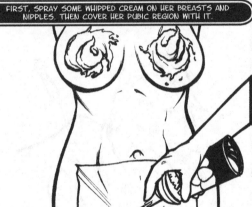

FIRST, SPRAY SOME WHIPPED CREAM ON HER BREASTS AND NIPPLES. THEN COVER HER PUBIC REGION WITH IT.

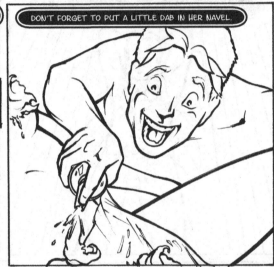

DON'T FORGET TO PUT A LITTLE DAB IN HER NAVEL.

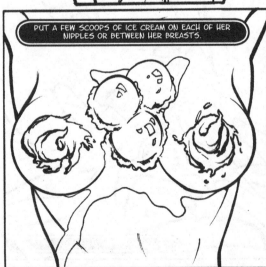

PUT A FEW SCOOPS OF ICE CREAM ON EACH OF HER NIPPLES OR BETWEEN HER BREASTS.

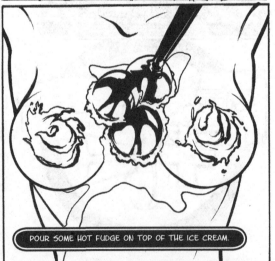

POUR SOME HOT FUDGE ON TOP OF THE ICE CREAM.

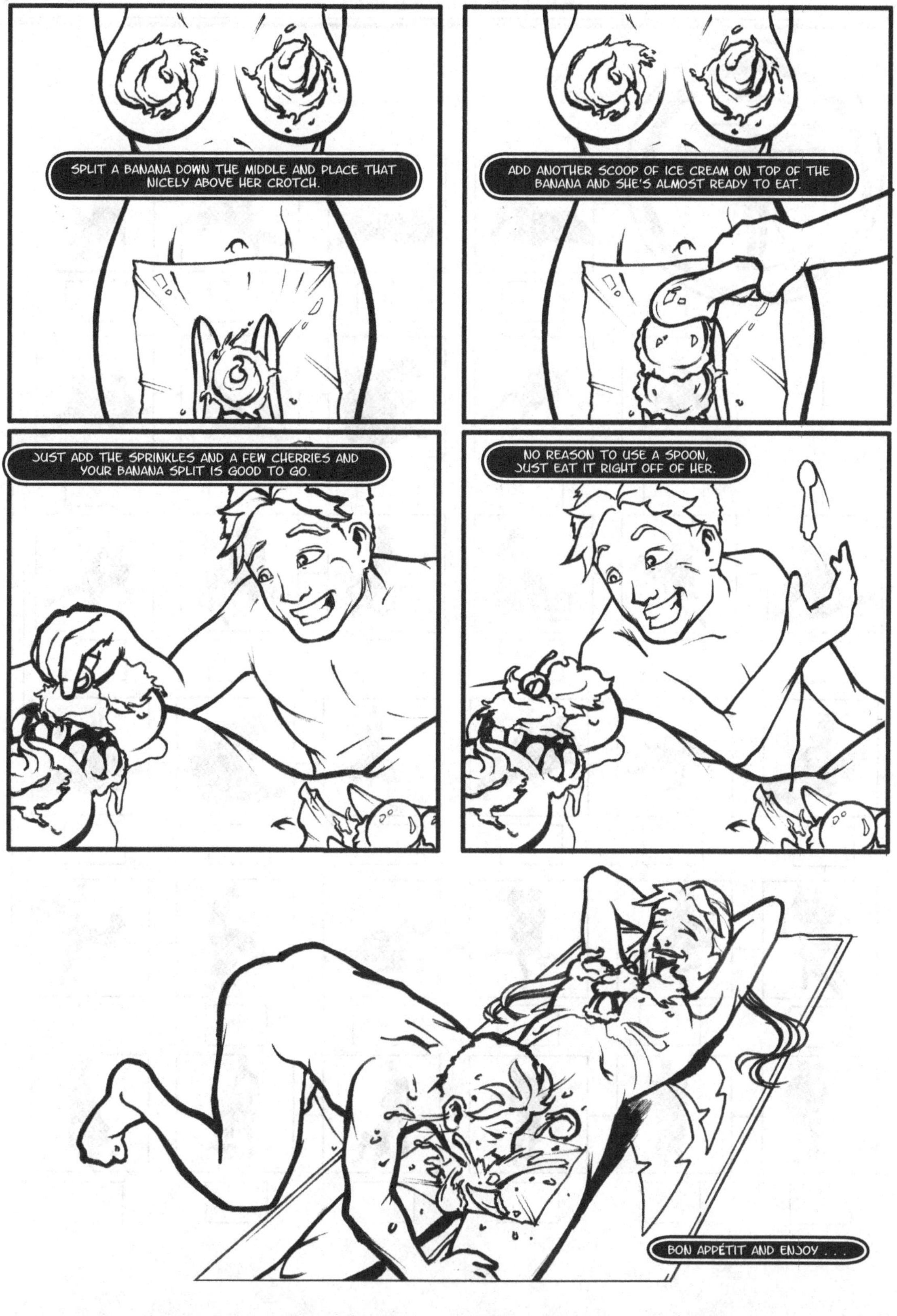
SPLIT A BANANA DOWN THE MIDDLE AND PLACE THAT NICELY ABOVE HER CROTCH.
ADD ANOTHER SCOOP OF ICE CREAM ON TOP OF THE BANANA AND SHE'S ALMOST READY TO EAT.
JUST ADD THE SPRINKLES AND A FEW CHERRIES AND YOUR BANANA SPLIT IS GOOD TO GO.
NO REASON TO USE A SPOON, JUST EAT IT RIGHT OFF OF HER.
BON APPÉTIT AND ENJOY . . .

LET'S DO IT ALL

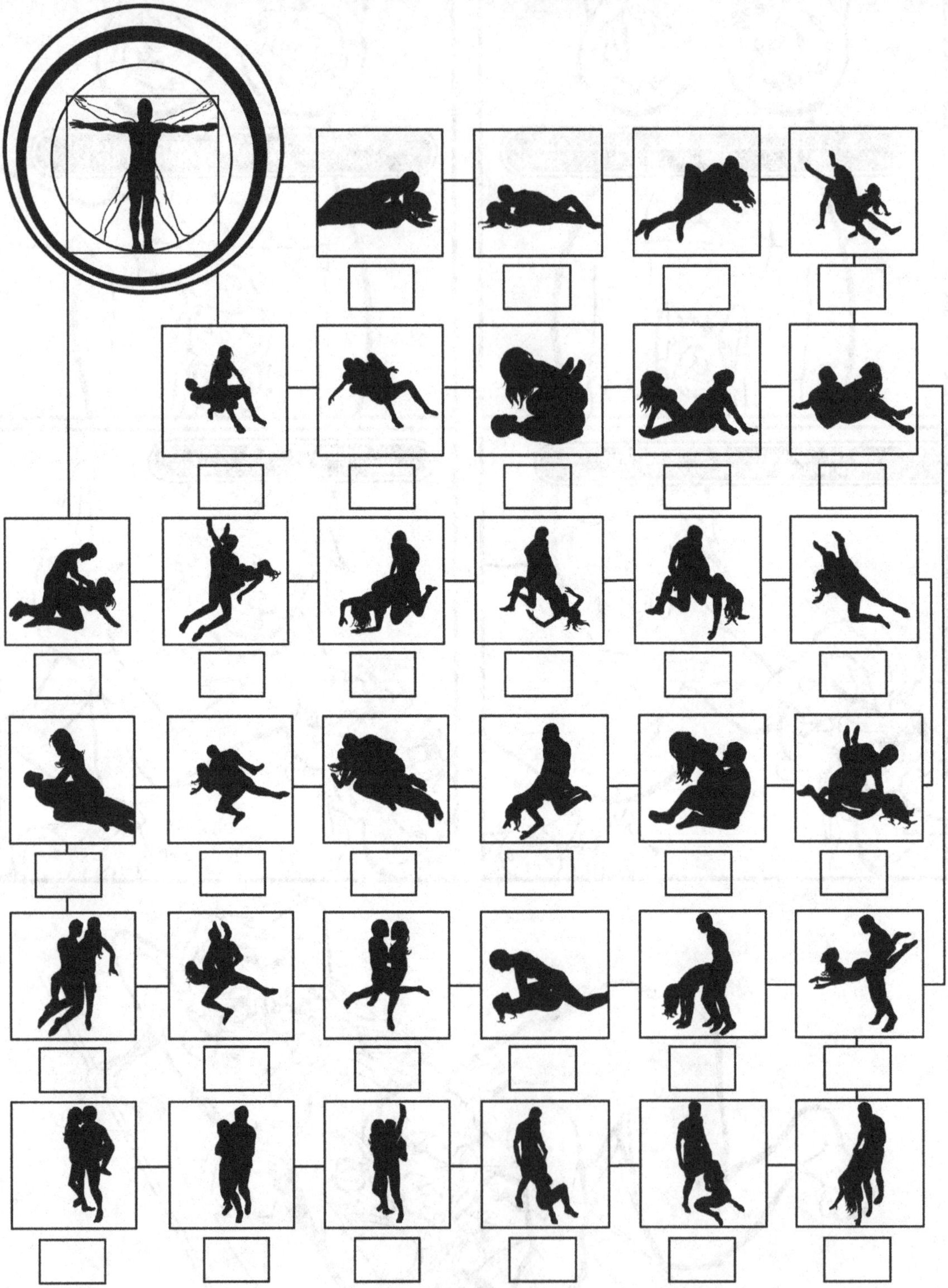

CHAPTER 24

ÜBERCOOL SEX POSITIONS FOR TWO

WHEN IT COMES TO INTERCOURSE, THE POSSIBILITIES ARE NEARLY ENDLESS. IN THIS SECTION OF THE BOOK, WE'LL ILLUSTRATE SOME OF OUR FAVORITES.

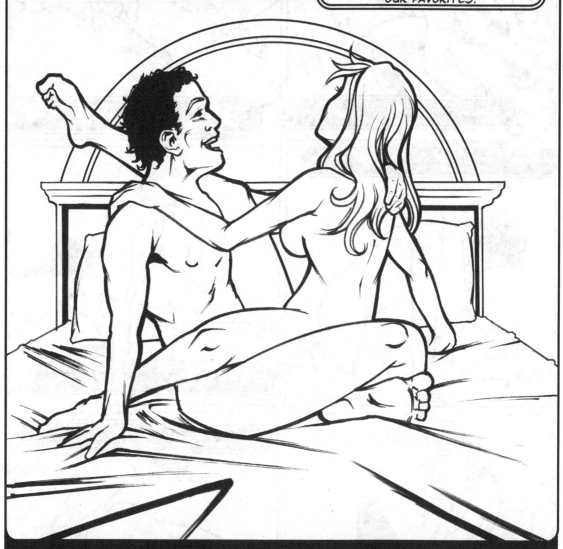

WE'LL SHOW YOU HOW . . .

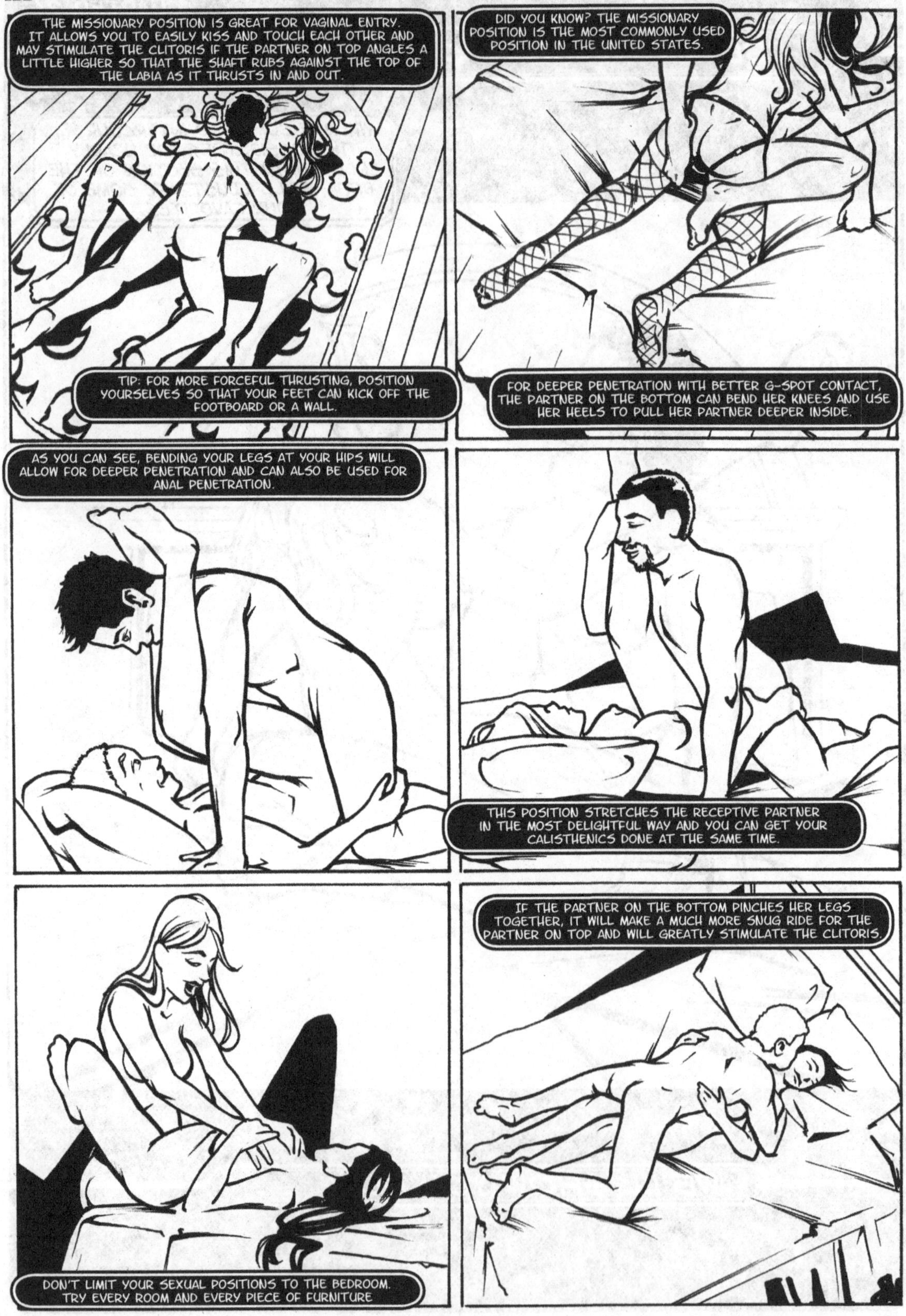
THE MISSIONARY POSITION IS GREAT FOR VAGINAL ENTRY. IT ALLOWS YOU TO EASILY KISS AND TOUCH EACH OTHER AND MAY STIMULATE THE CLITORIS IF THE PARTNER ON TOP ANGLES A LITTLE HIGHER SO THAT THE SHAFT RUBS AGAINST THE TOP OF THE LABIA AS IT THRUSTS IN AND OUT.
TIP: FOR MORE FORCEFUL THRUSTING, POSITION YOURSELVES SO THAT YOUR FEET CAN KICK OFF THE FOOTBOARD OR A WALL.
DID YOU KNOW? THE MISSIONARY POSITION IS THE MOST COMMONLY USED POSITION IN THE UNITED STATES.
FOR DEEPER PENETRATION WITH BETTER G-SPOT CONTACT, THE PARTNER ON THE BOTTOM CAN BEND HER KNEES AND USE HER HEELS TO PULL HER PARTNER DEEPER INSIDE.
AS YOU CAN SEE, BENDING YOUR LEGS AT YOUR HIPS WILL ALLOW FOR DEEPER PENETRATION AND CAN ALSO BE USED FOR ANAL PENETRATION.
THIS POSITION STRETCHES THE RECEPTIVE PARTNER IN THE MOST DELIGHTFUL WAY AND YOU CAN GET YOUR CALISTHENICS DONE AT THE SAME TIME.
DON'T LIMIT YOUR SEXUAL POSITIONS TO THE BEDROOM. TRY EVERY ROOM AND EVERY PIECE OF FURNITURE
IF THE PARTNER ON THE BOTTOM PINCHES HER LEGS TOGETHER, IT WILL MAKE A MUCH MORE SNUG RIDE FOR THE PARTNER ON TOP AND WILL GREATLY STIMULATE THE CLITORIS.

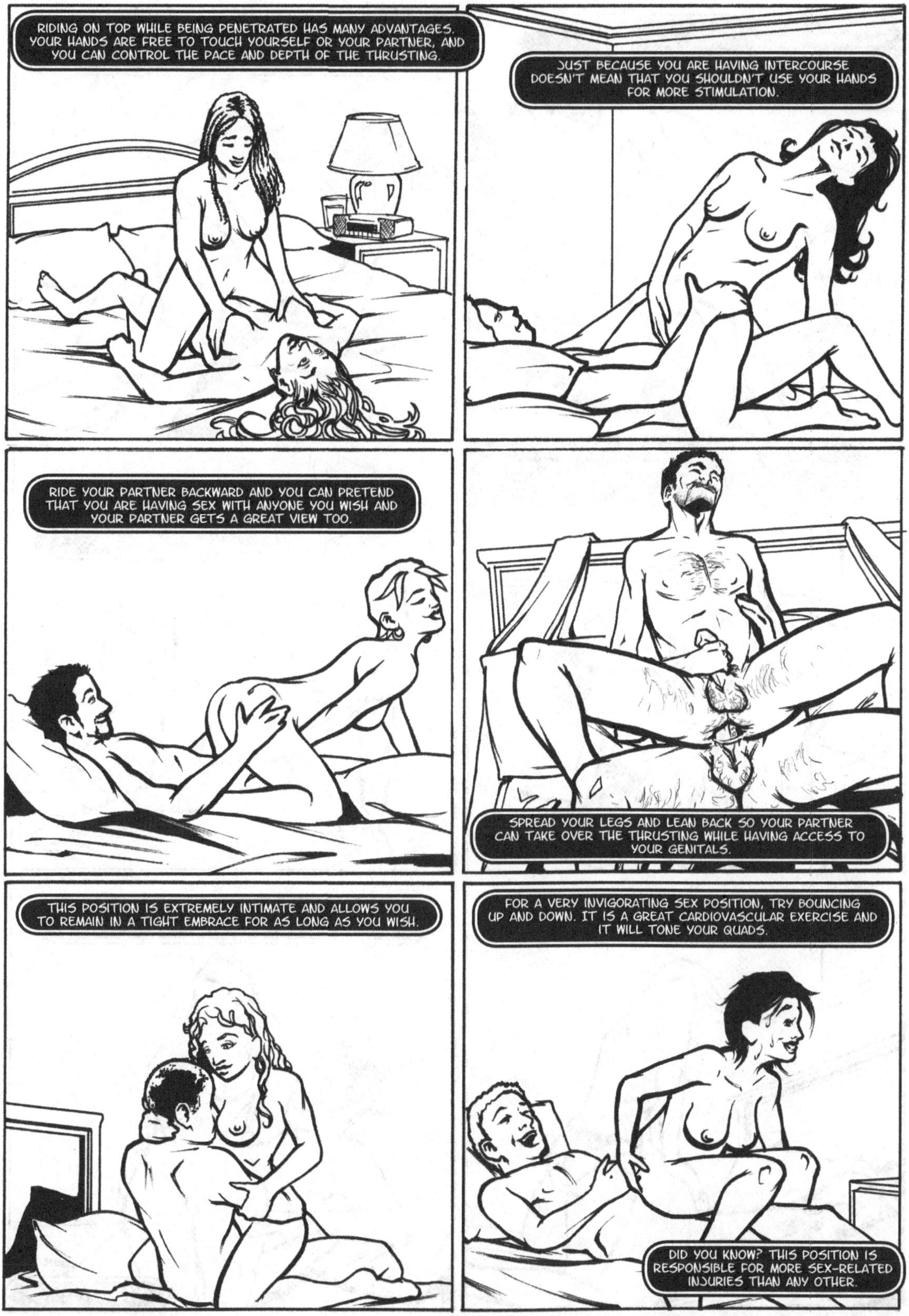
RIDING ON TOP WHILE BEING PENETRATED HAS MANY ADVANTAGES. YOUR HANDS ARE FREE TO TOUCH YOURSELF OR YOUR PARTNER, AND YOU CAN CONTROL THE PACE AND DEPTH OF THE THRUSTING.
JUST BECAUSE YOU ARE HAVING INTERCOURSE DOESN'T MEAN THAT YOU SHOULDN'T USE YOUR HANDS FOR MORE STIMULATION.
RIDE YOUR PARTNER BACKWARD AND YOU CAN PRETEND THAT YOU ARE HAVING SEX WITH ANYONE YOU WISH AND YOUR PARTNER GETS A GREAT VIEW TOO.
SPREAD YOUR LEGS AND LEAN BACK SO YOUR PARTNER CAN TAKE OVER THE THRUSTING WHILE HAVING ACCESS TO YOUR GENITALS.
THIS POSITION IS EXTREMELY INTIMATE AND ALLOWS YOU TO REMAIN IN A TIGHT EMBRACE FOR AS LONG AS YOU WISH.
FOR A VERY INVIGORATING SEX POSITION, TRY BOUNCING UP AND DOWN. IT IS A GREAT CARDIOVASCULAR EXERCISE AND IT WILL TONE YOUR QUADS.
DID YOU KNOW? THIS POSITION IS RESPONSIBLE FOR MORE SEX-RELATED INJURIES THAN ANY OTHER.

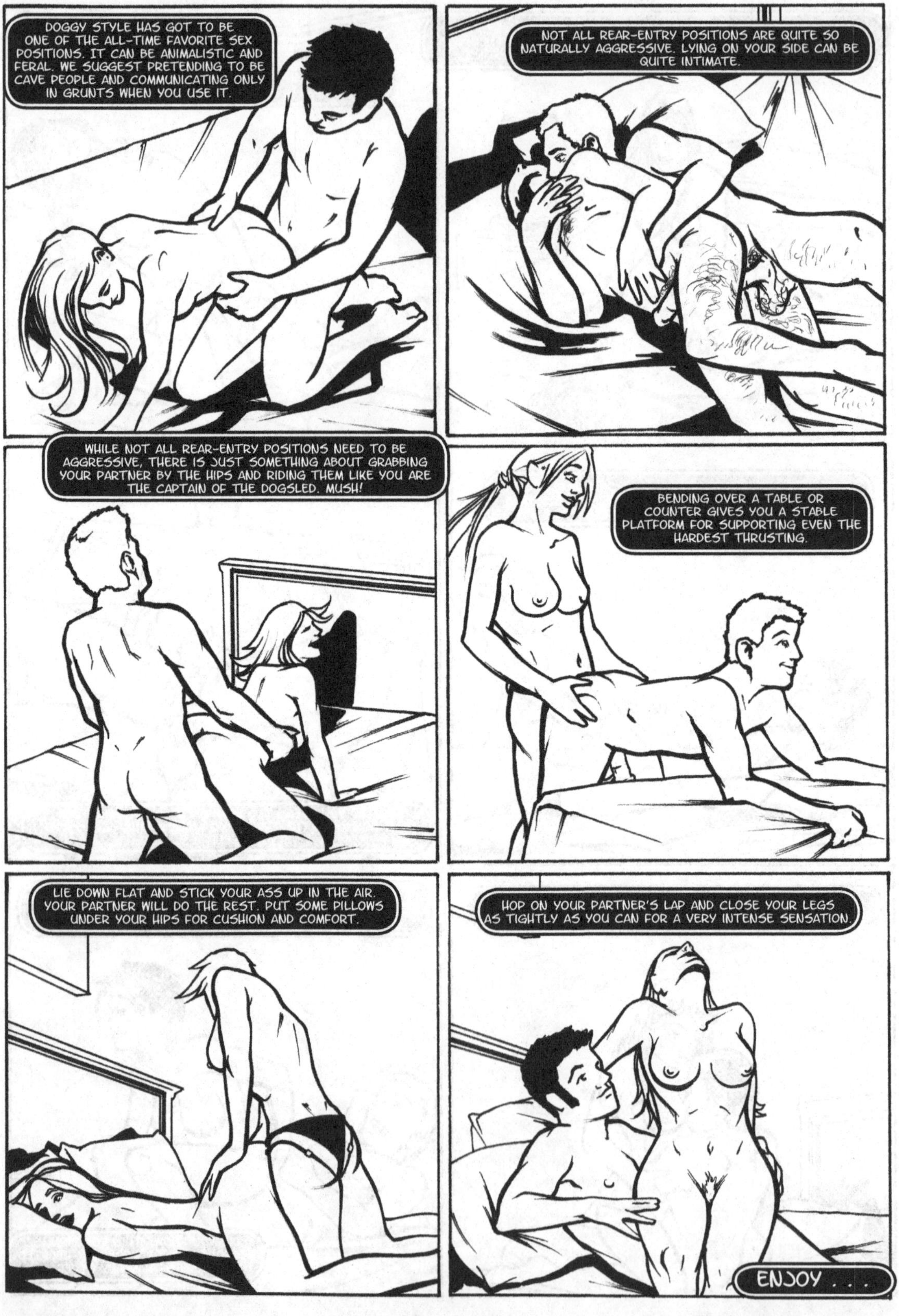
DOGGY STYLE HAS GOT TO BE ONE OF THE ALL-TIME FAVORITE SEX POSITIONS. IT CAN BE ANIMALISTIC AND FERAL. WE SUGGEST PRETENDING TO BE CAVE PEOPLE AND COMMUNICATING ONLY IN GRUNTS WHEN YOU USE IT.
NOT ALL REAR-ENTRY POSITIONS ARE QUITE SO NATURALLY AGGRESSIVE. LYING ON YOUR SIDE CAN BE QUITE INTIMATE.
WHILE NOT ALL REAR-ENTRY POSITIONS NEED TO BE AGGRESSIVE, THERE IS JUST SOMETHING ABOUT GRABBING YOUR PARTNER BY THE HIPS AND RIDING THEM LIKE YOU ARE THE CAPTAIN OF THE DOGSLED. MUSH!
BENDING OVER A TABLE OR COUNTER GIVES YOU A STABLE PLATFORM FOR SUPPORTING EVEN THE HARDEST THRUSTING.
LIE DOWN FLAT AND STICK YOUR ASS UP IN THE AIR. YOUR PARTNER WILL DO THE REST. PUT SOME PILLOWS UNDER YOUR HIPS FOR CUSHION AND COMFORT.
HOP ON YOUR PARTNER'S LAP AND CLOSE YOUR LEGS AS TIGHTLY AS YOU CAN FOR A VERY INTENSE SENSATION.
ENJOY . . .

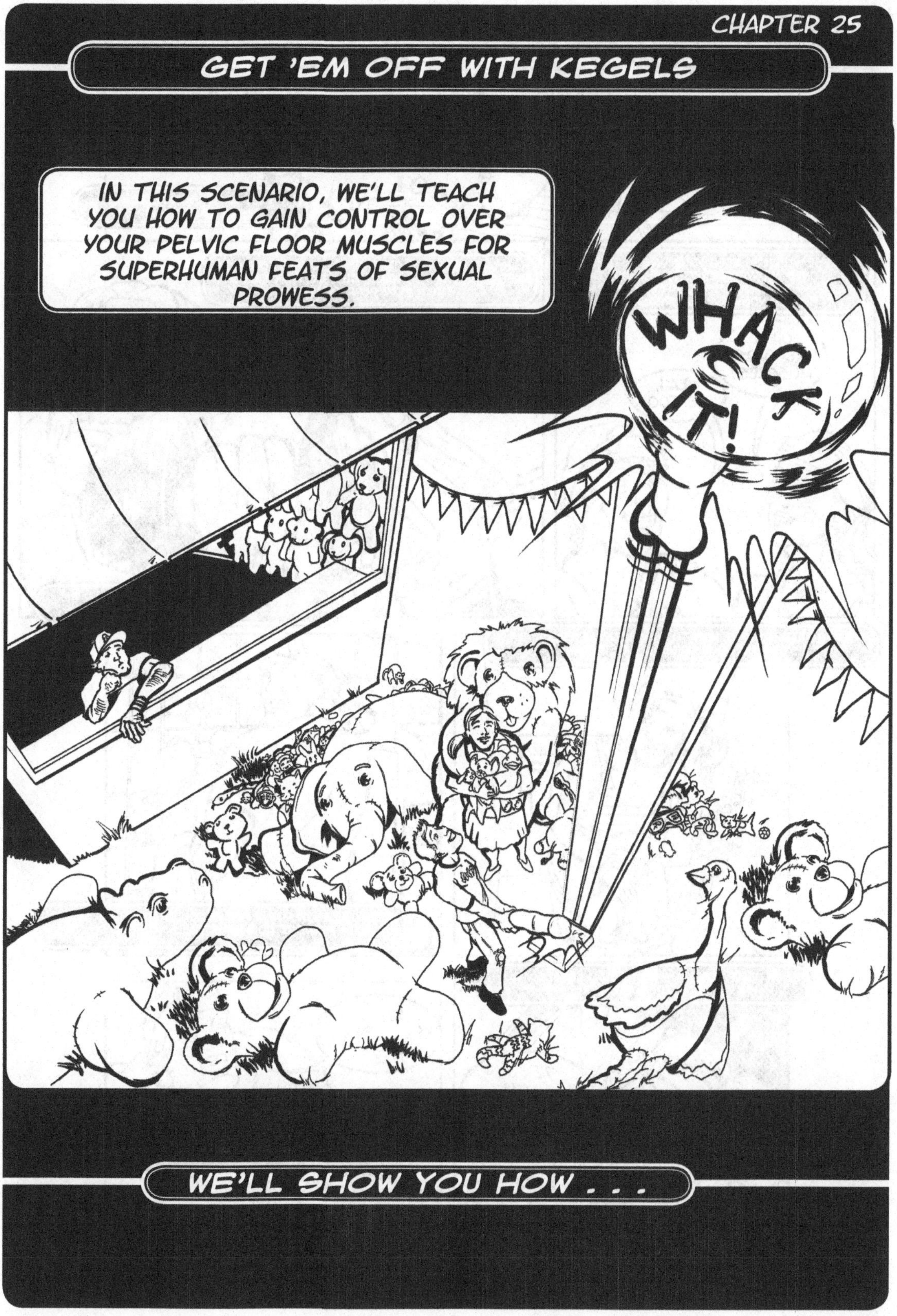

CHAPTER 25
GET 'EM OFF WITH KEGELS
IN THIS SCENARIO, WE'LL TEACH YOU HOW TO GAIN CONTROL OVER YOUR PELVIC FLOOR MUSCLES FOR SUPERHUMAN FEATS OF SEXUAL PROWESS.
WHACK IT!
WE'LL SHOW YOU HOW . . .

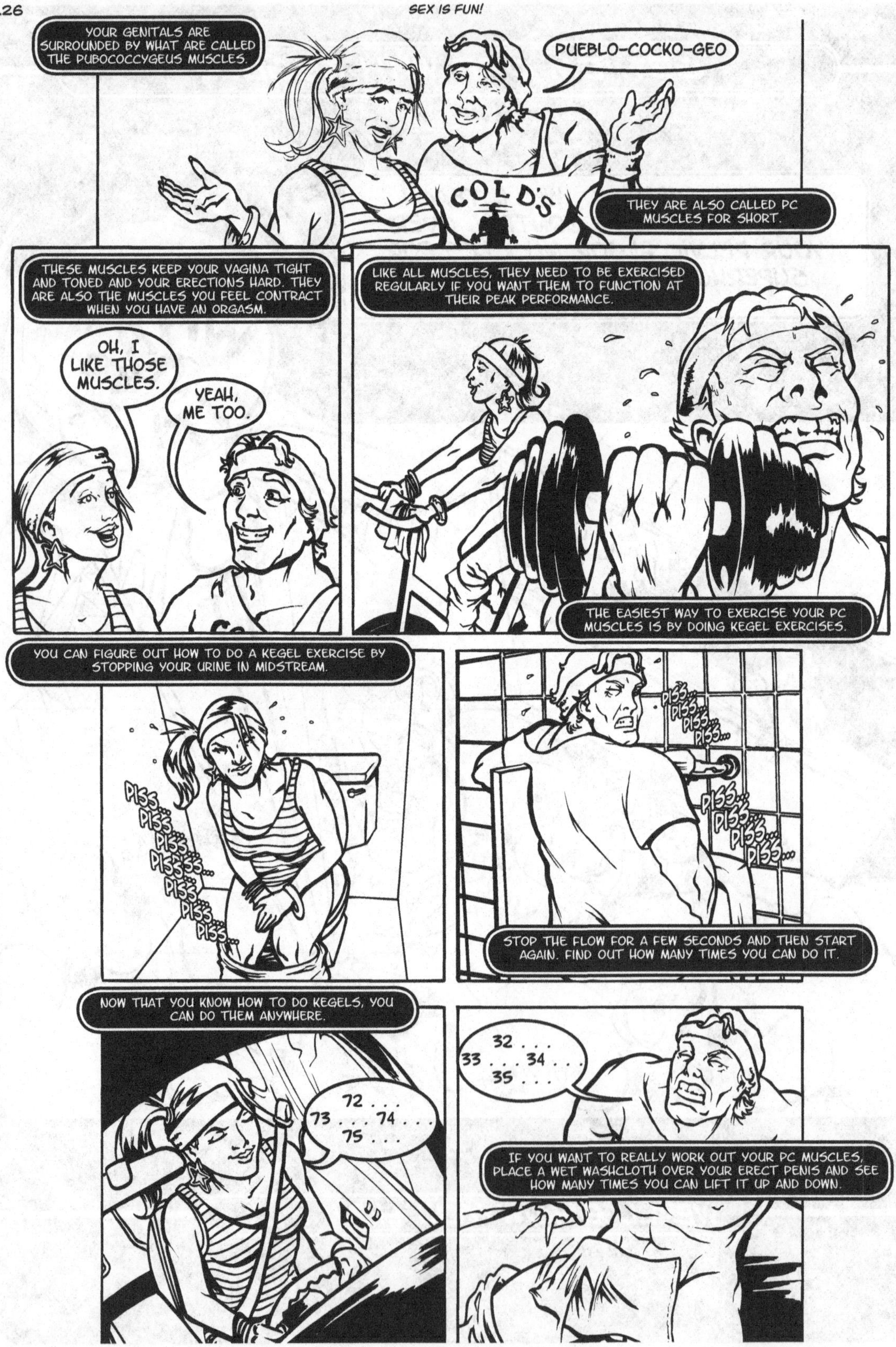
YOUR GENITALS ARE SURROUNDED BY WHAT ARE CALLED THE PUBOCOCCYGEUS MUSCLES.
PUEBLO-COCKO-GEO
COLD'S
THEY ARE ALSO CALLED PC MUSCLES FOR SHORT.
THESE MUSCLES KEEP YOUR VAGINA TIGHT AND TONED AND YOUR ERECTIONS HARD. THEY ARE ALSO THE MUSCLES YOU FEEL CONTRACT WHEN YOU HAVE AN ORGASM.
OH, I LIKE THOSE MUSCLES.
YEAH, ME TOO.
LIKE ALL MUSCLES, THEY NEED TO BE EXERCISED REGULARLY IF YOU WANT THEM TO FUNCTION AT THEIR PEAK PERFORMANCE.
THE EASIEST WAY TO EXERCISE YOUR PC MUSCLES IS BY DOING KEGEL EXERCISES.
YOU CAN FIGURE OUT HOW TO DO A KEGEL EXERCISE BY STOPPING YOUR URINE IN MIDSTREAM.
PISS... PISS... PISS... PISSSS... PISS... PISS... PISS...
PISS... PISS... PISS... PISS...
PISS... PISS... PISS... PISS...
STOP THE FLOW FOR A FEW SECONDS AND THEN START AGAIN. FIND OUT HOW MANY TIMES YOU CAN DO IT.
NOW THAT YOU KNOW HOW TO DO KEGELS, YOU CAN DO THEM ANYWHERE.
72 . . . 73 . . . 74 . . . 75 . . .
32 . . . 33 . . . 34 . . . 35 . . .
IF YOU WANT TO REALLY WORK OUT YOUR PC MUSCLES, PLACE A WET WASHCLOTH OVER YOUR ERECT PENIS AND SEE HOW MANY TIMES YOU CAN LIFT IT UP AND DOWN.

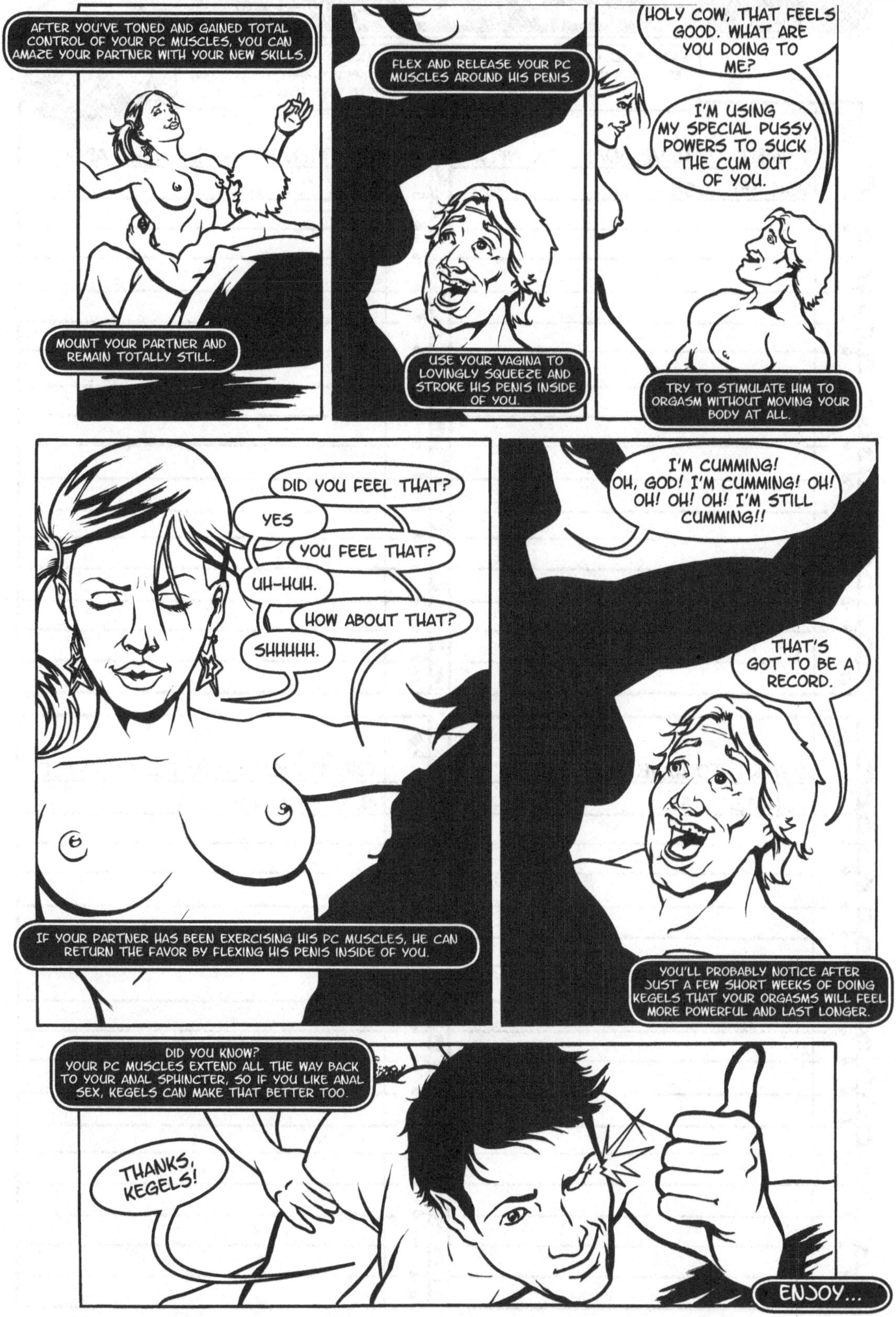
AFTER YOU'VE TONED AND GAINED TOTAL CONTROL OF YOUR PC MUSCLES, YOU CAN AMAZE YOUR PARTNER WITH YOUR NEW SKILLS.
MOUNT YOUR PARTNER AND REMAIN TOTALLY STILL.
FLEX AND RELEASE YOUR PC MUSCLES AROUND HIS PENIS.
USE YOUR VAGINA TO LOVINGLY SQUEEZE AND STROKE HIS PENIS INSIDE OF YOU.
HOLY COW, THAT FEELS GOOD. WHAT ARE YOU DOING TO ME?
I'M USING MY SPECIAL PUSSY POWERS TO SUCK THE CUM OUT OF YOU.
TRY TO STIMULATE HIM TO ORGASM WITHOUT MOVING YOUR BODY AT ALL.
DID YOU FEEL THAT?
YES
YOU FEEL THAT?
UH-HUH.
HOW ABOUT THAT?
SHHHHH.
IF YOUR PARTNER HAS BEEN EXERCISING HIS PC MUSCLES, HE CAN RETURN THE FAVOR BY FLEXING HIS PENIS INSIDE OF YOU.
I'M CUMMING! OH, GOD! I'M CUMMING! OH! OH! OH! OH! I'M STILL CUMMING!!
THAT'S GOT TO BE A RECORD.
YOU'LL PROBABLY NOTICE AFTER JUST A FEW SHORT WEEKS OF DOING KEGELS THAT YOUR ORGASMS WILL FEEL MORE POWERFUL AND LAST LONGER.
DID YOU KNOW? YOUR PC MUSCLES EXTEND ALL THE WAY BACK TO YOUR ANAL SPHINCTER, SO IF YOU LIKE ANAL SEX, KEGELS CAN MAKE THAT BETTER TOO.
THANKS, KEGELS!
ENJOY...

TAKING IT IN THE POOPER

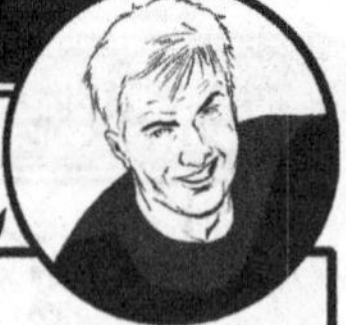

SOME PEOPLE LOVE ANAL SEX AND OTHERS DON'T LIKE IT (YET). IN THE SPACES BELOW, EXPLAIN TO YOUR PARTNER THE REASONS WHY YOU WANT TO HAVE ANAL SEX AND THE REASONS YOU DON'T WANT TO HAVE ANAL SEX.

I WANT TO HAVE ANAL SEX WITH YOU BECAUSE . . .

THE THINGS I DON'T LIKE ABOUT ANAL SEX ARE . . .

I WANT TO HAVE ANAL SEX WITH YOU BECAUSE . . .

THE THINGS I DON'T LIKE ABOUT ANAL SEX ARE . . .

CHAPTER 26

BUTT SEX

WHETHER YOU ARE AN ANAL VIRGIN, A DABBLER OR A FULLY FLEDGED BUTT-PACKING PAIR, THIS CHAPTER WILL SHOW YOU THE PLEASURE POSSIBILITIES OF BREACHING THE BACK DOOR.

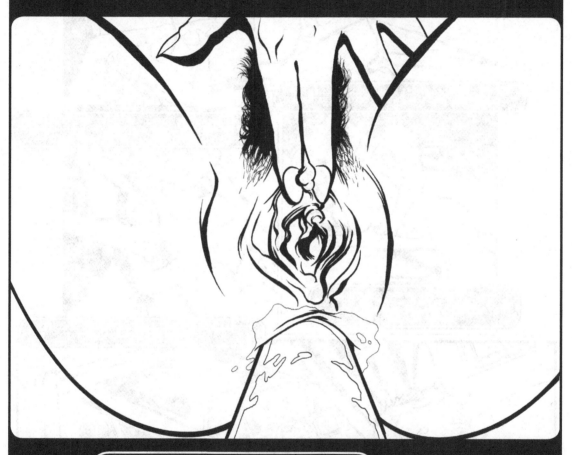

WHAT YOU'LL NEED . . .

LOTS OF LUBRICATION

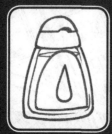

LOTS OF TIME

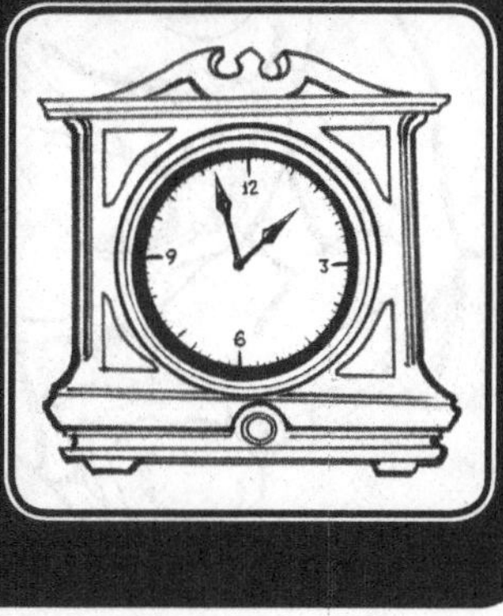

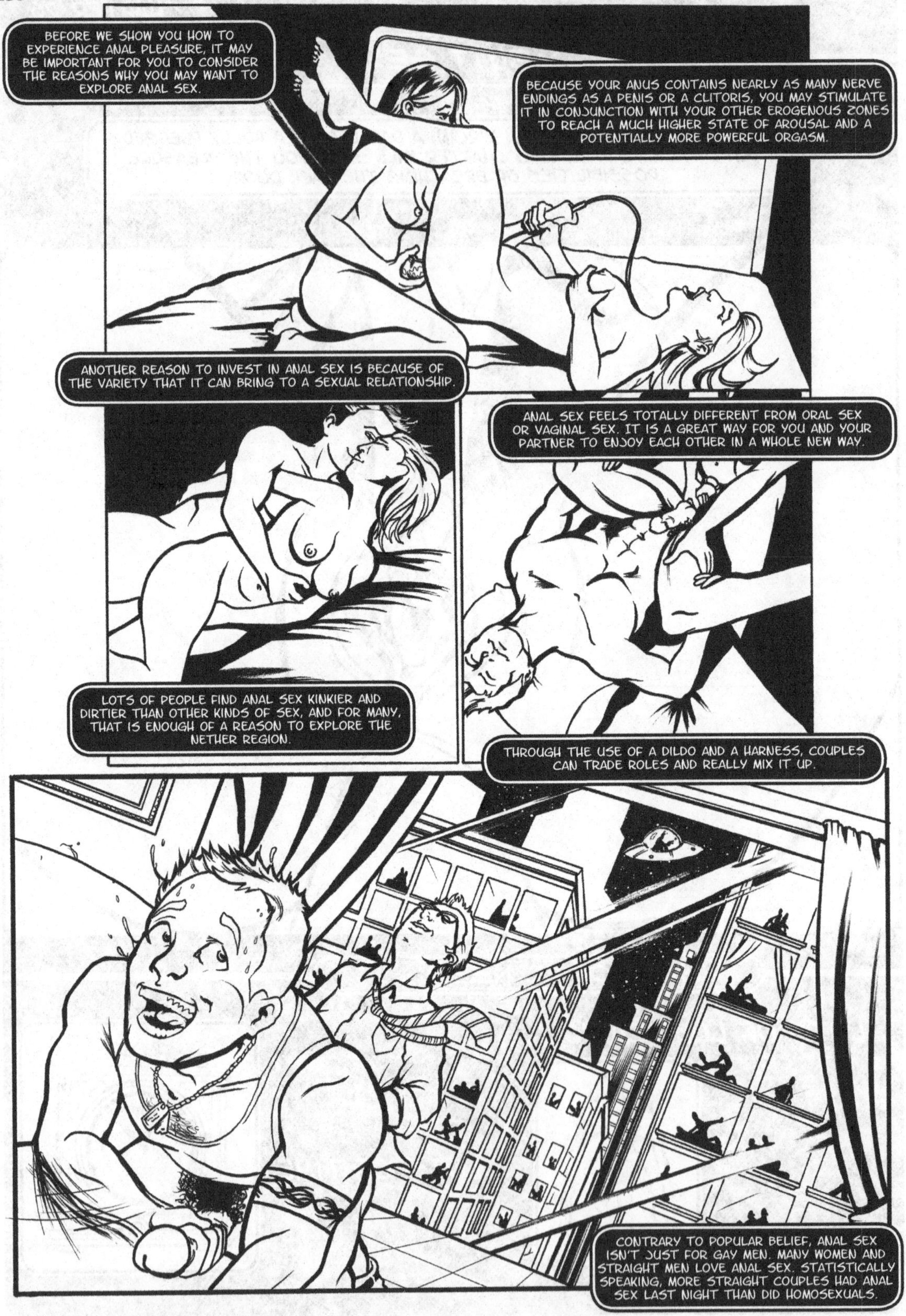
BEFORE WE SHOW YOU HOW TO EXPERIENCE ANAL PLEASURE, IT MAY BE IMPORTANT FOR YOU TO CONSIDER THE REASONS WHY YOU MAY WANT TO EXPLORE ANAL SEX.
BECAUSE YOUR ANUS CONTAINS NEARLY AS MANY NERVE ENDINGS AS A PENIS OR A CLITORIS, YOU MAY STIMULATE IT IN CONJUNCTION WITH YOUR OTHER EROGENOUS ZONES TO REACH A MUCH HIGHER STATE OF AROUSAL AND A POTENTIALLY MORE POWERFUL ORGASM.
ANOTHER REASON TO INVEST IN ANAL SEX IS BECAUSE OF THE VARIETY THAT IT CAN BRING TO A SEXUAL RELATIONSHIP.
ANAL SEX FEELS TOTALLY DIFFERENT FROM ORAL SEX OR VAGINAL SEX. IT IS A GREAT WAY FOR YOU AND YOUR PARTNER TO ENJOY EACH OTHER IN A WHOLE NEW WAY.
LOTS OF PEOPLE FIND ANAL SEX KINKIER AND DIRTIER THAN OTHER KINDS OF SEX, AND FOR MANY, THAT IS ENOUGH OF A REASON TO EXPLORE THE NETHER REGION.
THROUGH THE USE OF A DILDO AND A HARNESS, COUPLES CAN TRADE ROLES AND REALLY MIX IT UP.
CONTRARY TO POPULAR BELIEF, ANAL SEX ISN'T JUST FOR GAY MEN. MANY WOMEN AND STRAIGHT MEN LOVE ANAL SEX. STATISTICALLY SPEAKING, MORE STRAIGHT COUPLES HAD ANAL SEX LAST NIGHT THAN DID HOMOSEXUALS.

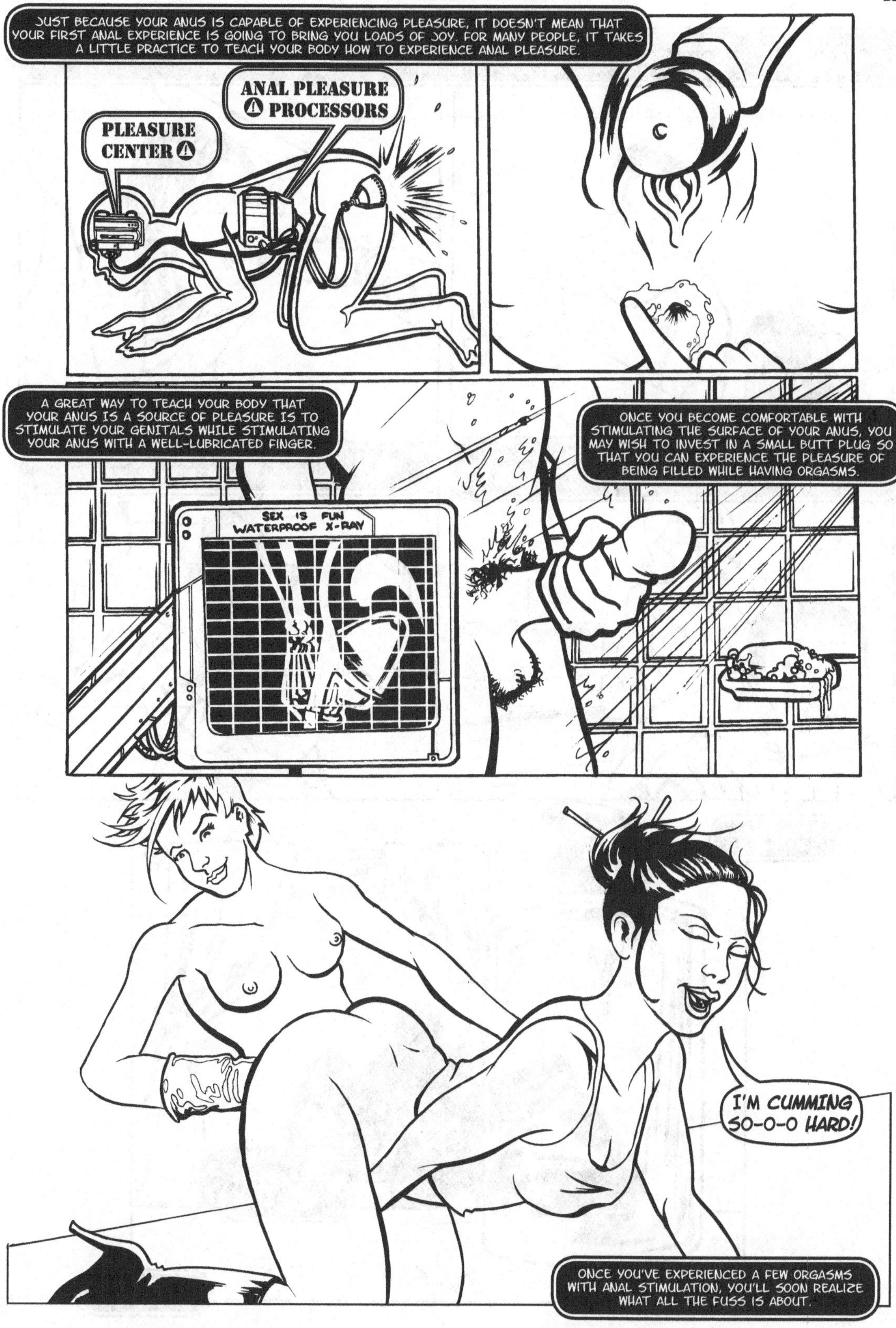
JUST BECAUSE YOUR ANUS IS CAPABLE OF EXPERIENCING PLEASURE, IT DOESN'T MEAN THAT YOUR FIRST ANAL EXPERIENCE IS GOING TO BRING YOU LOADS OF JOY. FOR MANY PEOPLE, IT TAKES A LITTLE PRACTICE TO TEACH YOUR BODY HOW TO EXPERIENCE ANAL PLEASURE.
PLEASURE CENTER
ANAL PLEASURE PROCESSORS
A GREAT WAY TO TEACH YOUR BODY THAT YOUR ANUS IS A SOURCE OF PLEASURE IS TO STIMULATE YOUR GENITALS WHILE STIMULATING YOUR ANUS WITH A WELL-LUBRICATED FINGER.
ONCE YOU BECOME COMFORTABLE WITH STIMULATING THE SURFACE OF YOUR ANUS, YOU MAY WISH TO INVEST IN A SMALL BUTT PLUG SO THAT YOU CAN EXPERIENCE THE PLEASURE OF BEING FILLED WHILE HAVING ORGASMS.
SEX IS FUN WATERPROOF X-RAY
I'M CUMMING SO-O-O HARD!
ONCE YOU'VE EXPERIENCED A FEW ORGASMS WITH ANAL STIMULATION, YOU'LL SOON REALIZE WHAT ALL THE FUSS IS ABOUT.

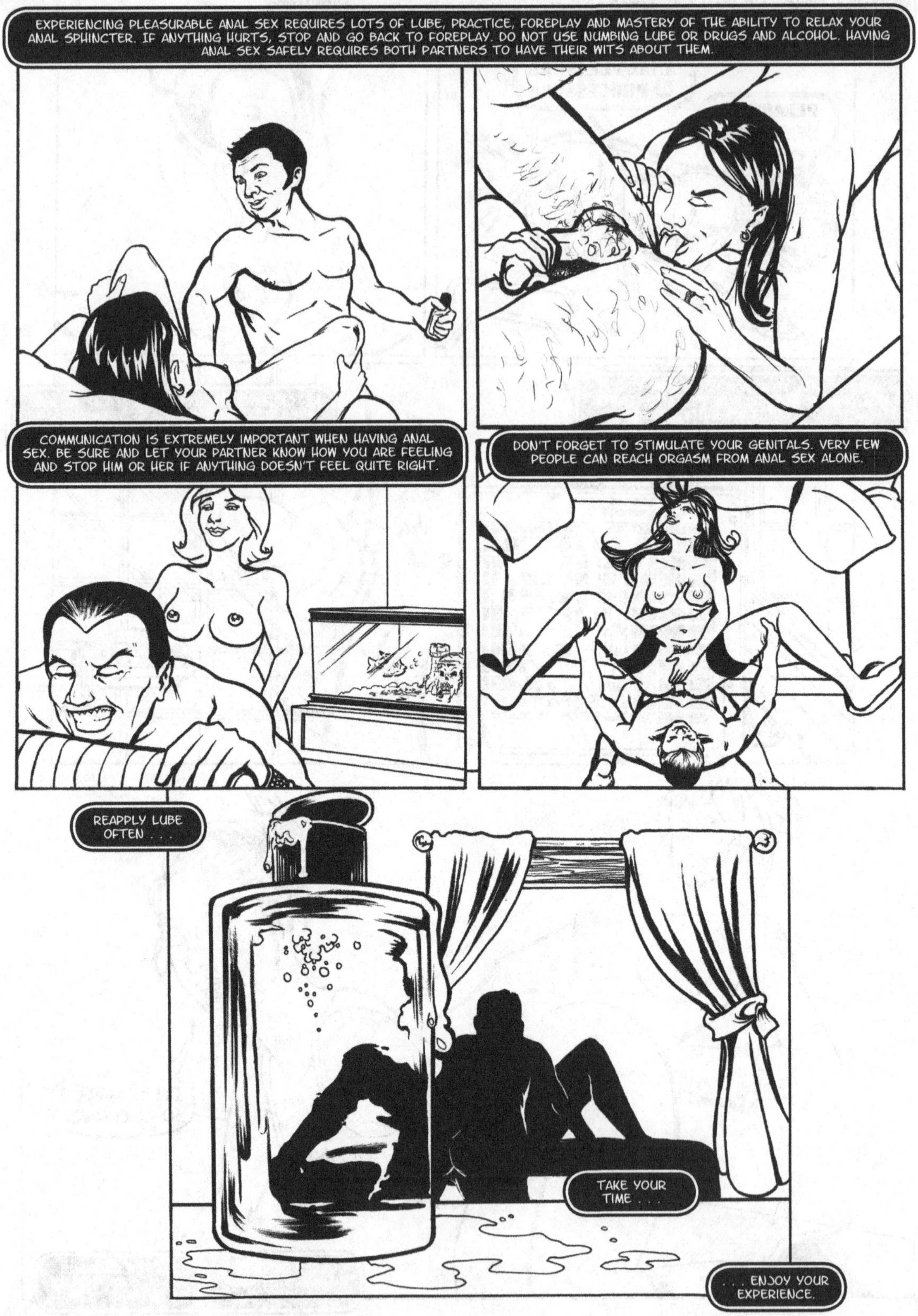
EXPERIENCING PLEASURABLE ANAL SEX REQUIRES LOTS OF LUBE, PRACTICE, FOREPLAY AND MASTERY OF THE ABILITY TO RELAX YOUR ANAL SPHINCTER. IF ANYTHING HURTS, STOP AND GO BACK TO FOREPLAY. DO NOT USE NUMBING LUBE OR DRUGS AND ALCOHOL. HAVING ANAL SEX SAFELY REQUIRES BOTH PARTNERS TO HAVE THEIR WITS ABOUT THEM.
COMMUNICATION IS EXTREMELY IMPORTANT WHEN HAVING ANAL SEX. BE SURE AND LET YOUR PARTNER KNOW HOW YOU ARE FEELING AND STOP HIM OR HER IF ANYTHING DOESN'T FEEL QUITE RIGHT.
DON'T FORGET TO STIMULATE YOUR GENITALS. VERY FEW PEOPLE CAN REACH ORGASM FROM ANAL SEX ALONE.
REAPPLY LUBE OFTEN . . .
TAKE YOUR TIME . . .
. . . ENJOY YOUR EXPERIENCE.

CHAPTER 27

CUMMING ON CUE

HAVE YOU EVER FELT AS THOUGH SEX JUST DOESN'T LAST LONG ENOUGH? OR THAT IT TAKES YOU TOO LONG TO REACH ORGASM? IN THIS SCENARIO, WE'LL TEACH YOU HOW YOU CAN GAIN SOME CONTROL OVER THE TIMING OF YOUR ORGASM SO THAT YOU'LL LAST LONG ENOUGH TO PLEASURE YOUR PARTNER AND REACH CLIMAX BEFORE YOU GET SORE.

ITS GONNA BLOW!
CUM SQUAD

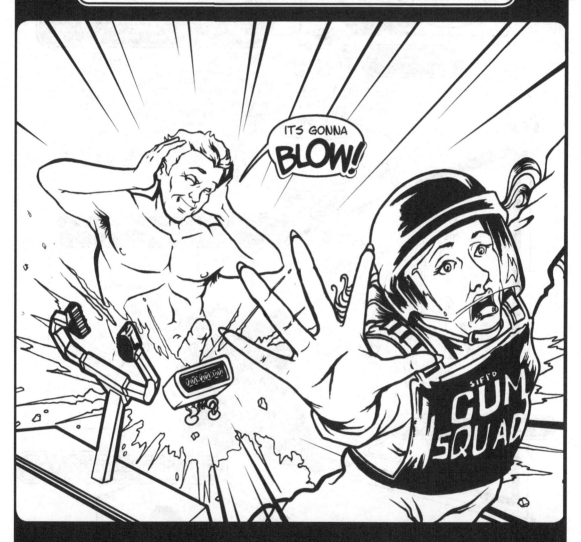

WE'LL SHOW YOU HOW . . .

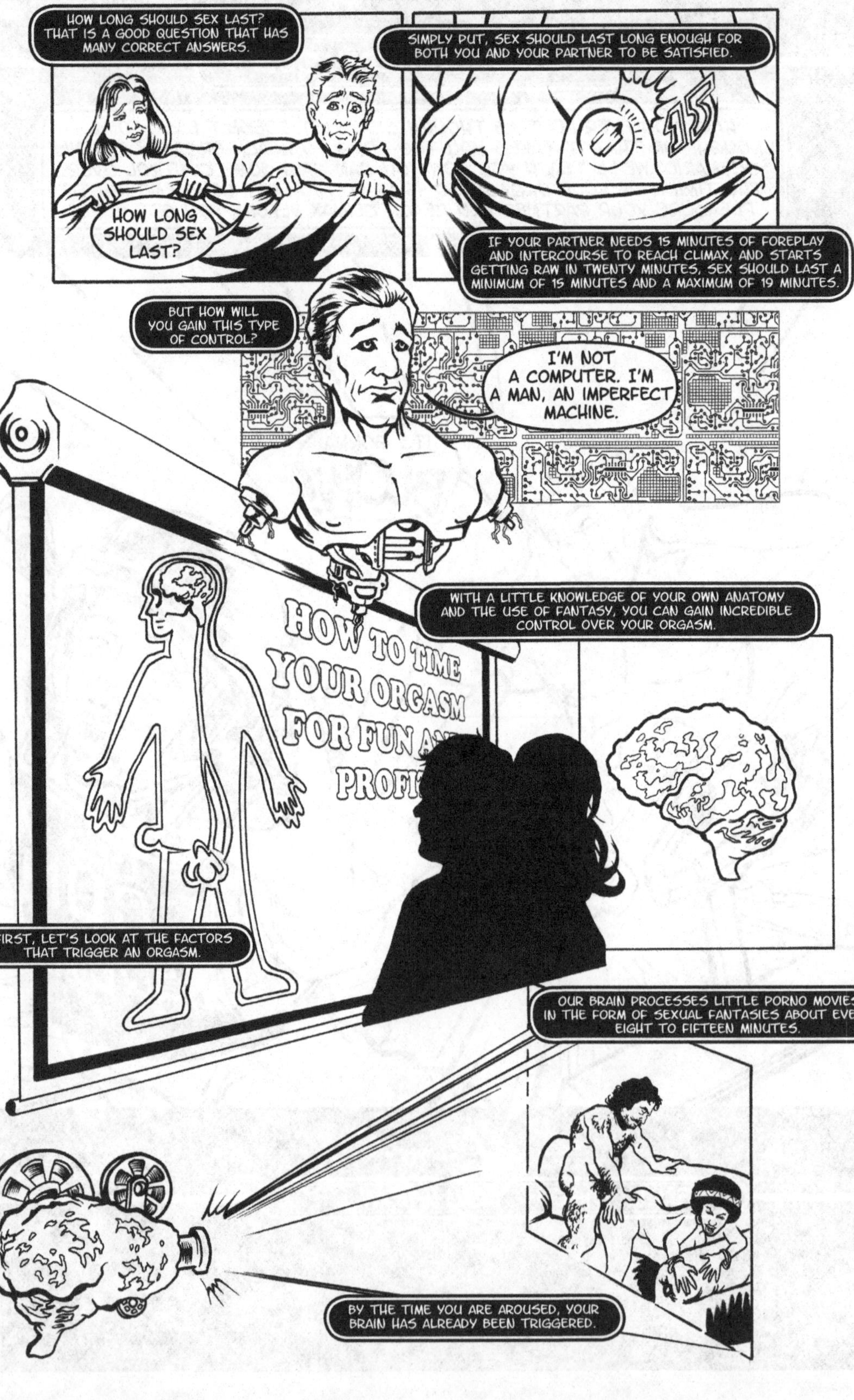
HOW LONG SHOULD SEX LAST? THAT IS A GOOD QUESTION THAT HAS MANY CORRECT ANSWERS.
HOW LONG SHOULD SEX LAST?
SIMPLY PUT, SEX SHOULD LAST LONG ENOUGH FOR BOTH YOU AND YOUR PARTNER TO BE SATISFIED.
15
IF YOUR PARTNER NEEDS 15 MINUTES OF FOREPLAY AND INTERCOURSE TO REACH CLIMAX, AND STARTS GETTING RAW IN TWENTY MINUTES, SEX SHOULD LAST A MINIMUM OF 15 MINUTES AND A MAXIMUM OF 19 MINUTES.
BUT HOW WILL YOU GAIN THIS TYPE OF CONTROL?
I'M NOT A COMPUTER. I'M A MAN, AN IMPERFECT MACHINE.
WITH A LITTLE KNOWLEDGE OF YOUR OWN ANATOMY AND THE USE OF FANTASY, YOU CAN GAIN INCREDIBLE CONTROL OVER YOUR ORGASM.
HOW TO TIME YOUR ORGASM FOR FUN A
PROFI
FIRST, LET'S LOOK AT THE FACTORS THAT TRIGGER AN ORGASM.
OUR BRAIN PROCESSES LITTLE PORNO MOVIES IN THE FORM OF SEXUAL FANTASIES ABOUT EVERY EIGHT TO FIFTEEN MINUTES.
BY THE TIME YOU ARE AROUSED, YOUR BRAIN HAS ALREADY BEEN TRIGGERED.

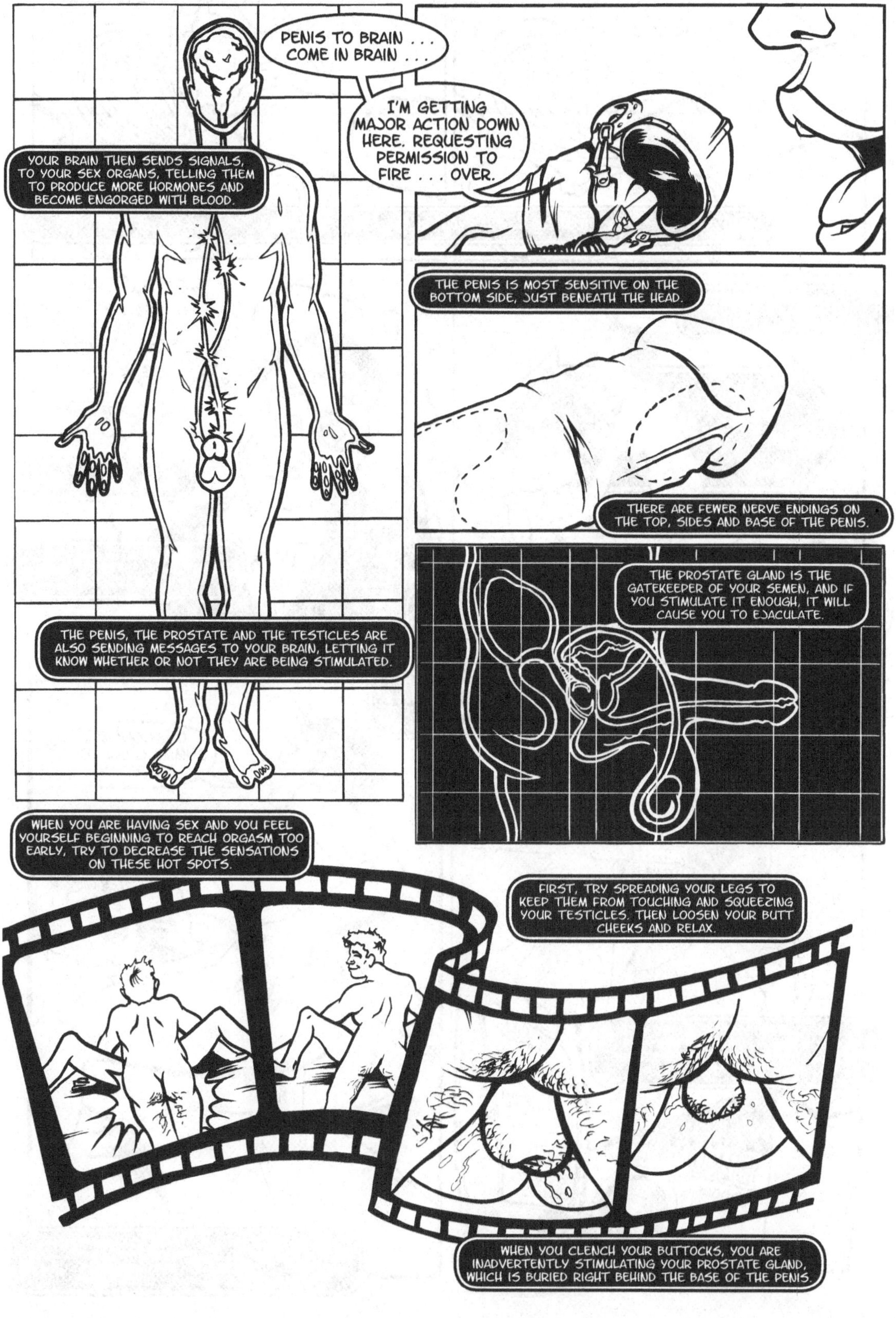
PENIS TO BRAIN . . . COME IN BRAIN . . .
I'M GETTING MAJOR ACTION DOWN HERE. REQUESTING PERMISSION TO FIRE . . . OVER.
YOUR BRAIN THEN SENDS SIGNALS, TO YOUR SEX ORGANS, TELLING THEM TO PRODUCE MORE HORMONES AND BECOME ENGORGED WITH BLOOD.
THE PENIS, THE PROSTATE AND THE TESTICLES ARE ALSO SENDING MESSAGES TO YOUR BRAIN, LETTING IT KNOW WHETHER OR NOT THEY ARE BEING STIMULATED.
THE PENIS IS MOST SENSITIVE ON THE BOTTOM SIDE, JUST BENEATH THE HEAD.
THERE ARE FEWER NERVE ENDINGS ON THE TOP, SIDES AND BASE OF THE PENIS.
THE PROSTATE GLAND IS THE GATEKEEPER OF YOUR SEMEN, AND IF YOU STIMULATE IT ENOUGH, IT WILL CAUSE YOU TO EJACULATE.
WHEN YOU ARE HAVING SEX AND YOU FEEL YOURSELF BEGINNING TO REACH ORGASM TOO EARLY, TRY TO DECREASE THE SENSATIONS ON THESE HOT SPOTS.
FIRST, TRY SPREADING YOUR LEGS TO KEEP THEM FROM TOUCHING AND SQUEEZING YOUR TESTICLES. THEN LOOSEN YOUR BUTT CHEEKS AND RELAX.
WHEN YOU CLENCH YOUR BUTTOCKS, YOU ARE INADVERTENTLY STIMULATING YOUR PROSTATE GLAND, WHICH IS BURIED RIGHT BEHIND THE BASE OF THE PENIS.

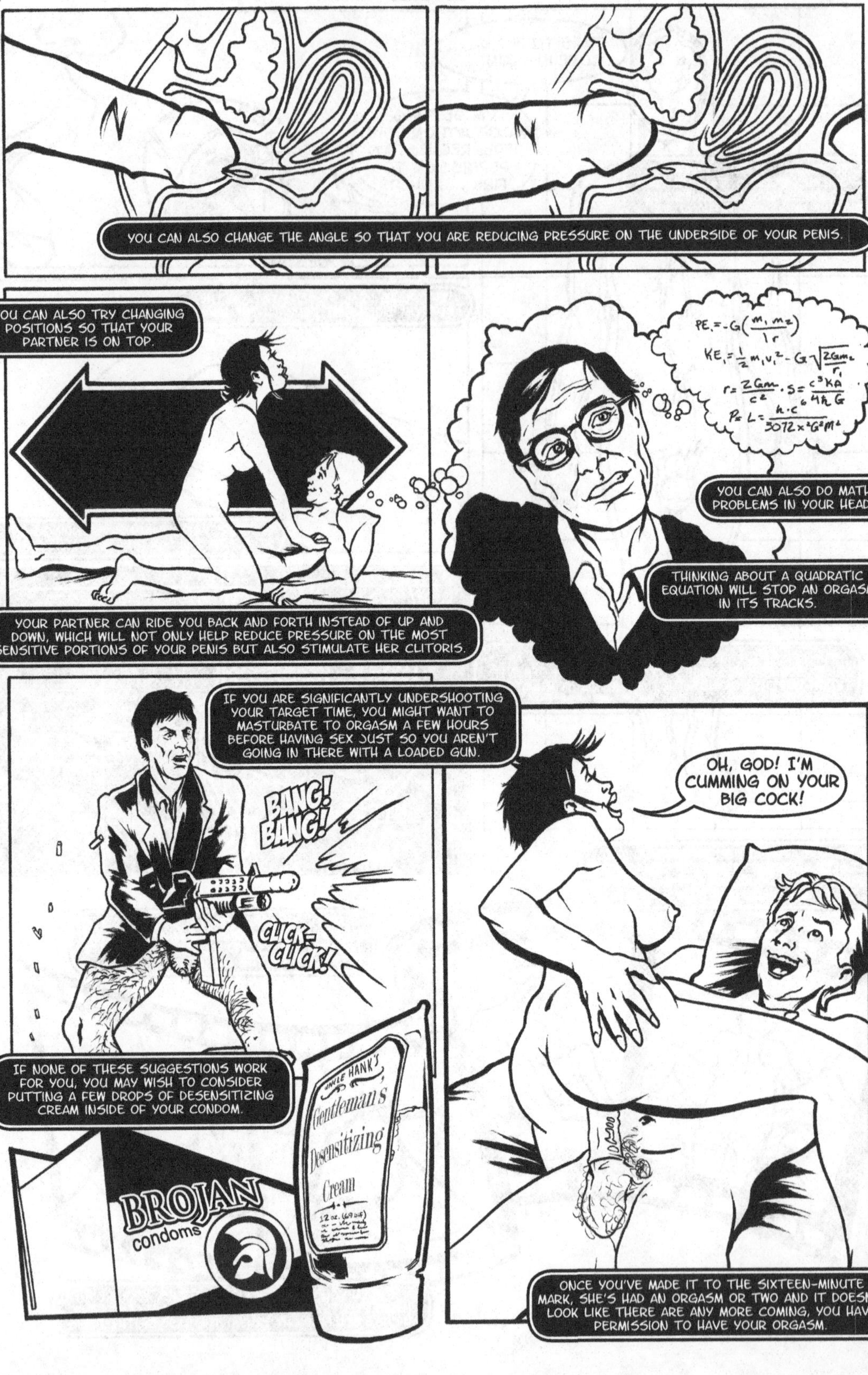
YOU CAN ALSO CHANGE THE ANGLE SO THAT YOU ARE REDUCING PRESSURE ON THE UNDERSIDE OF YOUR PENIS.
YOU CAN ALSO TRY CHANGING POSITIONS SO THAT YOUR PARTNER IS ON TOP.
YOUR PARTNER CAN RIDE YOU BACK AND FORTH INSTEAD OF UP AND DOWN, WHICH WILL NOT ONLY HELP REDUCE PRESSURE ON THE MOST SENSITIVE PORTIONS OF YOUR PENIS BUT ALSO STIMULATE HER CLITORIS.
YOU CAN ALSO DO MATH PROBLEMS IN YOUR HEAD.
THINKING ABOUT A QUADRATIC EQUATION WILL STOP AN ORGASM IN ITS TRACKS.
IF YOU ARE SIGNIFICANTLY UNDERSHOOTING YOUR TARGET TIME, YOU MIGHT WANT TO MASTURBATE TO ORGASM A FEW HOURS BEFORE HAVING SEX JUST SO YOU AREN'T GOING IN THERE WITH A LOADED GUN.
BANG! BANG!
CLICK-CLICK!
IF NONE OF THESE SUGGESTIONS WORK FOR YOU, YOU MAY WISH TO CONSIDER PUTTING A FEW DROPS OF DESENSITIZING CREAM INSIDE OF YOUR CONDOM.
UNCLE HANK'S
Gentleman's
Desensitizing
Cream
BROJAN
condoms
OH, GOD! I'M CUMMING ON YOUR BIG COCK!
ONCE YOU'VE MADE IT TO THE SIXTEEN-MINUTE MARK, SHE'S HAD AN ORGASM OR TWO AND IT DOESN'T LOOK LIKE THERE ARE ANY MORE COMING, YOU HAVE PERMISSION TO HAVE YOUR ORGASM.

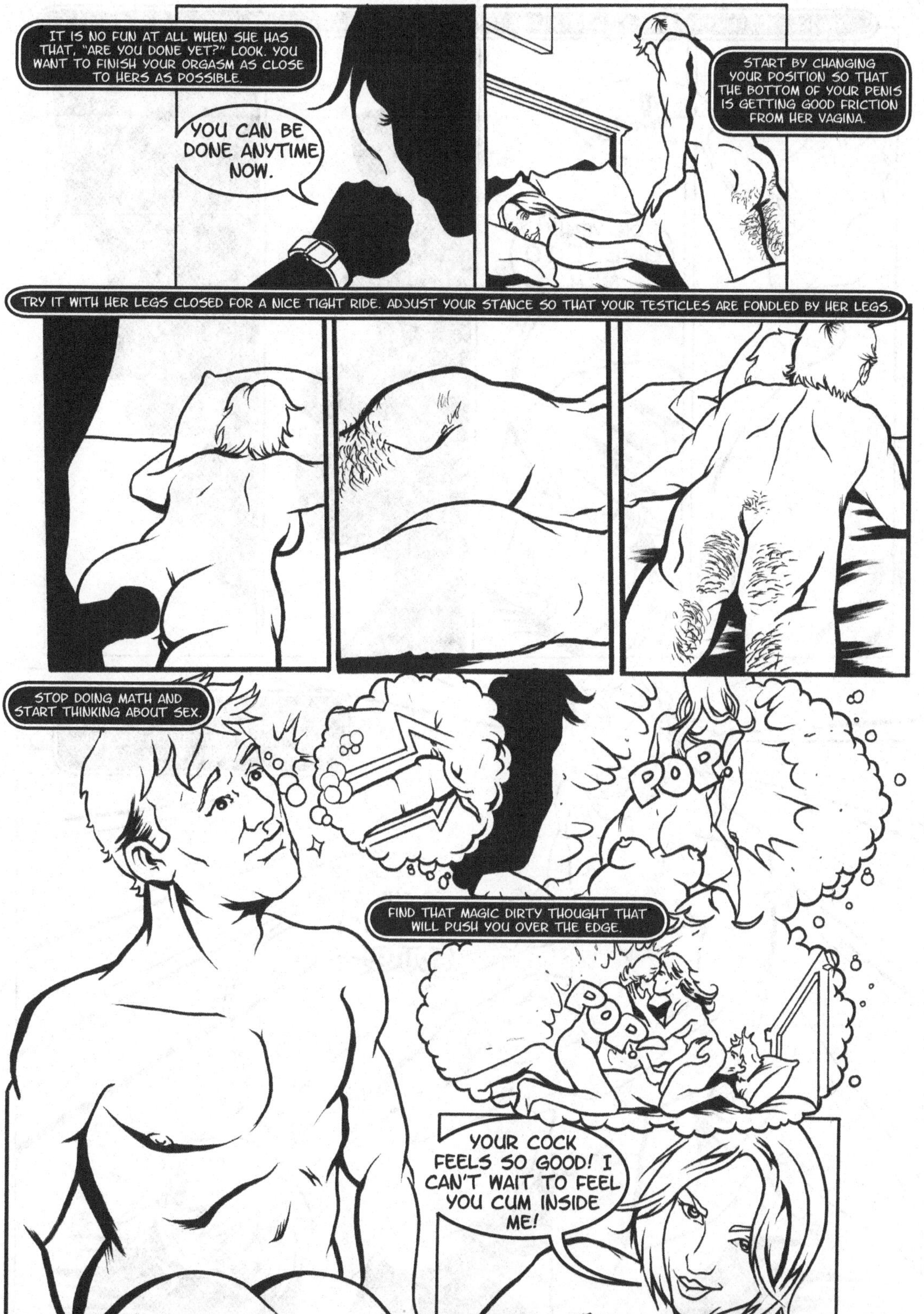
IT IS NO FUN AT ALL WHEN SHE HAS THAT, "ARE YOU DONE YET?" LOOK. YOU WANT TO FINISH YOUR ORGASM AS CLOSE TO HERS AS POSSIBLE.
YOU CAN BE DONE ANYTIME NOW.
START BY CHANGING YOUR POSITION SO THAT THE BOTTOM OF YOUR PENIS IS GETTING GOOD FRICTION FROM HER VAGINA.
TRY IT WITH HER LEGS CLOSED FOR A NICE TIGHT RIDE. ADJUST YOUR STANCE SO THAT YOUR TESTICLES ARE FONDLED BY HER LEGS.
STOP DOING MATH AND START THINKING ABOUT SEX.
POP
FIND THAT MAGIC DIRTY THOUGHT THAT WILL PUSH YOU OVER THE EDGE.
POP
YOUR COCK FEELS SO GOOD! I CAN'T WAIT TO FEEL YOU CUM INSIDE ME!
YOUR PARTNER CAN HELP YOU OUT WITH A LITTLE DIRTY TALK TOO.

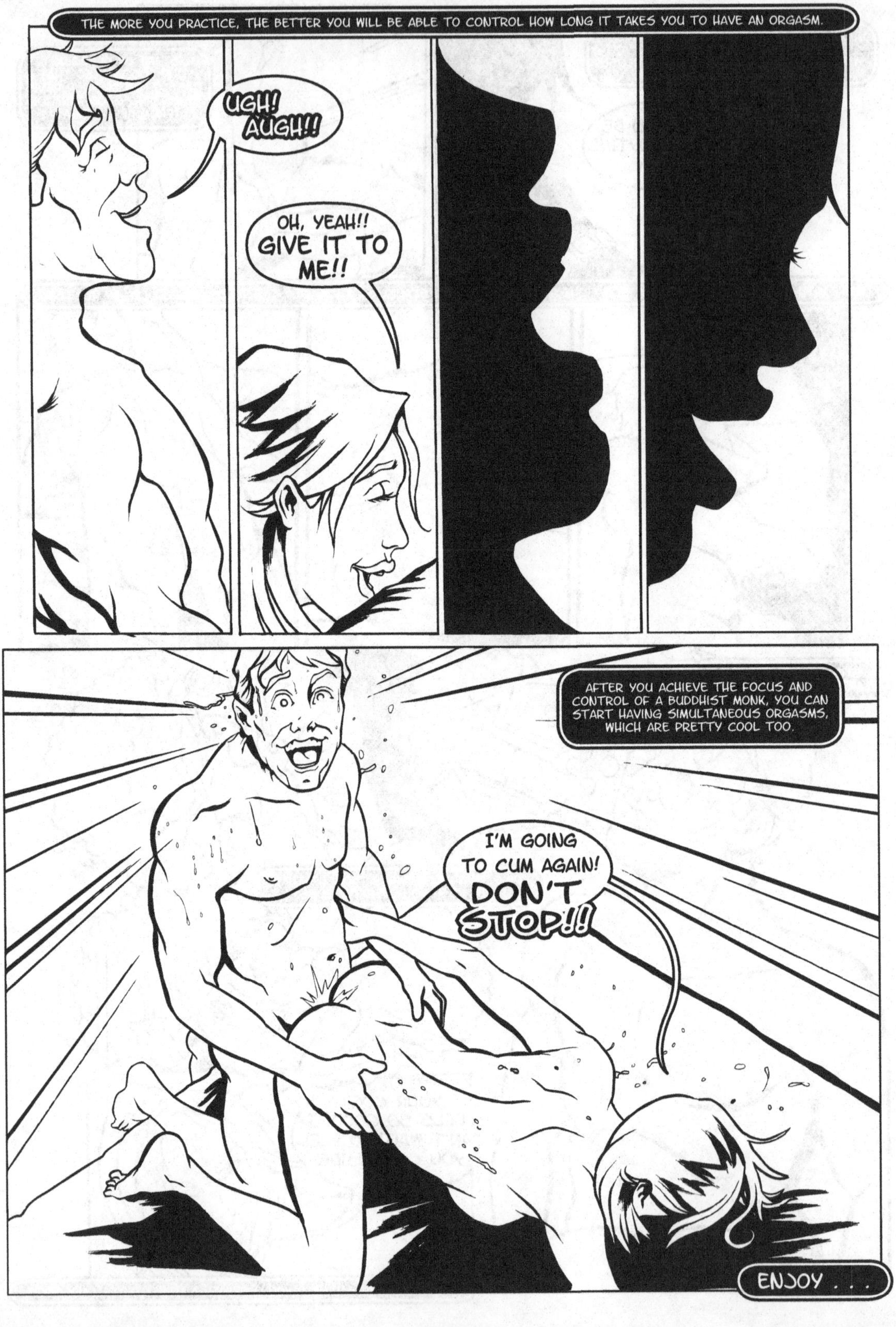
THE MORE YOU PRACTICE, THE BETTER YOU WILL BE ABLE TO CONTROL HOW LONG IT TAKES YOU TO HAVE AN ORGASM.
UGH! AUGH!!
OH, YEAH!! GIVE IT TO ME!!
AFTER YOU ACHIEVE THE FOCUS AND CONTROL OF A BUDDHIST MONK, YOU CAN START HAVING SIMULTANEOUS ORGASMS, WHICH ARE PRETTY COOL TOO.
I'M GOING TO CUM AGAIN! DON'T STOP!!
ENJOY . . .

CHAPTER 28

WET SEX

IF YOU ARE LUCKY ENOUGH TO HAVE ACCESS TO A PRIVATE BODY OF WATER, THIS SCENARIO WILL SHOW YOU HOW TO FULLY EXPLOIT IT FOR MAXIMUM SEXUAL FUN.

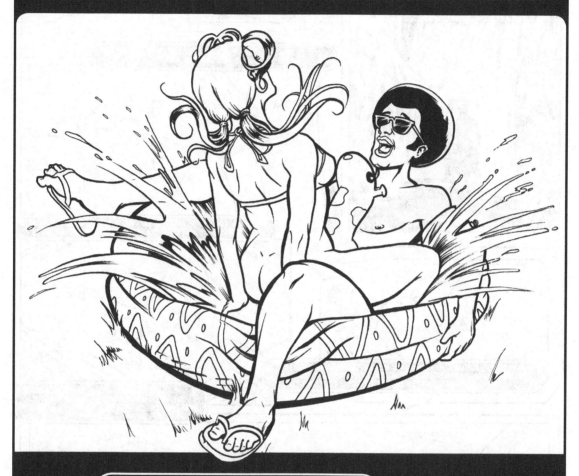

WHAT YOU'LL NEED . . .

PRIVATE BODY OF WATER

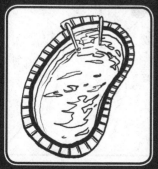

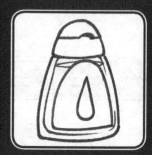

SILICONE-BASED LUBRICATION

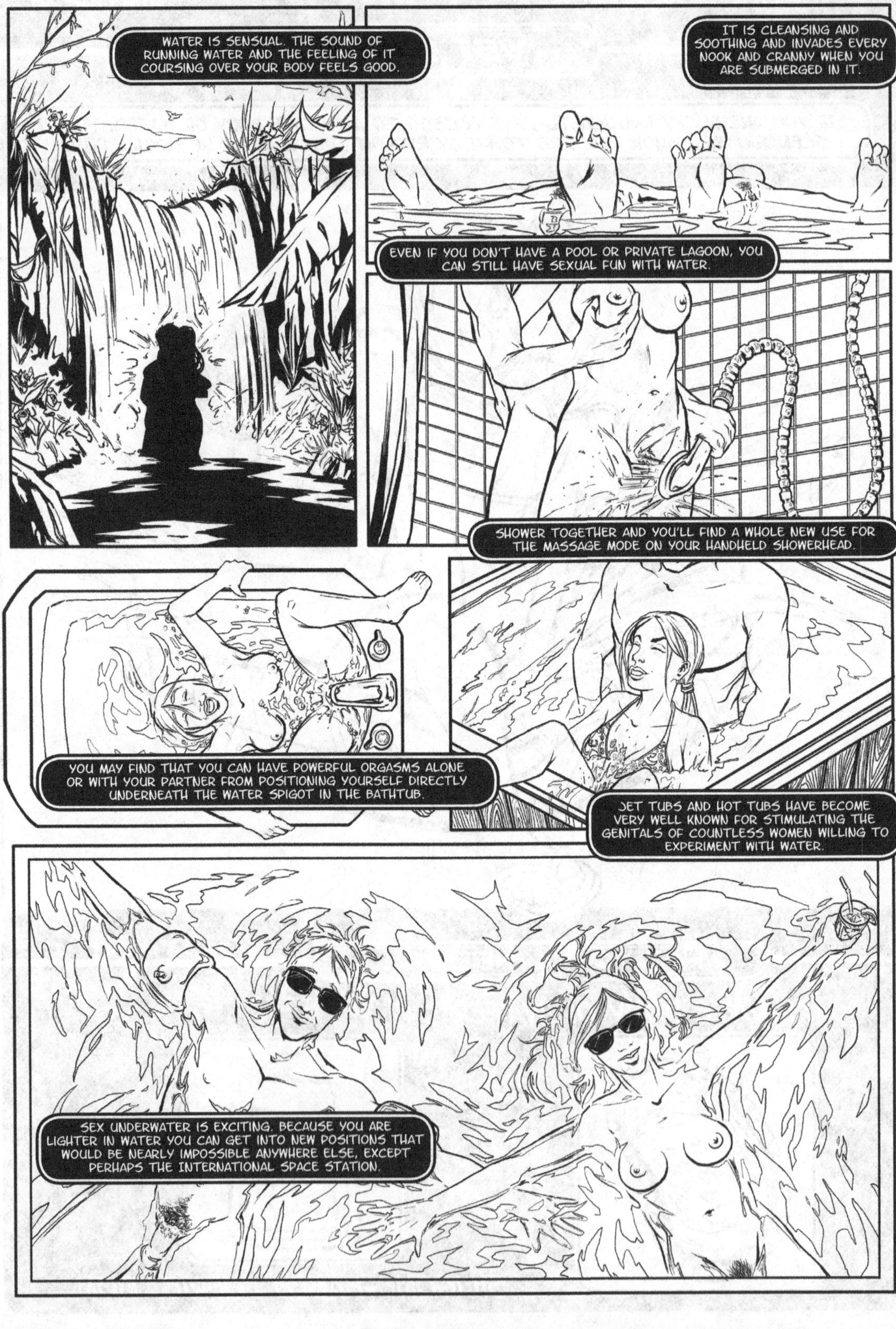
WATER IS SENSUAL. THE SOUND OF RUNNING WATER AND THE FEELING OF IT COURSING OVER YOUR BODY FEELS GOOD.
IT IS CLEANSING AND SOOTHING AND INVADES EVERY NOOK AND CRANNY WHEN YOU ARE SUBMERGED IN IT.
EVEN IF YOU DON'T HAVE A POOL OR PRIVATE LAGOON, YOU CAN STILL HAVE SEXUAL FUN WITH WATER.
SHOWER TOGETHER AND YOU'LL FIND A WHOLE NEW USE FOR THE MASSAGE MODE ON YOUR HANDHELD SHOWERHEAD.
YOU MAY FIND THAT YOU CAN HAVE POWERFUL ORGASMS ALONE OR WITH YOUR PARTNER FROM POSITIONING YOURSELF DIRECTLY UNDERNEATH THE WATER SPIGOT IN THE BATHTUB.
JET TUBS AND HOT TUBS HAVE BECOME VERY WELL KNOWN FOR STIMULATING THE GENITALS OF COUNTLESS WOMEN WILLING TO EXPERIMENT WITH WATER.
SEX UNDERWATER IS EXCITING. BECAUSE YOU ARE LIGHTER IN WATER YOU CAN GET INTO NEW POSITIONS THAT WOULD BE NEARLY IMPOSSIBLE ANYWHERE ELSE, EXCEPT PERHAPS THE INTERNATIONAL SPACE STATION.

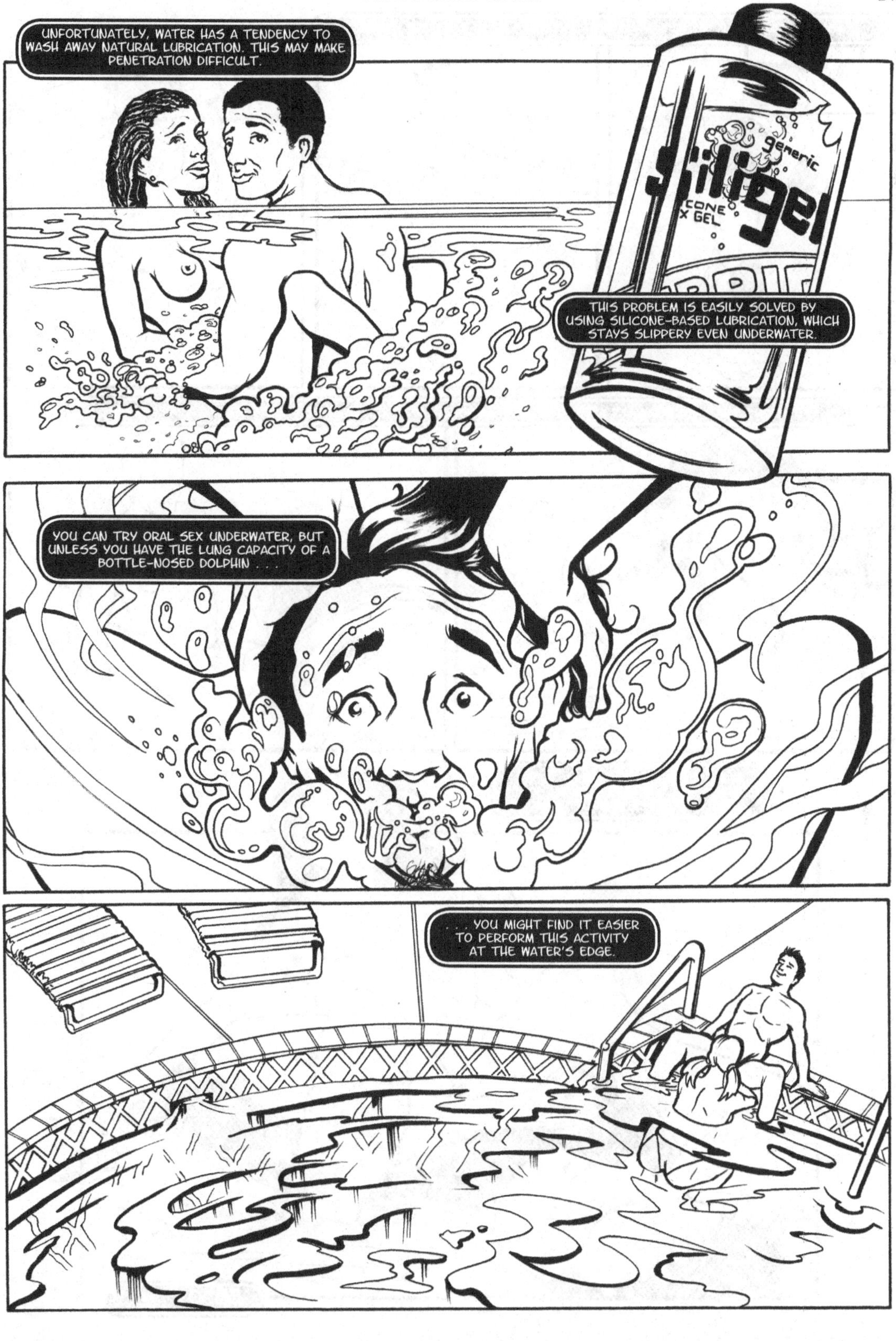
UNFORTUNATELY, WATER HAS A TENDENCY TO WASH AWAY NATURAL LUBRICATION. THIS MAY MAKE PENETRATION DIFFICULT.
generic
Siligel
THIS PROBLEM IS EASILY SOLVED BY USING SILICONE-BASED LUBRICATION, WHICH STAYS SLIPPERY EVEN UNDERWATER.
YOU CAN TRY ORAL SEX UNDERWATER, BUT UNLESS YOU HAVE THE LUNG CAPACITY OF A BOTTLE-NOSED DOLPHIN . . .
. . . YOU MIGHT FIND IT EASIER TO PERFORM THIS ACTIVITY AT THE WATER'S EDGE.

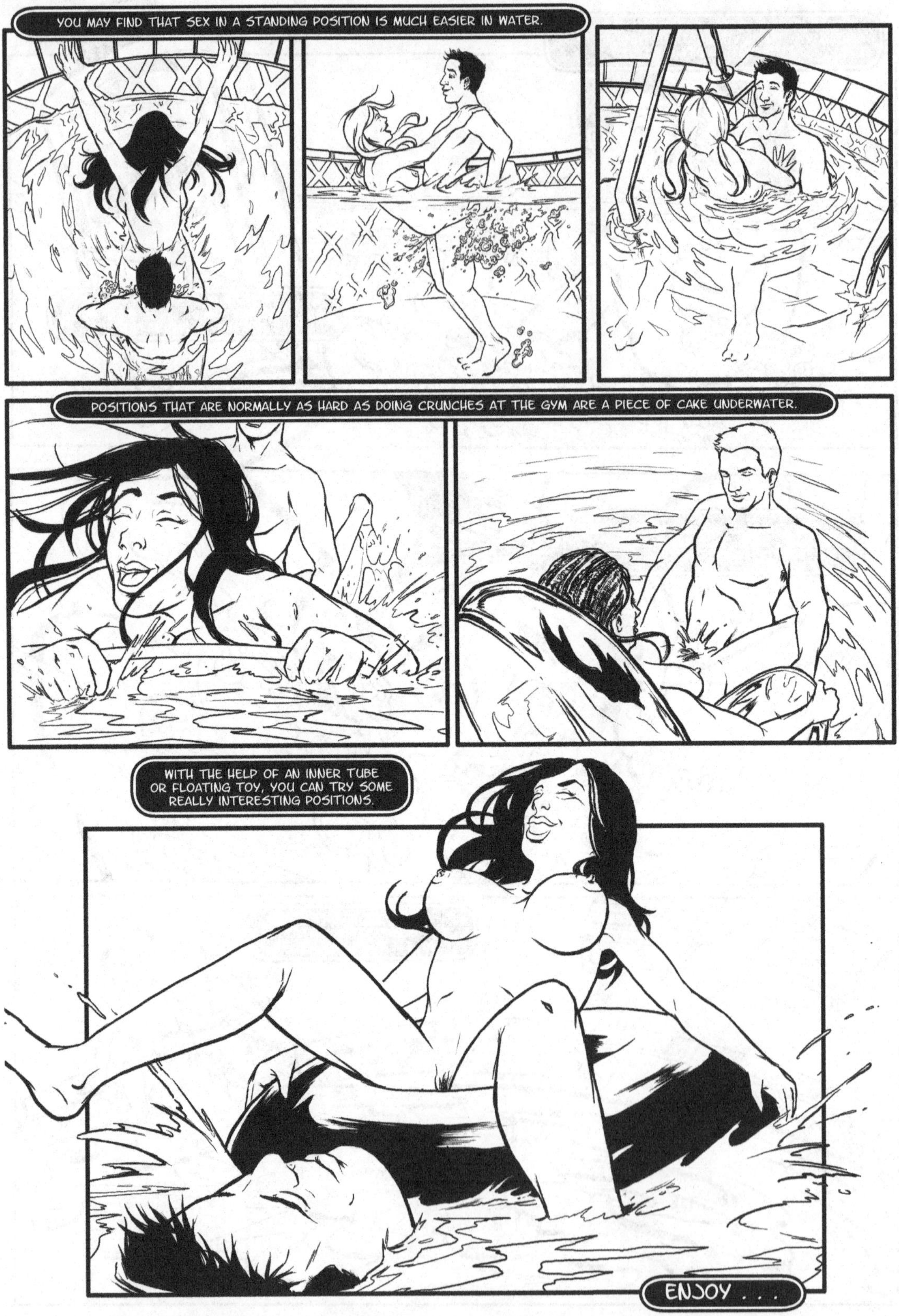
YOU MAY FIND THAT SEX IN A STANDING POSITION IS MUCH EASIER IN WATER.
POSITIONS THAT ARE NORMALLY AS HARD AS DOING CRUNCHES AT THE GYM ARE A PIECE OF CAKE UNDERWATER.
WITH THE HELP OF AN INNER TUBE OR FLOATING TOY, YOU CAN TRY SOME REALLY INTERESTING POSITIONS.
ENJOY . . .

CHAPTER 29

BEND OVER, BABY

WHEN YOU ARE IN THE MOOD FOR SOMETHING A LITTLE ROUGHER THAN THE USUAL SEX PLAY, TRY THIS IDEA.

WHAT YOU'LL NEED . . .

LUBRICATION

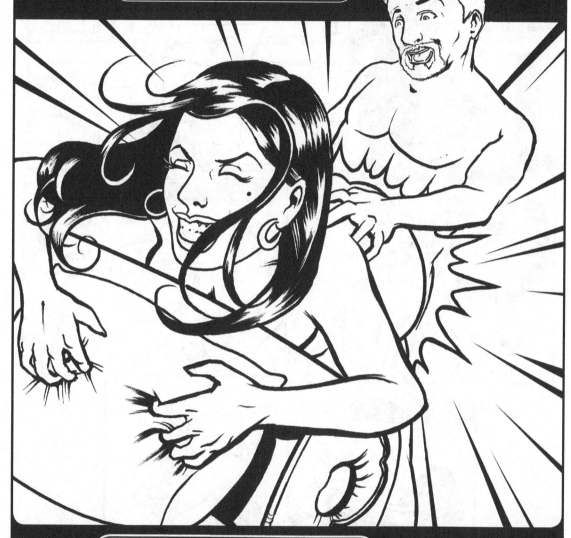

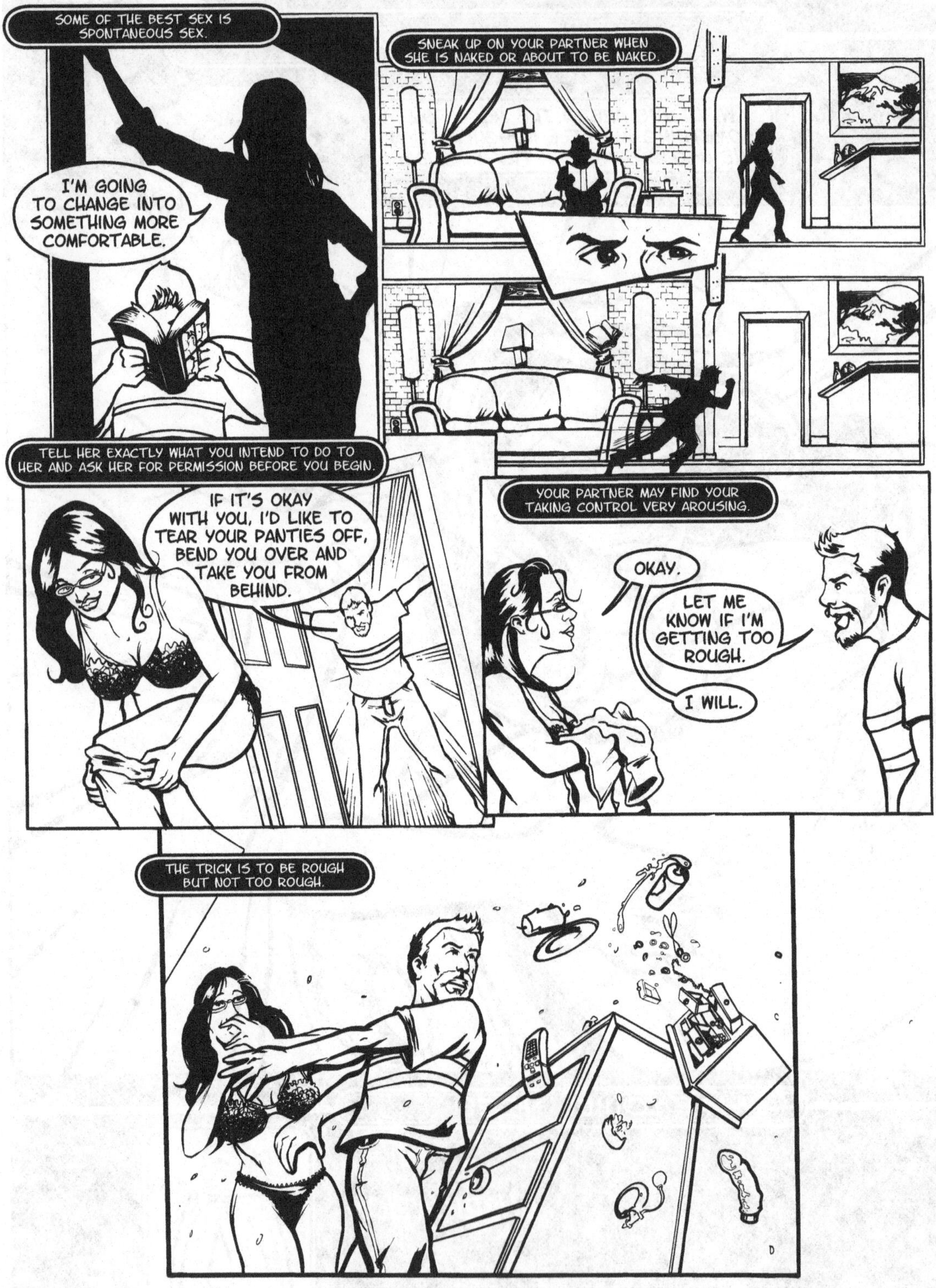
SOME OF THE BEST SEX IS SPONTANEOUS SEX.
I'M GOING TO CHANGE INTO SOMETHING MORE COMFORTABLE.
SNEAK UP ON YOUR PARTNER WHEN SHE IS NAKED OR ABOUT TO BE NAKED.
TELL HER EXACTLY WHAT YOU INTEND TO DO TO HER AND ASK HER FOR PERMISSION BEFORE YOU BEGIN.
IF IT'S OKAY WITH YOU, I'D LIKE TO TEAR YOUR PANTIES OFF, BEND YOU OVER AND TAKE YOU FROM BEHIND.
YOUR PARTNER MAY FIND YOUR TAKING CONTROL VERY AROUSING.
OKAY.
LET ME KNOW IF I'M GETTING TOO ROUGH.
I WILL.
THE TRICK IS TO BE ROUGH BUT NOT TOO ROUGH.

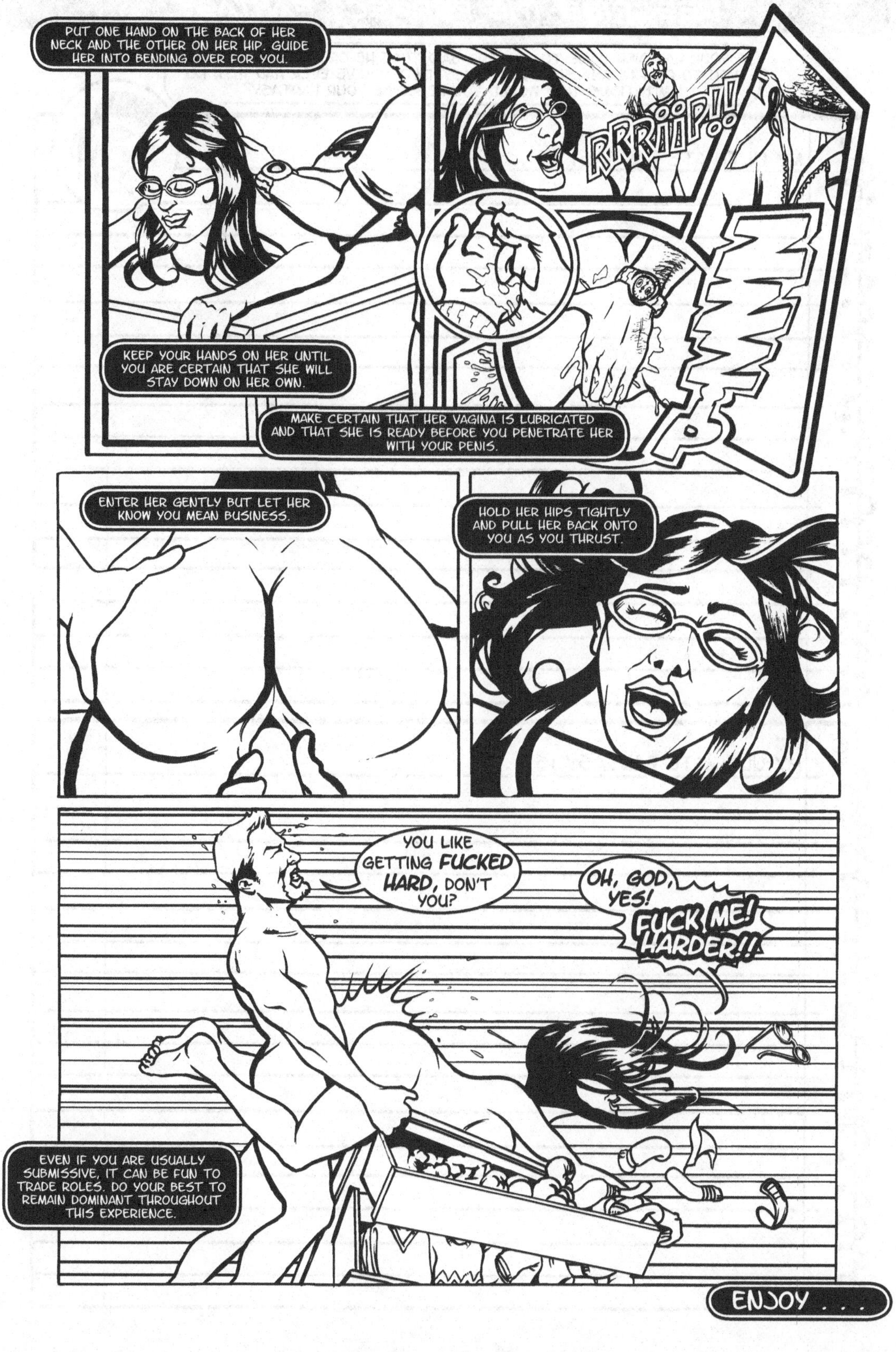
PUT ONE HAND ON THE BACK OF HER NECK AND THE OTHER ON HER HIP. GUIDE HER INTO BENDING OVER FOR YOU.
KEEP YOUR HANDS ON HER UNTIL YOU ARE CERTAIN THAT SHE WILL STAY DOWN ON HER OWN.
RRRIIIP!!
MAKE CERTAIN THAT HER VAGINA IS LUBRICATED AND THAT SHE IS READY BEFORE YOU PENETRATE HER WITH YOUR PENIS.
ENTER HER GENTLY BUT LET HER KNOW YOU MEAN BUSINESS.
HOLD HER HIPS TIGHTLY AND PULL HER BACK ONTO YOU AS YOU THRUST.
YOU LIKE GETTING FUCKED HARD, DON'T YOU?
OH, GOD, YES!
FUCK ME! HARDER!!
EVEN IF YOU ARE USUALLY SUBMISSIVE, IT CAN BE FUN TO TRADE ROLES. DO YOUR BEST TO REMAIN DOMINANT THROUGHOUT THIS EXPERIENCE.
ENJOY . . .

DESCRIBE THE PERFECT FANTASY

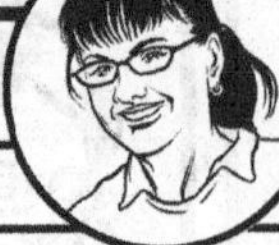
IF YOUR PARTNER CAME TO YOU AND SAID THAT HE OR SHE WOULD ALLOW YOU TO FULFILL ANY SEXUAL FANTASY THAT YOU'VE EVER HAD WITH NO LIMITATIONS, HOW WOULD YOU DESCRIBE YOUR FANTASY?

MY ULTIMATE FANTASY IS . . .

MY ULTIMATE FANTASY IS . . .

CHAPTER 30

BDSM AND SENSATION PLAY

IF YOU ARE ASKING YOURSELF WHAT BDSM MEANS OR WHY YOU WOULD WANT BDSM IN YOUR SEX LIFE, YOU'VE COME TO THE RIGHT CHAPTER.

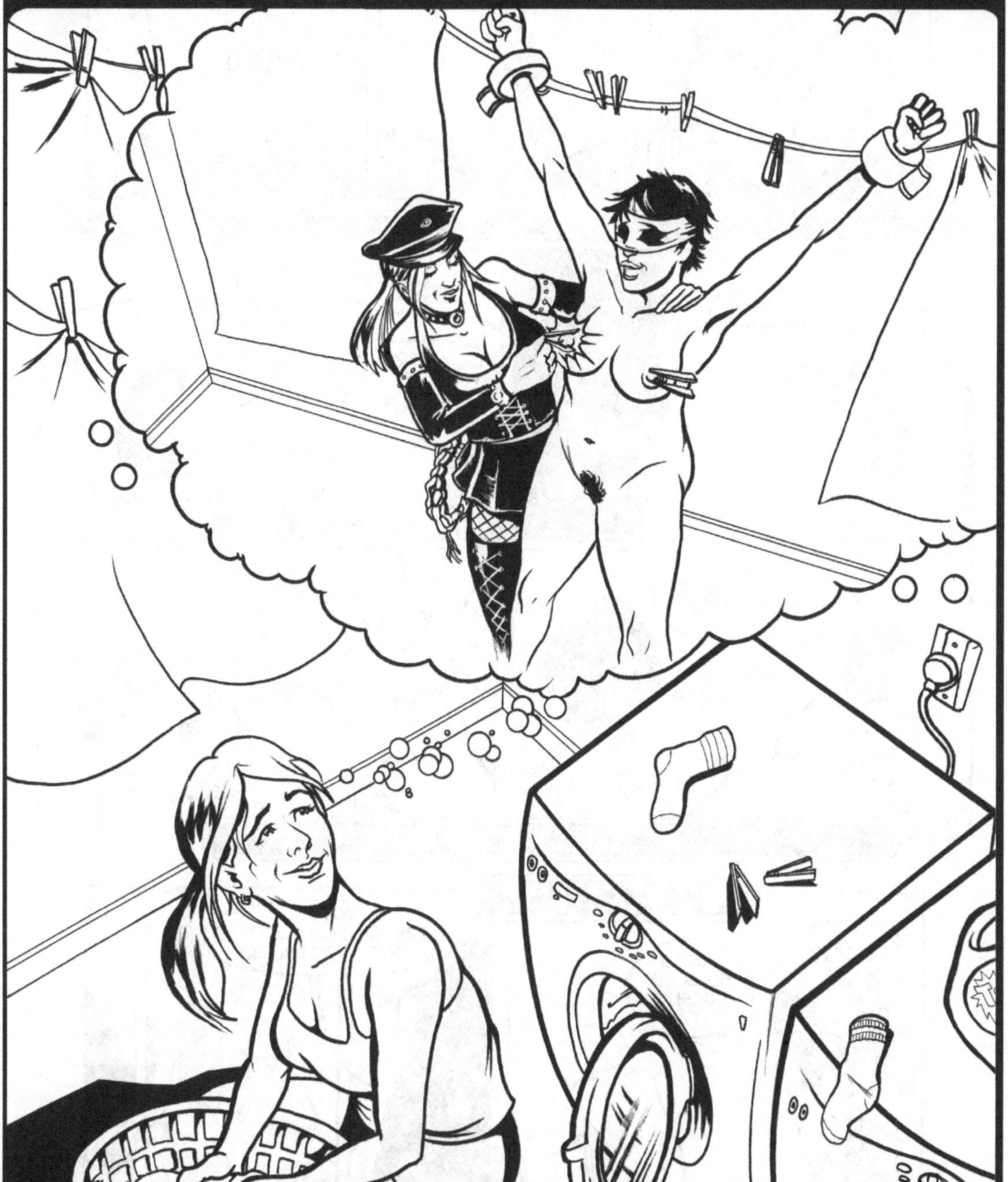

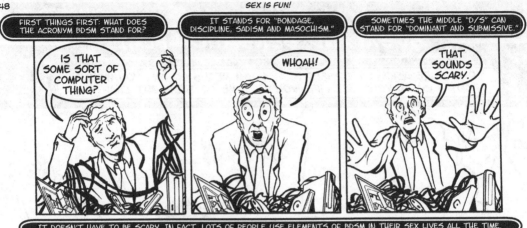

FIRST THINGS FIRST: WHAT DOES THE ACRONYM BDSM STAND FOR?

IS THAT SOME SORT OF COMPUTER THING?

IT STANDS FOR "BONDAGE, DISCIPLINE, SADISM AND MASOCHISM."

WHOAH!

SOMETIMES THE MIDDLE "D/S" CAN STAND FOR "DOMINANT AND SUBMISSIVE."

THAT SOUNDS SCARY.

IT DOESN'T HAVE TO BE SCARY. IN FACT, LOTS OF PEOPLE USE ELEMENTS OF BDSM IN THEIR SEX LIVES ALL THE TIME.

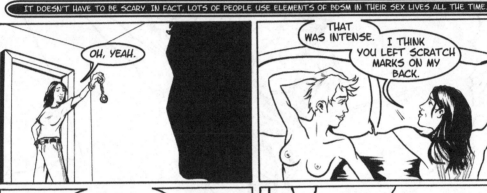

OH, YEAH.

THAT WAS INTENSE. I THINK YOU LEFT SCRATCH MARKS ON MY BACK.

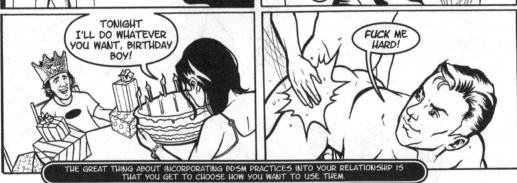

TONIGHT I'LL DO WHATEVER YOU WANT, BIRTHDAY BOY!

FUCK ME HARD!

THE GREAT THING ABOUT INCORPORATING BDSM PRACTICES INTO YOUR RELATIONSHIP IS THAT YOU GET TO CHOOSE HOW YOU WANT TO USE THEM.

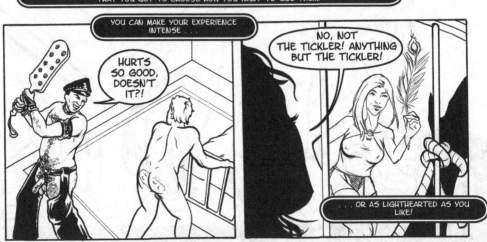

YOU CAN MAKE YOUR EXPERIENCE INTENSE . . .

HURTS SO GOOD, DOESN'T IT?!

NO, NOT THE TICKLER! ANYTHING BUT THE TICKLER!

. . . OR AS LIGHTHEARTED AS YOU LIKE!

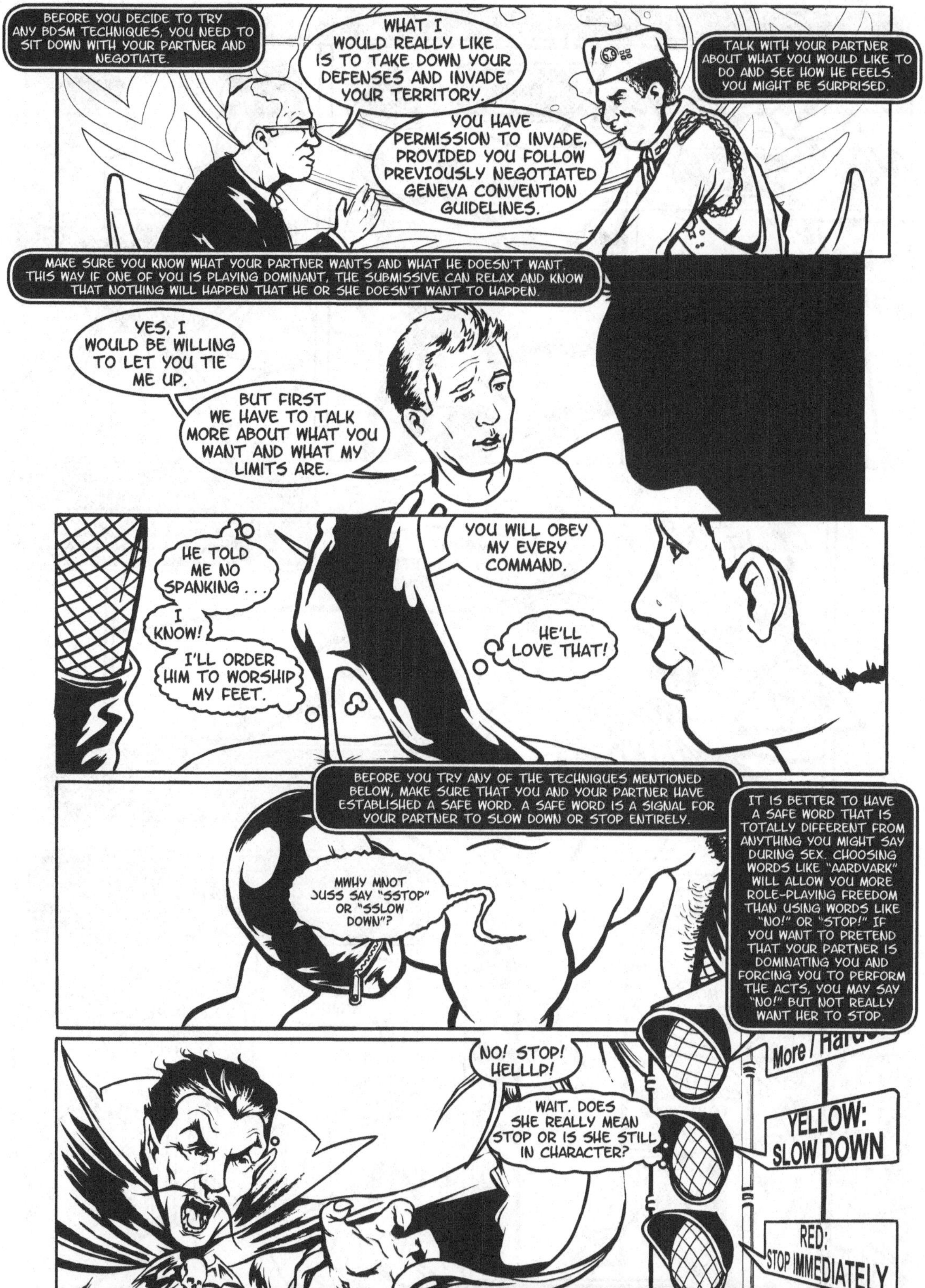
BEFORE YOU DECIDE TO TRY ANY BDSM TECHNIQUES, YOU NEED TO SIT DOWN WITH YOUR PARTNER AND NEGOTIATE.
WHAT I WOULD REALLY LIKE IS TO TAKE DOWN YOUR DEFENSES AND INVADE YOUR TERRITORY.
YOU HAVE PERMISSION TO INVADE, PROVIDED YOU FOLLOW PREVIOUSLY NEGOTIATED GENEVA CONVENTION GUIDELINES.
TALK WITH YOUR PARTNER ABOUT WHAT YOU WOULD LIKE TO DO AND SEE HOW HE FEELS. YOU MIGHT BE SURPRISED.
MAKE SURE YOU KNOW WHAT YOUR PARTNER WANTS AND WHAT HE DOESN'T WANT. THIS WAY IF ONE OF YOU IS PLAYING DOMINANT, THE SUBMISSIVE CAN RELAX AND KNOW THAT NOTHING WILL HAPPEN THAT HE OR SHE DOESN'T WANT TO HAPPEN.
YES, I WOULD BE WILLING TO LET YOU TIE ME UP.
BUT FIRST WE HAVE TO TALK MORE ABOUT WHAT YOU WANT AND WHAT MY LIMITS ARE.
HE TOLD ME NO SPANKING . . .
I KNOW!
I'LL ORDER HIM TO WORSHIP MY FEET.
YOU WILL OBEY MY EVERY COMMAND.
HE'LL LOVE THAT!
BEFORE YOU TRY ANY OF THE TECHNIQUES MENTIONED BELOW, MAKE SURE THAT YOU AND YOUR PARTNER HAVE ESTABLISHED A SAFE WORD. A SAFE WORD IS A SIGNAL FOR YOUR PARTNER TO SLOW DOWN OR STOP ENTIRELY.
MWHY MNOT JUSS SAY "SSTOP" OR "SSLOW DOWN"?
IT IS BETTER TO HAVE A SAFE WORD THAT IS TOTALLY DIFFERENT FROM ANYTHING YOU MIGHT SAY DURING SEX. CHOOSING WORDS LIKE "AARDVARK" WILL ALLOW YOU MORE ROLE-PLAYING FREEDOM THAN USING WORDS LIKE "NO!" OR "STOP!" IF YOU WANT TO PRETEND THAT YOUR PARTNER IS DOMINATING YOU AND FORCING YOU TO PERFORM THE ACTS, YOU MAY SAY "NO!" BUT NOT REALLY WANT HER TO STOP.
NO! STOP! HELLLP!
WAIT. DOES SHE REALLY MEAN STOP OR IS SHE STILL IN CHARACTER?
YELLOW: SLOW DOWN
RED: STOP IMMEDIATELY
MANY PEOPLE USE THE COLORS OF TRAFFIC LIGHTS AS SAFE WORDS. YELLOW MEANS "SLOW DOWN" AND RED MEANS "STOP NOW."

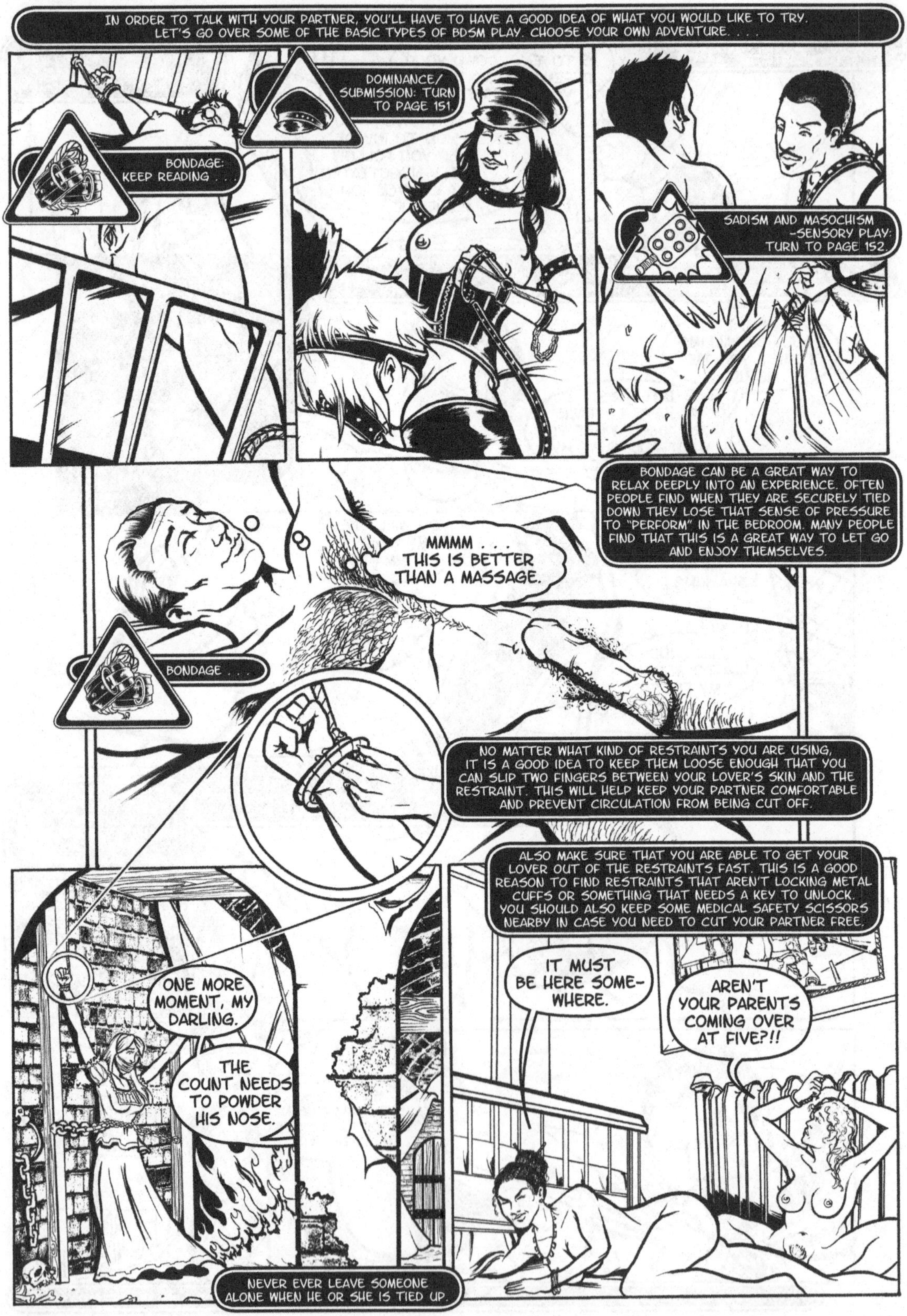
IN ORDER TO TALK WITH YOUR PARTNER, YOU'LL HAVE TO HAVE A GOOD IDEA OF WHAT YOU WOULD LIKE TO TRY. LET'S GO OVER SOME OF THE BASIC TYPES OF BDSM PLAY. CHOOSE YOUR OWN ADVENTURE . . . .
BONDAGE: KEEP READING . . .
DOMINANCE/ SUBMISSION: TURN TO PAGE 151.
SADISM AND MASOCHISM -SENSORY PLAY: TURN TO PAGE 152.
BONDAGE CAN BE A GREAT WAY TO RELAX DEEPLY INTO AN EXPERIENCE. OFTEN PEOPLE FIND WHEN THEY ARE SECURELY TIED DOWN THEY LOSE THAT SENSE OF PRESSURE TO "PERFORM" IN THE BEDROOM. MANY PEOPLE FIND THAT THIS IS A GREAT WAY TO LET GO AND ENJOY THEMSELVES.
MMMM . . . THIS IS BETTER THAN A MASSAGE.
BONDAGE . . .
NO MATTER WHAT KIND OF RESTRAINTS YOU ARE USING, IT IS A GOOD IDEA TO KEEP THEM LOOSE ENOUGH THAT YOU CAN SLIP TWO FINGERS BETWEEN YOUR LOVER'S SKIN AND THE RESTRAINT. THIS WILL HELP KEEP YOUR PARTNER COMFORTABLE AND PREVENT CIRCULATION FROM BEING CUT OFF.
ONE MORE MOMENT, MY DARLING.
THE COUNT NEEDS TO POWDER HIS NOSE.
NEVER EVER LEAVE SOMEONE ALONE WHEN HE OR SHE IS TIED UP.
ALSO MAKE SURE THAT YOU ARE ABLE TO GET YOUR LOVER OUT OF THE RESTRAINTS FAST. THIS IS A GOOD REASON TO FIND RESTRAINTS THAT AREN'T LOCKING METAL CUFFS OR SOMETHING THAT NEEDS A KEY TO UNLOCK. YOU SHOULD ALSO KEEP SOME MEDICAL SAFETY SCISSORS NEARBY IN CASE YOU NEED TO CUT YOUR PARTNER FREE.
IT MUST BE HERE SOME-WHERE.
AREN'T YOUR PARENTS COMING OVER AT FIVE?!!

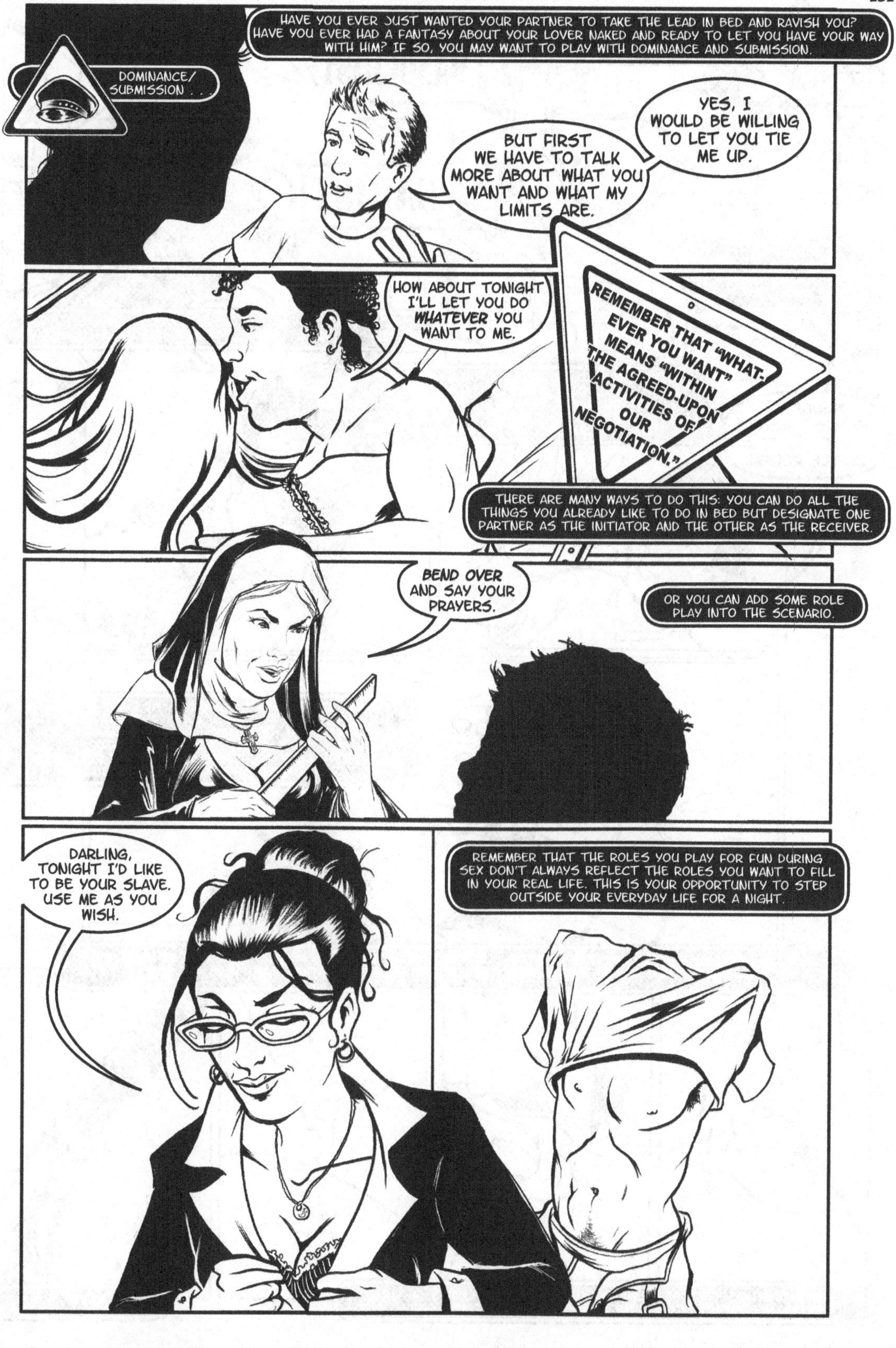
HAVE YOU EVER JUST WANTED YOUR PARTNER TO TAKE THE LEAD IN BED AND RAVISH YOU? HAVE YOU EVER HAD A FANTASY ABOUT YOUR LOVER NAKED AND READY TO LET YOU HAVE YOUR WAY WITH HIM? IF SO, YOU MAY WANT TO PLAY WITH DOMINANCE AND SUBMISSION.
DOMINANCE/ SUBMISSION . . .
YES, I WOULD BE WILLING TO LET YOU TIE ME UP.
BUT FIRST WE HAVE TO TALK MORE ABOUT WHAT YOU WANT AND WHAT MY LIMITS ARE.
HOW ABOUT TONIGHT I'LL LET YOU DO WHATEVER YOU WANT TO ME.
REMEMBER THAT "WHATEVER YOU WANT" MEANS "WITHIN THE AGREED-UPON ACTIVITIES OF OUR NEGOTIATION."
THERE ARE MANY WAYS TO DO THIS: YOU CAN DO ALL THE THINGS YOU ALREADY LIKE TO DO IN BED BUT DESIGNATE ONE PARTNER AS THE INITIATOR AND THE OTHER AS THE RECEIVER.
BEND OVER AND SAY YOUR PRAYERS.
OR YOU CAN ADD SOME ROLE PLAY INTO THE SCENARIO.
DARLING, TONIGHT I'D LIKE TO BE YOUR SLAVE. USE ME AS YOU WISH.
REMEMBER THAT THE ROLES YOU PLAY FOR FUN DURING SEX DON'T ALWAYS REFLECT THE ROLES YOU WANT TO FILL IN YOUR REAL LIFE. THIS IS YOUR OPPORTUNITY TO STEP OUTSIDE YOUR EVERYDAY LIFE FOR A NIGHT.

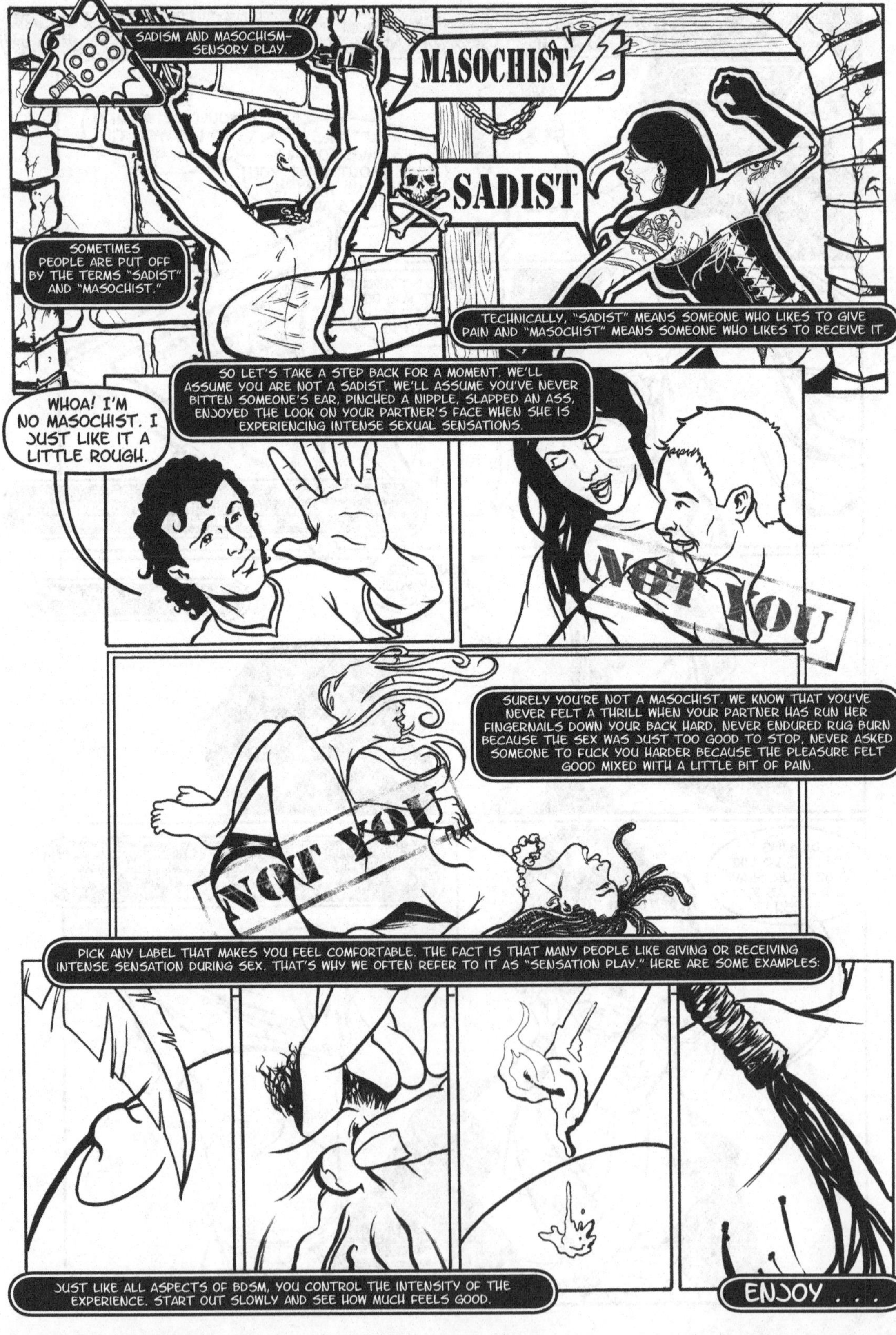
SADISM AND MASOCHISM- SENSORY PLAY.
MASOCHIST
SADIST
SOMETIMES PEOPLE ARE PUT OFF BY THE TERMS "SADIST" AND "MASOCHIST."
TECHNICALLY, "SADIST" MEANS SOMEONE WHO LIKES TO GIVE PAIN AND "MASOCHIST" MEANS SOMEONE WHO LIKES TO RECEIVE IT.
WHOA! I'M NO MASOCHIST. I JUST LIKE IT A LITTLE ROUGH.
SO LET'S TAKE A STEP BACK FOR A MOMENT. WE'LL ASSUME YOU ARE NOT A SADIST. WE'LL ASSUME YOU'VE NEVER BITTEN SOMEONE'S EAR, PINCHED A NIPPLE, SLAPPED AN ASS, ENJOYED THE LOOK ON YOUR PARTNER'S FACE WHEN SHE IS EXPERIENCING INTENSE SEXUAL SENSATIONS.
NOT YOU
SURELY YOU'RE NOT A MASOCHIST. WE KNOW THAT YOU'VE NEVER FELT A THRILL WHEN YOUR PARTNER HAS RUN HER FINGERNAILS DOWN YOUR BACK HARD, NEVER ENDURED RUG BURN BECAUSE THE SEX WAS JUST TOO GOOD TO STOP, NEVER ASKED SOMEONE TO FUCK YOU HARDER BECAUSE THE PLEASURE FELT GOOD MIXED WITH A LITTLE BIT OF PAIN.
NOT YOU
PICK ANY LABEL THAT MAKES YOU FEEL COMFORTABLE. THE FACT IS THAT MANY PEOPLE LIKE GIVING OR RECEIVING INTENSE SENSATION DURING SEX. THAT'S WHY WE OFTEN REFER TO IT AS "SENSATION PLAY." HERE ARE SOME EXAMPLES:
JUST LIKE ALL ASPECTS OF BDSM, YOU CONTROL THE INTENSITY OF THE EXPERIENCE. START OUT SLOWLY AND SEE HOW MUCH FEELS GOOD.
ENJOY . . .

CHAPTER 31

BUY HIM A FRENCH MAID FOR THE EVENING

PLAN A SPECIAL EVENING JUST FOR THE TWO OF YOU.

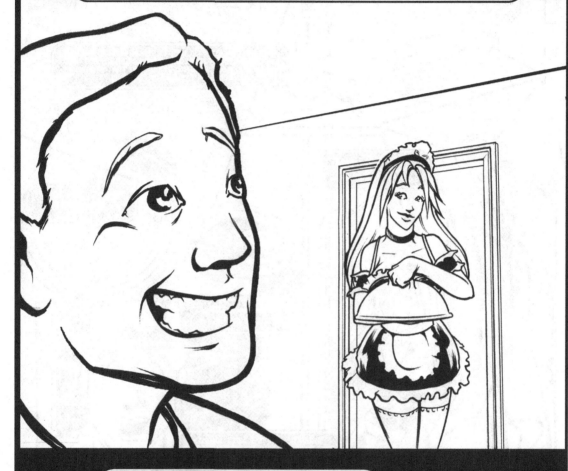

WHAT YOU'LL NEED . . .

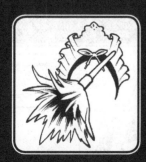

FRENCH MAID COSTUME

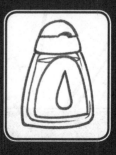

LUBRICATION

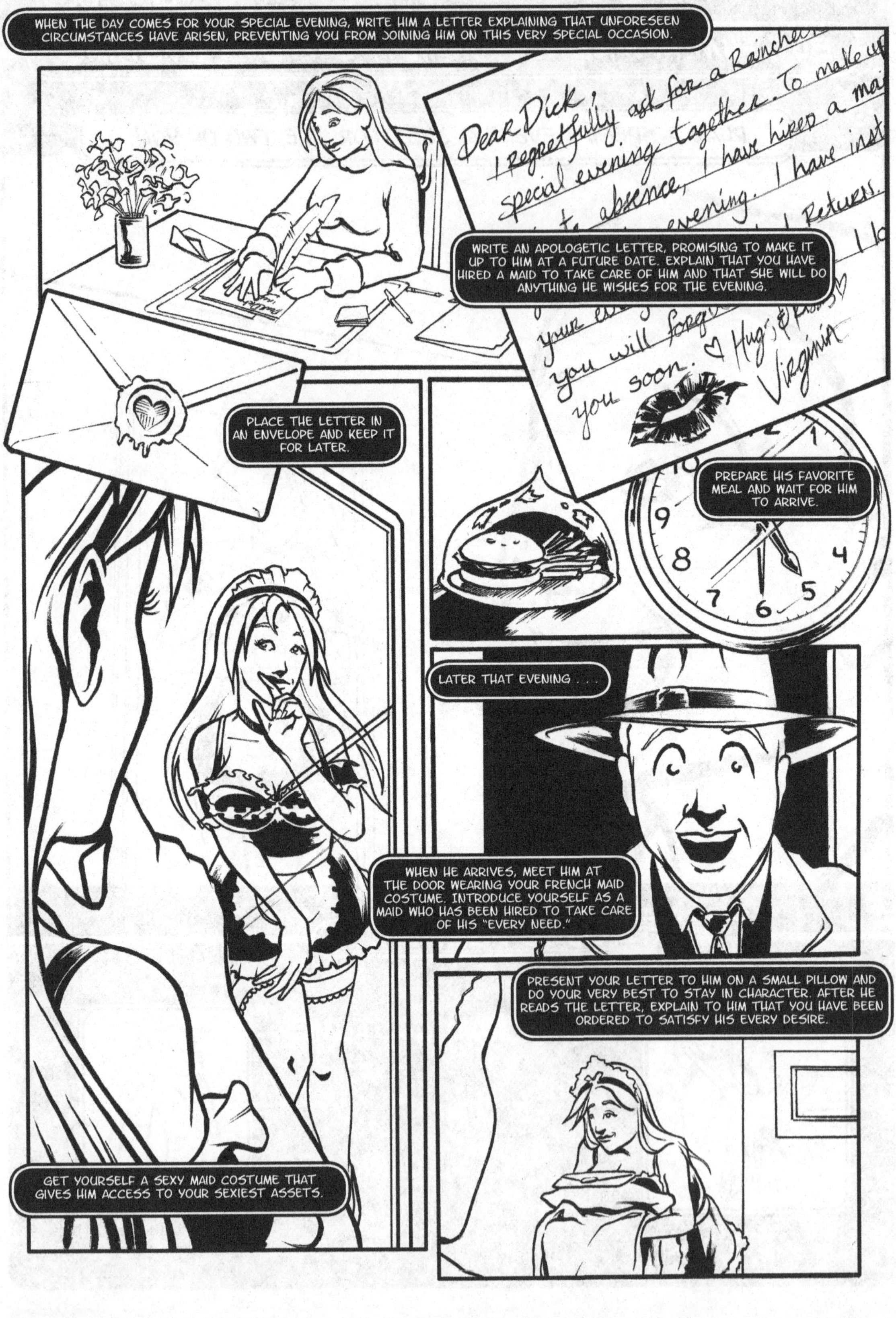

WHEN THE DAY COMES FOR YOUR SPECIAL EVENING, WRITE HIM A LETTER EXPLAINING THAT UNFORESEEN CIRCUMSTANCES HAVE ARISEN, PREVENTING YOU FROM JOINING HIM ON THIS VERY SPECIAL OCCASION.
Dear Dick,
I regretfully ask for a Rainche
special evening together. To make up
absence, I have hired a mai
evening. I have inst
Returns.
you will forg
you soon. ♥ Hugs
Virginia
WRITE AN APOLOGETIC LETTER, PROMISING TO MAKE IT UP TO HIM AT A FUTURE DATE. EXPLAIN THAT YOU HAVE HIRED A MAID TO TAKE CARE OF HIM AND THAT SHE WILL DO ANYTHING HE WISHES FOR THE EVENING.
PLACE THE LETTER IN AN ENVELOPE AND KEEP IT FOR LATER.
PREPARE HIS FAVORITE MEAL AND WAIT FOR HIM TO ARRIVE.
GET YOURSELF A SEXY MAID COSTUME THAT GIVES HIM ACCESS TO YOUR SEXIEST ASSETS.
LATER THAT EVENING . . .
WHEN HE ARRIVES, MEET HIM AT THE DOOR WEARING YOUR FRENCH MAID COSTUME. INTRODUCE YOURSELF AS A MAID WHO HAS BEEN HIRED TO TAKE CARE OF HIS "EVERY NEED."
PRESENT YOUR LETTER TO HIM ON A SMALL PILLOW AND DO YOUR VERY BEST TO STAY IN CHARACTER. AFTER HE READS THE LETTER, EXPLAIN TO HIM THAT YOU HAVE BEEN ORDERED TO SATISFY HIS EVERY DESIRE.

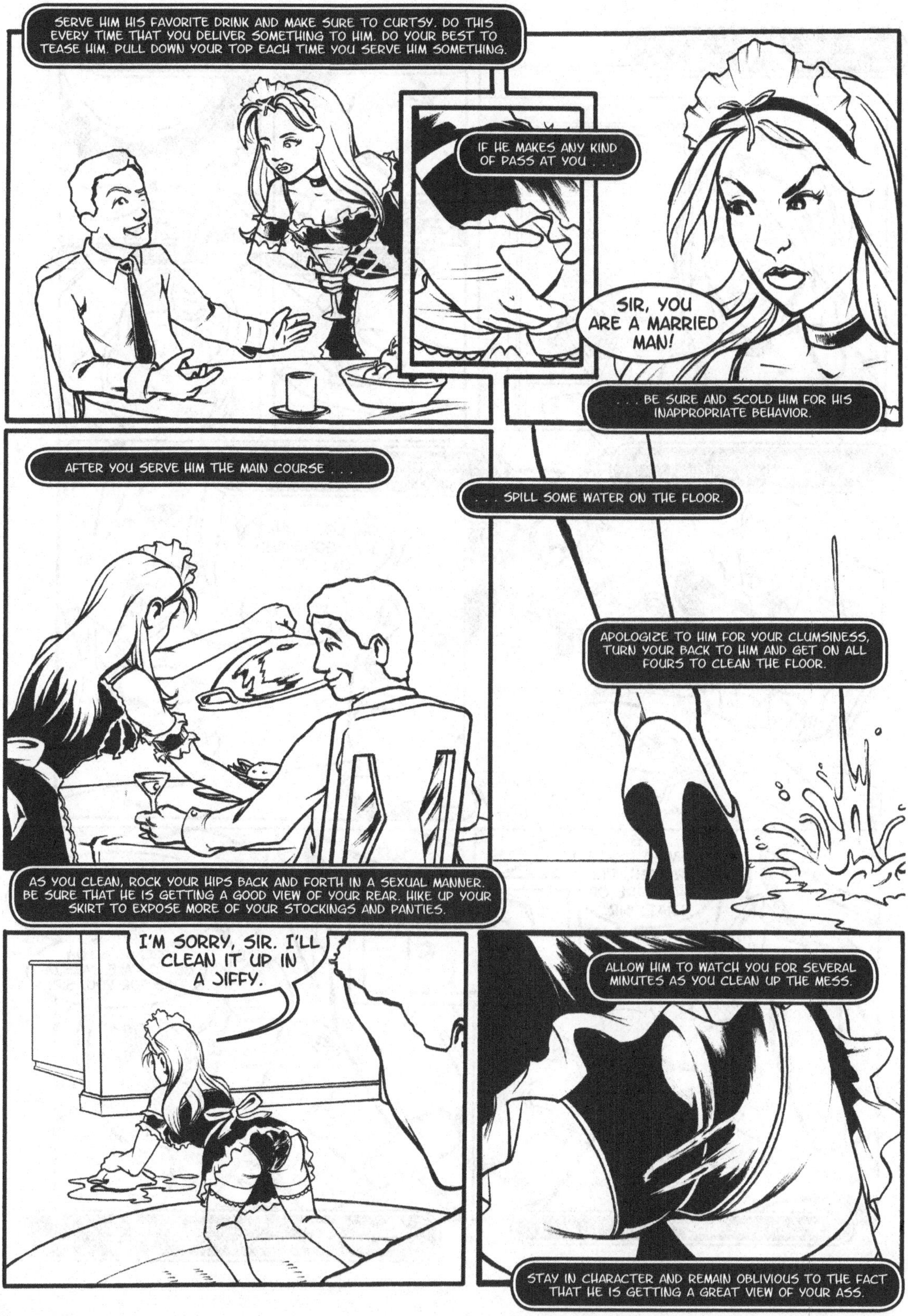
SERVE HIM HIS FAVORITE DRINK AND MAKE SURE TO CURTSY. DO THIS EVERY TIME THAT YOU DELIVER SOMETHING TO HIM. DO YOUR BEST TO TEASE HIM. PULL DOWN YOUR TOP EACH TIME YOU SERVE HIM SOMETHING.
IF HE MAKES ANY KIND OF PASS AT YOU . . .
SIR, YOU ARE A MARRIED MAN!
. . . BE SURE AND SCOLD HIM FOR HIS INAPPROPRIATE BEHAVIOR.
AFTER YOU SERVE HIM THE MAIN COURSE . . .
. . . SPILL SOME WATER ON THE FLOOR.
APOLOGIZE TO HIM FOR YOUR CLUMSINESS, TURN YOUR BACK TO HIM AND GET ON ALL FOURS TO CLEAN THE FLOOR.
AS YOU CLEAN, ROCK YOUR HIPS BACK AND FORTH IN A SEXUAL MANNER. BE SURE THAT HE IS GETTING A GOOD VIEW OF YOUR REAR. HIKE UP YOUR SKIRT TO EXPOSE MORE OF YOUR STOCKINGS AND PANTIES.
I'M SORRY, SIR. I'LL CLEAN IT UP IN A JIFFY.
ALLOW HIM TO WATCH YOU FOR SEVERAL MINUTES AS YOU CLEAN UP THE MESS.
STAY IN CHARACTER AND REMAIN OBLIVIOUS TO THE FACT THAT HE IS GETTING A GREAT VIEW OF YOUR ASS.

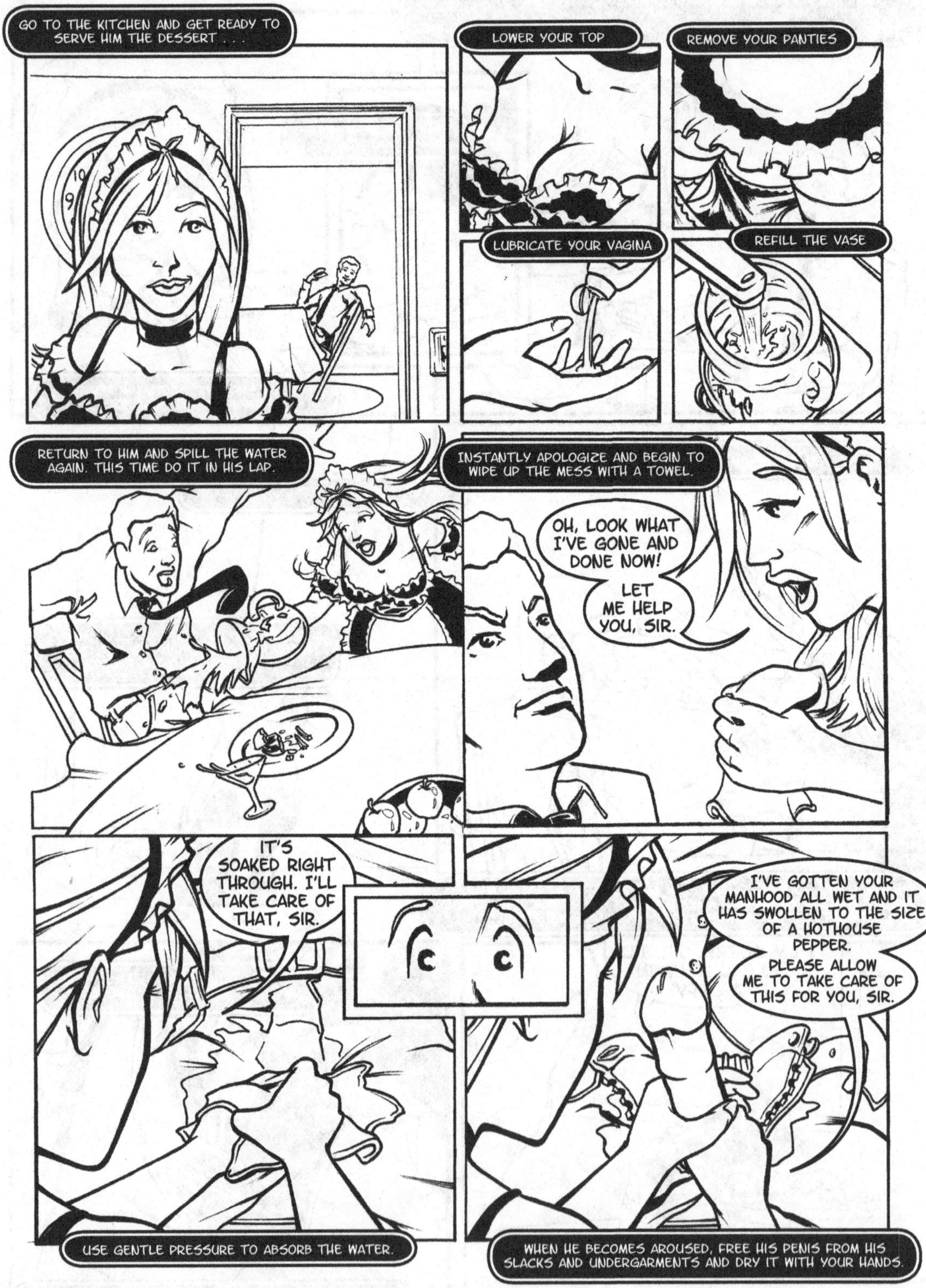
GO TO THE KITCHEN AND GET READY TO SERVE HIM THE DESSERT . . .
LOWER YOUR TOP
REMOVE YOUR PANTIES
LUBRICATE YOUR VAGINA
REFILL THE VASE
RETURN TO HIM AND SPILL THE WATER AGAIN. THIS TIME DO IT IN HIS LAP.
INSTANTLY APOLOGIZE AND BEGIN TO WIPE UP THE MESS WITH A TOWEL.
OH, LOOK WHAT I'VE GONE AND DONE NOW!
LET ME HELP YOU, SIR.
IT'S SOAKED RIGHT THROUGH. I'LL TAKE CARE OF THAT, SIR.
USE GENTLE PRESSURE TO ABSORB THE WATER.
I'VE GOTTEN YOUR MANHOOD ALL WET AND IT HAS SWOLLEN TO THE SIZE OF A HOTHOUSE PEPPER.
PLEASE ALLOW ME TO TAKE CARE OF THIS FOR YOU, SIR.
WHEN HE BECOMES AROUSED, FREE HIS PENIS FROM HIS SLACKS AND UNDERGARMENTS AND DRY IT WITH YOUR HANDS.

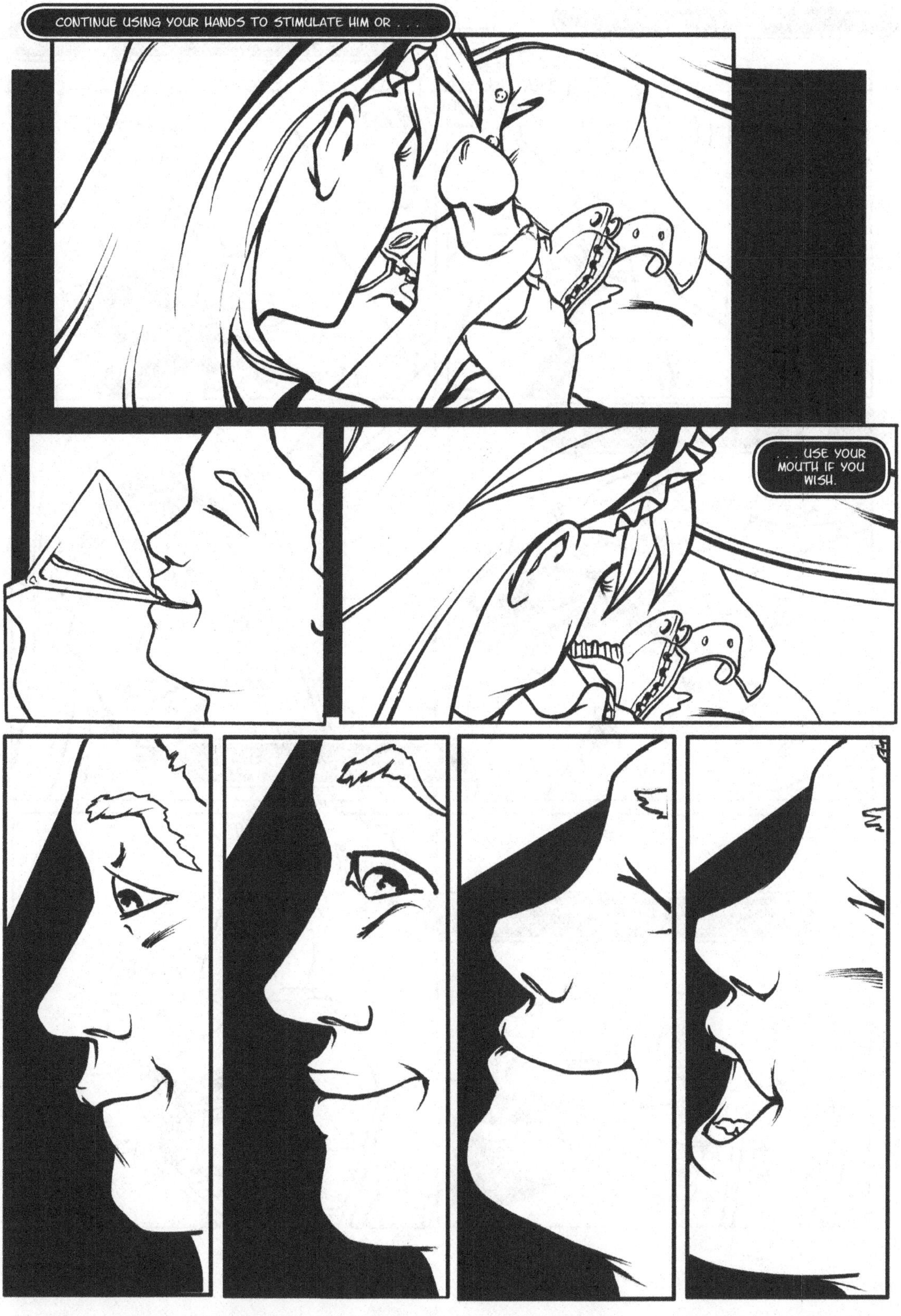
CONTINUE USING YOUR HANDS TO STIMULATE HIM OR . . .
. . . USE YOUR MOUTH IF YOU WISH.

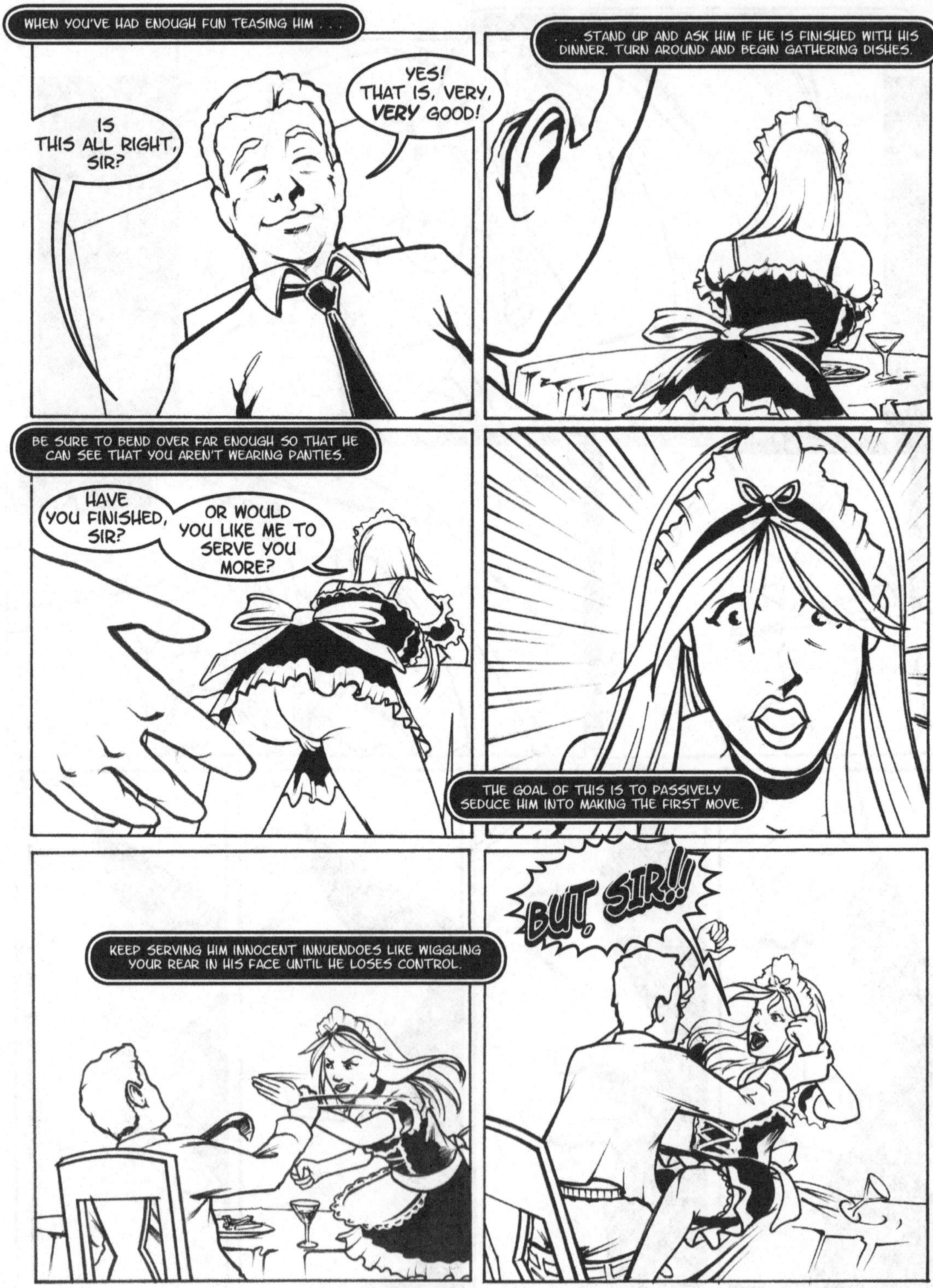
WHEN YOU'VE HAD ENOUGH FUN TEASING HIM . . .
IS THIS ALL RIGHT, SIR?
YES! THAT IS, VERY, VERY GOOD!
. . . . STAND UP AND ASK HIM IF HE IS FINISHED WITH HIS DINNER. TURN AROUND AND BEGIN GATHERING DISHES.
BE SURE TO BEND OVER FAR ENOUGH SO THAT HE CAN SEE THAT YOU AREN'T WEARING PANTIES.
HAVE YOU FINISHED, SIR?
OR WOULD YOU LIKE ME TO SERVE YOU MORE?
THE GOAL OF THIS IS TO PASSIVELY SEDUCE HIM INTO MAKING THE FIRST MOVE.
KEEP SERVING HIM INNOCENT INNUENDOES LIKE WIGGLING YOUR REAR IN HIS FACE UNTIL HE LOSES CONTROL.
BUT, SIR!!

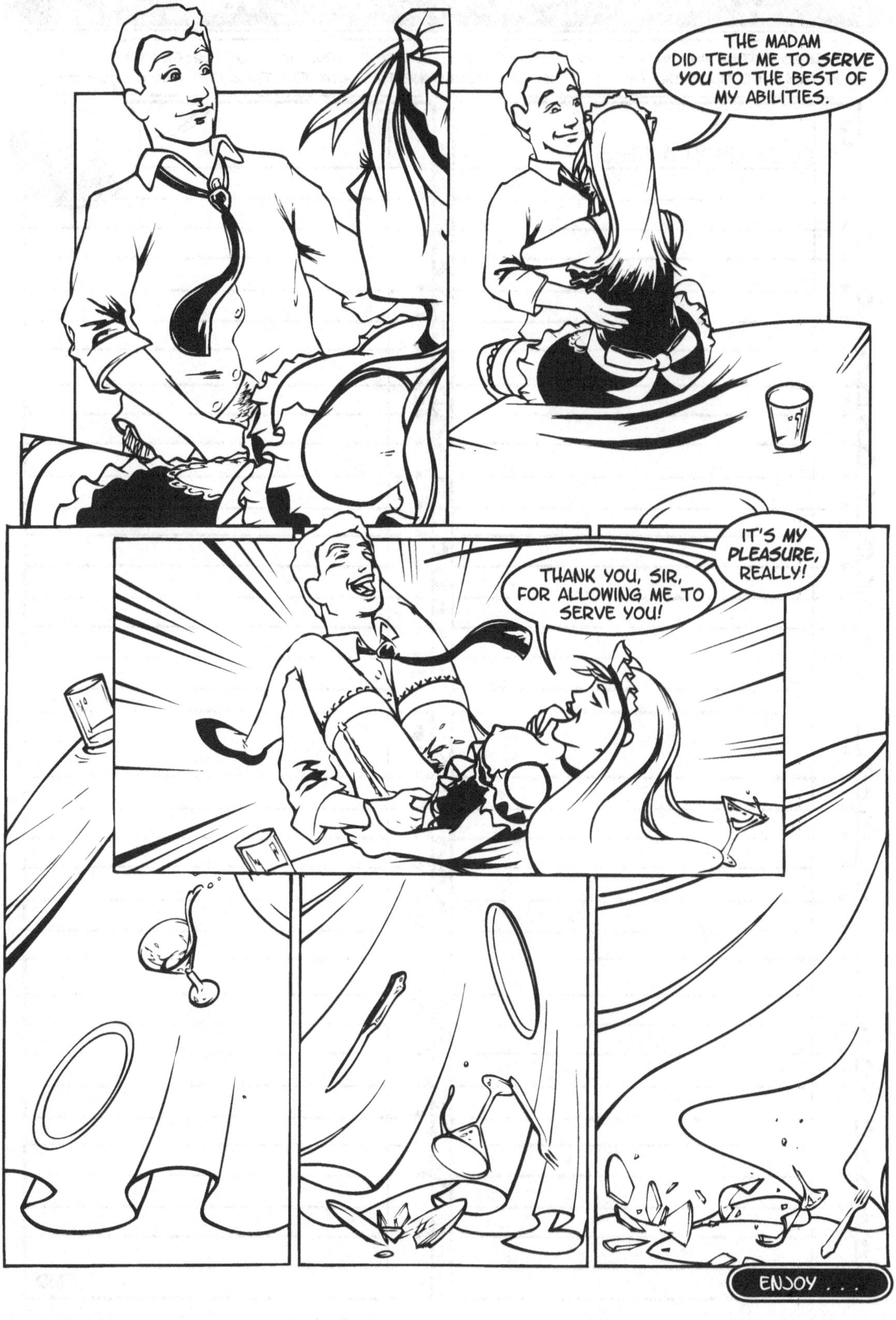
THE MADAM DID TELL ME TO *SERVE YOU* TO THE BEST OF MY ABILITIES.
THANK YOU, SIR, FOR ALLOWING ME TO SERVE YOU!
IT'S *MY PLEASURE*, REALLY!
ENJOY . . .

AN EROTIC STORY STARRING YOU

TAKE TURNS WRITING AN EROTIC STORY THAT FEATURES THE TWO OF YOU. THE FIRST PERSON WHO OPENS THIS PAGE WILL BEGIN THE STORY. IF YOU ARE READING THIS BOOK TOGETHER, FLIP A COIN.

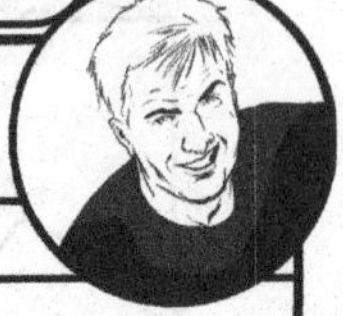

ONCE UPON A TIME . . .

THE END

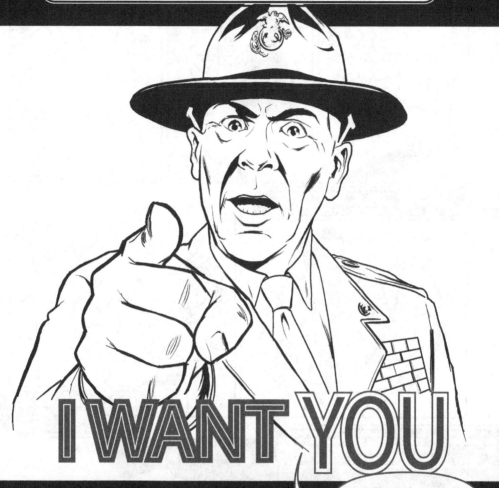

CHAPTER 32

THE SERGEANT AND THE NEW RECRUIT

IN THIS DOM/SUB ROLE-PLAY SCENARIO, WE'LL SHOW YOU HOW TO ADD A MILITARY FANTASY TO YOUR SEXUAL ARSENAL.

I WANT YOU

TO LICK MY BALLS!

WHAT YOU'LL NEED . . .

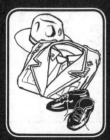

MILITARY UNIFORM

LUBRICATION

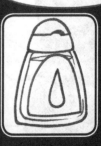

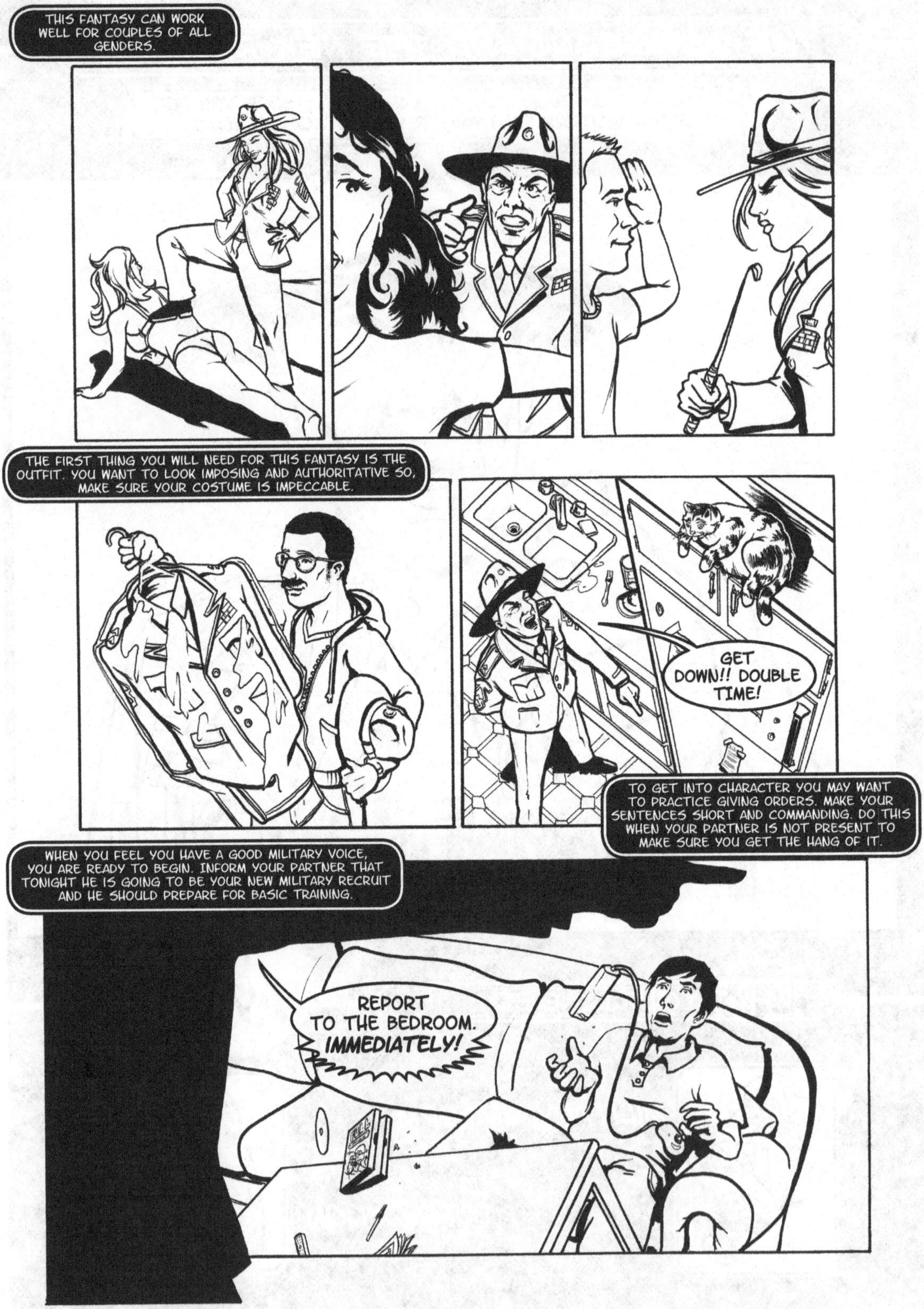
THIS FANTASY CAN WORK WELL FOR COUPLES OF ALL GENDERS.
THE FIRST THING YOU WILL NEED FOR THIS FANTASY IS THE OUTFIT. YOU WANT TO LOOK IMPOSING AND AUTHORITATIVE SO, MAKE SURE YOUR COSTUME IS IMPECCABLE.
GET DOWN!! DOUBLE TIME!
TO GET INTO CHARACTER YOU MAY WANT TO PRACTICE GIVING ORDERS. MAKE YOUR SENTENCES SHORT AND COMMANDING. DO THIS WHEN YOUR PARTNER IS NOT PRESENT TO MAKE SURE YOU GET THE HANG OF IT.
WHEN YOU FEEL YOU HAVE A GOOD MILITARY VOICE, YOU ARE READY TO BEGIN. INFORM YOUR PARTNER THAT TONIGHT HE IS GOING TO BE YOUR NEW MILITARY RECRUIT AND HE SHOULD PREPARE FOR BASIC TRAINING.
REPORT TO THE BEDROOM. *IMMEDIATELY!*

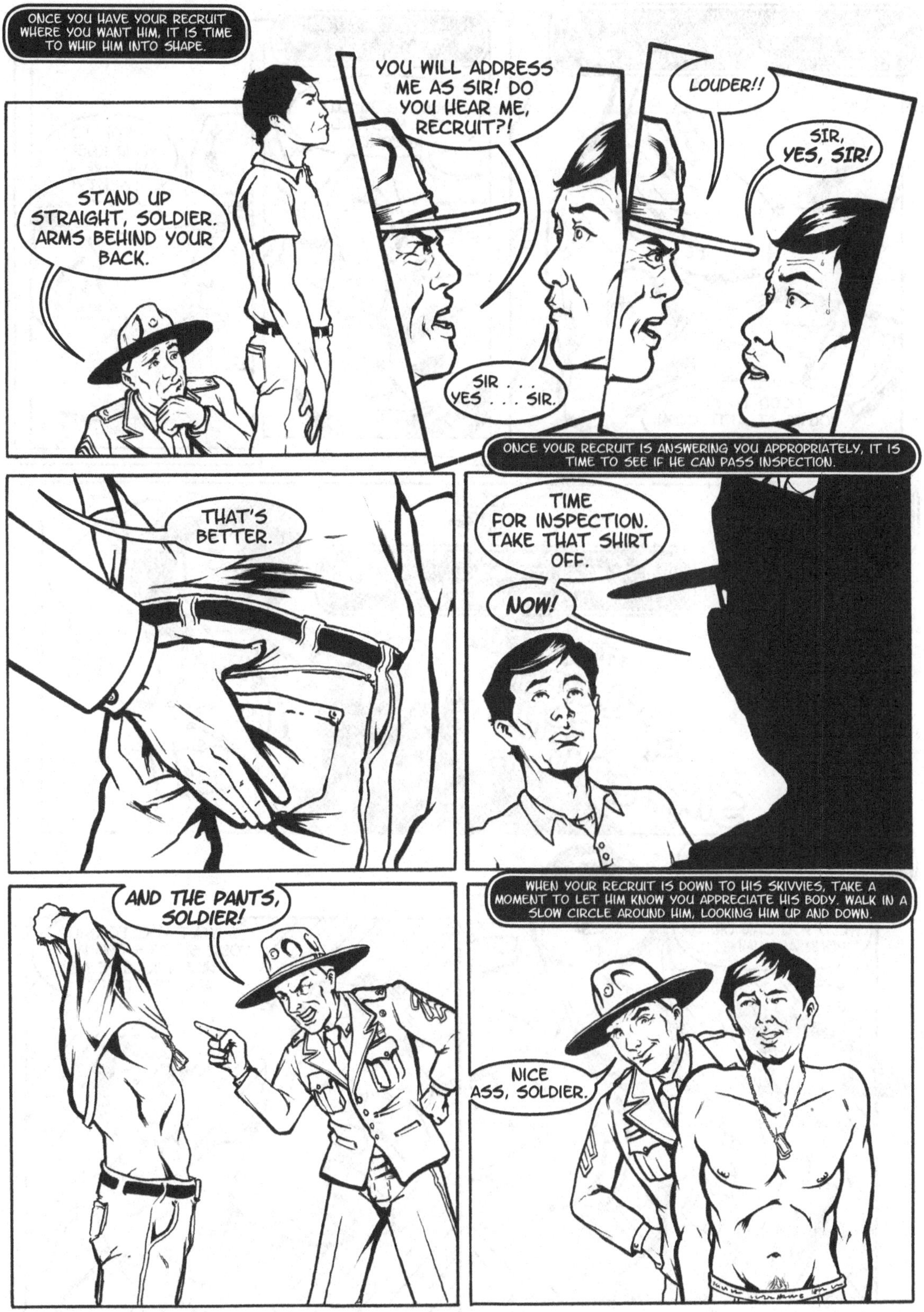
ONCE YOU HAVE YOUR RECRUIT WHERE YOU WANT HIM, IT IS TIME TO WHIP HIM INTO SHAPE.
STAND UP STRAIGHT, SOLDIER. ARMS BEHIND YOUR BACK.
YOU WILL ADDRESS ME AS SIR! DO YOU HEAR ME, RECRUIT?!
SIR . . . YES . . . SIR.
LOUDER!!
SIR, YES, SIR!
ONCE YOUR RECRUIT IS ANSWERING YOU APPROPRIATELY, IT IS TIME TO SEE IF HE CAN PASS INSPECTION.
THAT'S BETTER.
TIME FOR INSPECTION. TAKE THAT SHIRT OFF.
NOW!
AND THE PANTS, SOLDIER!
WHEN YOUR RECRUIT IS DOWN TO HIS SKIVVIES, TAKE A MOMENT TO LET HIM KNOW YOU APPRECIATE HIS BODY. WALK IN A SLOW CIRCLE AROUND HIM, LOOKING HIM UP AND DOWN.
NICE ASS, SOLDIER.

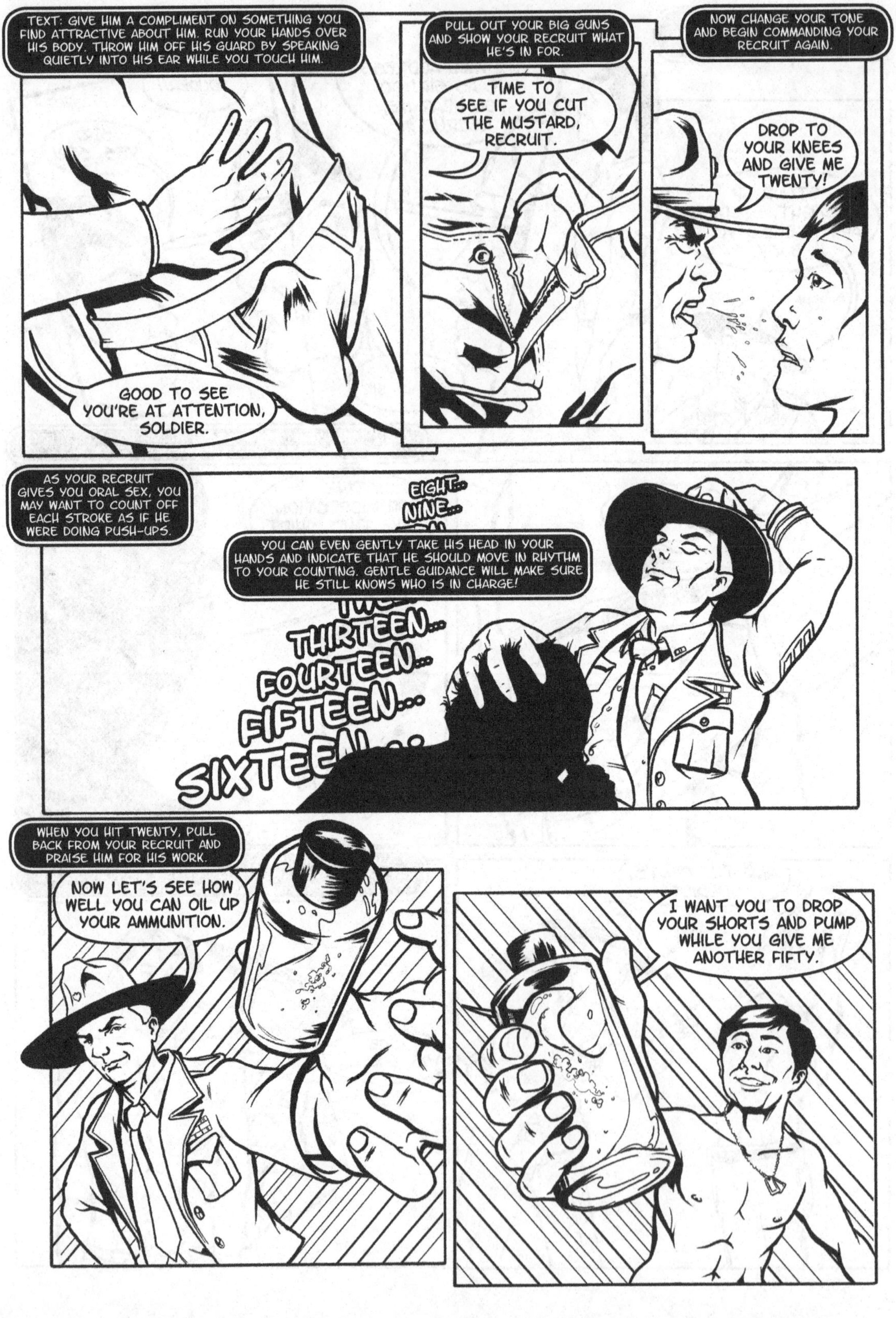
TEXT: GIVE HIM A COMPLIMENT ON SOMETHING YOU FIND ATTRACTIVE ABOUT HIM. RUN YOUR HANDS OVER HIS BODY. THROW HIM OFF HIS GUARD BY SPEAKING QUIETLY INTO HIS EAR WHILE YOU TOUCH HIM.
GOOD TO SEE YOU'RE AT ATTENTION, SOLDIER.
PULL OUT YOUR BIG GUNS AND SHOW YOUR RECRUIT WHAT HE'S IN FOR.
TIME TO SEE IF YOU CUT THE MUSTARD, RECRUIT.
NOW CHANGE YOUR TONE AND BEGIN COMMANDING YOUR RECRUIT AGAIN.
DROP TO YOUR KNEES AND GIVE ME TWENTY!
AS YOUR RECRUIT GIVES YOU ORAL SEX, YOU MAY WANT TO COUNT OFF EACH STROKE AS IF HE WERE DOING PUSH-UPS.
EIGHT... NINE...
YOU CAN EVEN GENTLY TAKE HIS HEAD IN YOUR HANDS AND INDICATE THAT HE SHOULD MOVE IN RHYTHM TO YOUR COUNTING. GENTLE GUIDANCE WILL MAKE SURE HE STILL KNOWS WHO IS IN CHARGE!
THIRTEEN... FOURTEEN... FIFTEEN...
WHEN YOU HIT TWENTY, PULL BACK FROM YOUR RECRUIT AND PRAISE HIM FOR HIS WORK.
NOW LET'S SEE HOW WELL YOU CAN OIL UP YOUR AMMUNITION.
I WANT YOU TO DROP YOUR SHORTS AND PUMP WHILE YOU GIVE ME ANOTHER FIFTY.

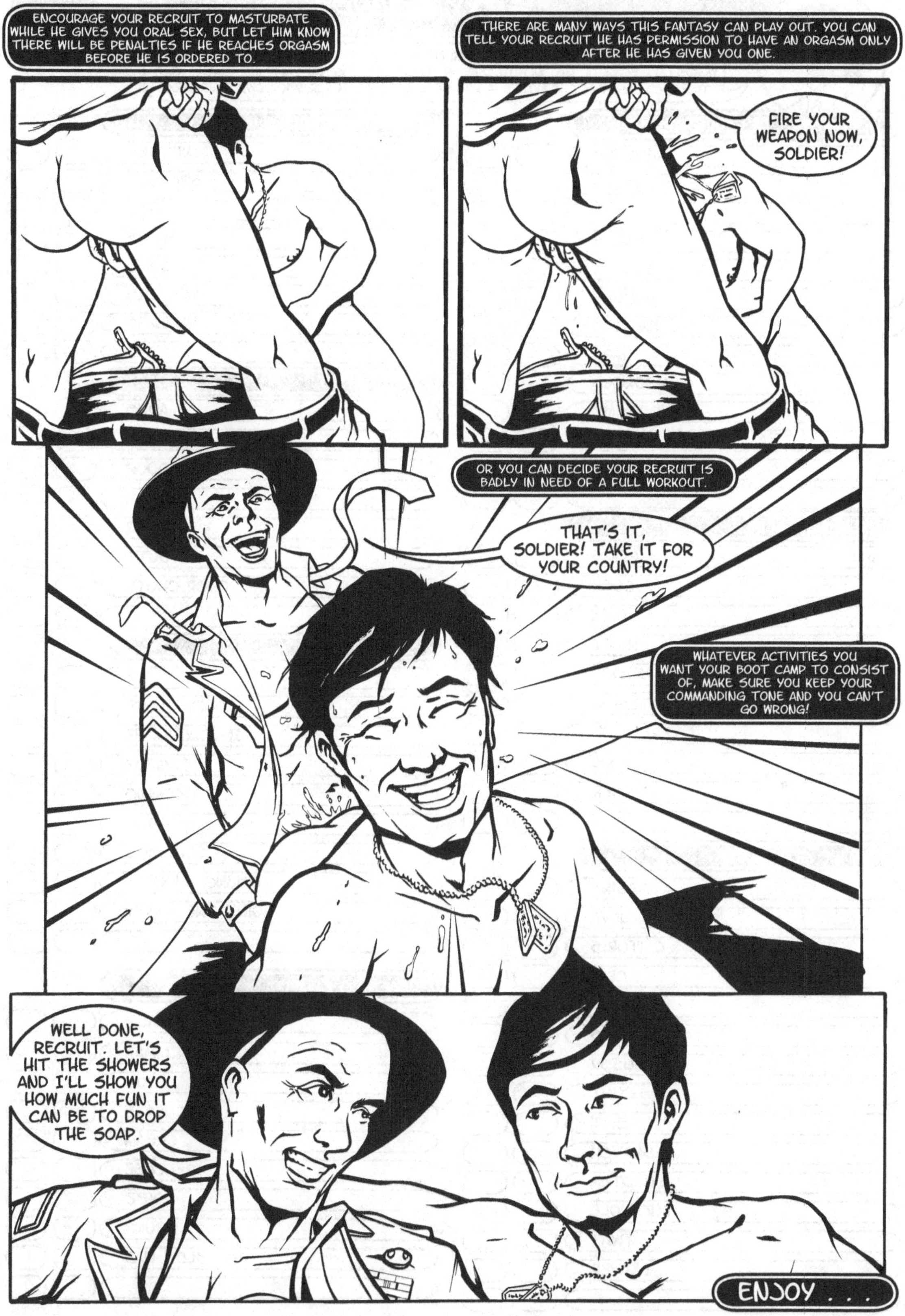
ENCOURAGE YOUR RECRUIT TO MASTURBATE WHILE HE GIVES YOU ORAL SEX, BUT LET HIM KNOW THERE WILL BE PENALTIES IF HE REACHES ORGASM BEFORE HE IS ORDERED TO.
THERE ARE MANY WAYS THIS FANTASY CAN PLAY OUT. YOU CAN TELL YOUR RECRUIT HE HAS PERMISSION TO HAVE AN ORGASM ONLY AFTER HE HAS GIVEN YOU ONE.
FIRE YOUR WEAPON NOW, SOLDIER!
OR YOU CAN DECIDE YOUR RECRUIT IS BADLY IN NEED OF A FULL WORKOUT.
THAT'S IT, SOLDIER! TAKE IT FOR YOUR COUNTRY!
WHATEVER ACTIVITIES YOU WANT YOUR BOOT CAMP TO CONSIST OF, MAKE SURE YOU KEEP YOUR COMMANDING TONE AND YOU CAN'T GO WRONG!
WELL DONE, RECRUIT. LET'S HIT THE SHOWERS AND I'LL SHOW YOU HOW MUCH FUN IT CAN BE TO DROP THE SOAP.
ENJOY . . .

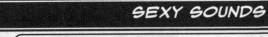

SEXY SOUNDS

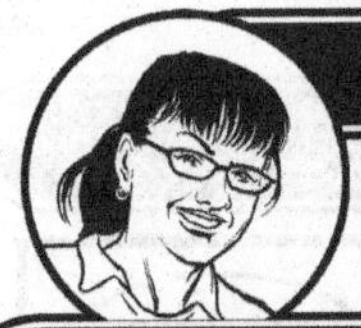

WHAT KINDS OF WORDS AROUSE YOU WHEN YOU HEAR THEM? RATE THE FOLLOWING WORDS ON A SCALE OF 1 TO 10, WITH 10 BEING SUPER-AROUSING AND 1 MEANING THAT IT KILLS THE MOOD. USE POST-IT NOTES IF YOU NEED MORE ROOM FOR YOUR OWN FAVORITES.

WORDS THAT DESCRIBE AROUSAL

- AROUSED
- HORNY
- WET
- RANDY
- TURNED ON
- HUNGRY
- EXCITED
- HARD
- ENGORGED
- THROBBING
- IN HEAT
- ACHING

MALE GENITALIA

- PENIS
- COCK
- DICK
- SHAFT
- MANHOOD
- HARD-ON
- ERECTION
- TOOL
- BONER

FEMALE GENITALIA

- VAGINA
- VULVA
- CLITORIS
- CLIT
- LABIA
- LIPS
- PUSSY
- CUNT
- SLIT
- SNATCH
- COOTER
- FUCKHOLE
- TWAT
- BEAVER

NIPPLES/BREASTS

- NIPPLES
- BREASTS
- TITS
- BOOBS
- JUGS
- KNOCKERS
- FUN BAGS

POSTERIOR

- ANUS
- ASS
- BACK DOOR
- BUM
- POOPER
- BUTT
- POOP CHUTE

SEX PLAY

- SEX
- MAKING LOVE
- INTERCOURSE
- FUCKING
- BONING
- DOING IT
- SCREWING
- MAKING WHOOPEE
- DOING THE NASTY

REACHING CLIMAX

- ORGASM
- CLIMAX
- CUM
- EJACULATE
- CREAM
- RELEASE
- JIZZ
- SPUNK
- BLOW WAD

CHAPTER 33

SLOPPY SECONDS

MANY PEOPLE ARE SEXUALLY AROUSED BY THE THOUGHT OF CATCHING THEIR PARTNER IN BED WITH ANOTHER PERSON. IN THIS SCENARIO, WE'LL SHOW YOU HOW TO SIMULATE AN AFFAIR FOR MAXIMUM FANTASY POTENTIAL WITH NONE OF THE REAL-WORLD RISKS.

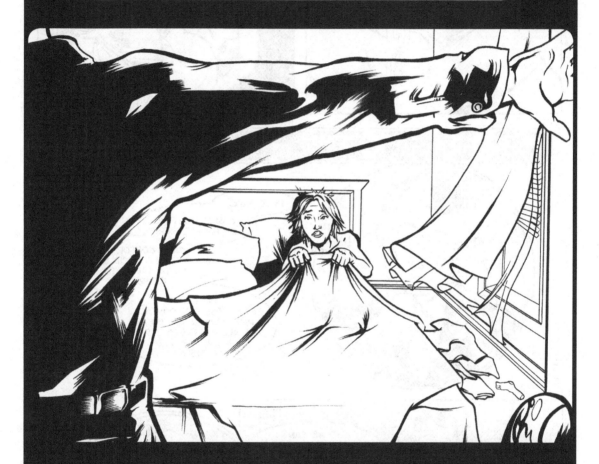

WHAT YOU'LL NEED . . .

LUBRICATION

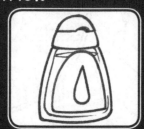

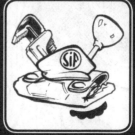

PROP CLOTHING

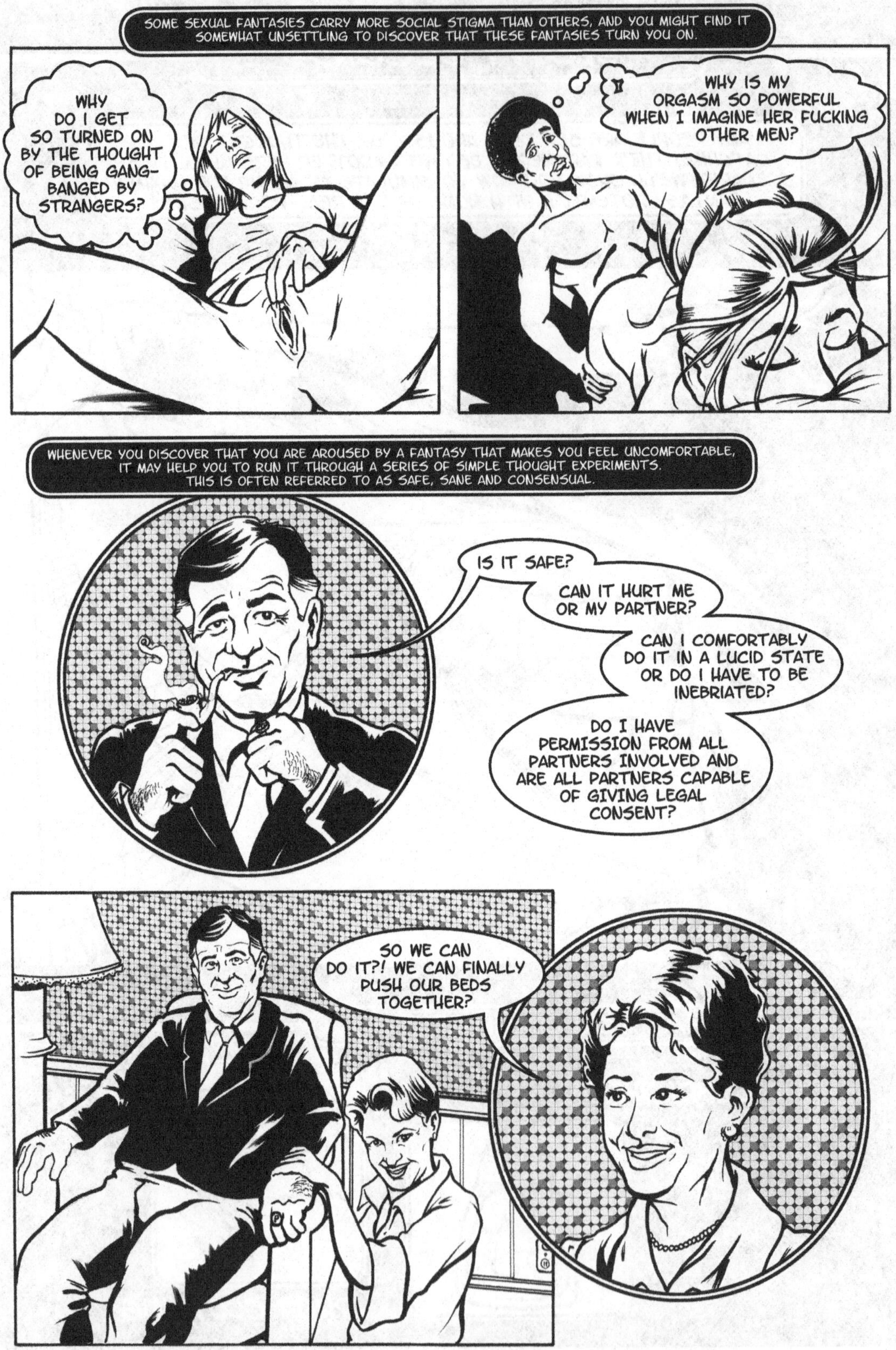
SOME SEXUAL FANTASIES CARRY MORE SOCIAL STIGMA THAN OTHERS, AND YOU MIGHT FIND IT SOMEWHAT UNSETTLING TO DISCOVER THAT THESE FANTASIES TURN YOU ON.
WHY DO I GET SO TURNED ON BY THE THOUGHT OF BEING GANG-BANGED BY STRANGERS?
WHY IS MY ORGASM SO POWERFUL WHEN I IMAGINE HER FUCKING OTHER MEN?
WHENEVER YOU DISCOVER THAT YOU ARE AROUSED BY A FANTASY THAT MAKES YOU FEEL UNCOMFORTABLE, IT MAY HELP YOU TO RUN IT THROUGH A SERIES OF SIMPLE THOUGHT EXPERIMENTS. THIS IS OFTEN REFERRED TO AS SAFE, SANE AND CONSENSUAL.
IS IT SAFE?
CAN IT HURT ME OR MY PARTNER?
CAN I COMFORTABLY DO IT IN A LUCID STATE OR DO I HAVE TO BE INEBRIATED?
DO I HAVE PERMISSION FROM ALL PARTNERS INVOLVED AND ARE ALL PARTNERS CAPABLE OF GIVING LEGAL CONSENT?
SO WE CAN DO IT?! WE CAN FINALLY PUSH OUR BEDS TOGETHER?

"CUCKOLD" OR "HOT-WIFE FANTASIES," AS THEY ARE OFTEN CALLED, ARE EXTREMELY COMMON FANTASIES FOR BOTH MEN AND WOMEN . . .

SOME COUPLES MIGHT ENJOY THE IDEA OF HAVING A NEW PERSON JOIN THEM IN THE FUN.

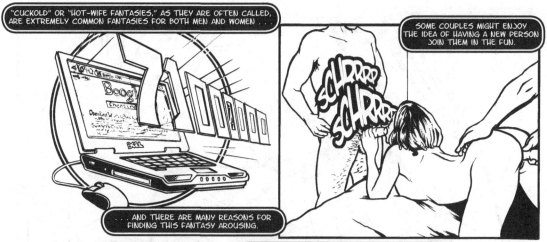

. . . AND THERE ARE MANY REASONS FOR FINDING THIS FANTASY AROUSING.

FOR SOME, THIS FANTASY MIGHT EXCITE BISEXUAL DESIRES.

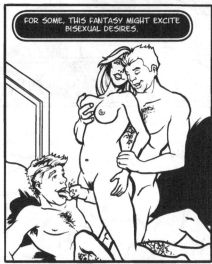

OTHERS MAY BE EXCITED BY THE CONCEPT OF HUMILIATION THAT A COMPETITOR MAY BRING.

OH! HIS COCK IS SO MUCH BIGGER THAN YOURS. WATCH HIM FUCK ME! WATCH HIM MAKE ME CUM!

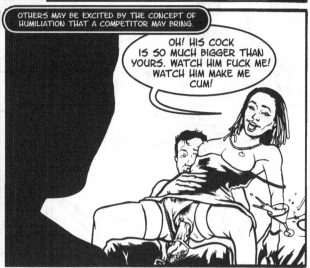

OTHER COUPLES MAY ENJOY THE IDEA OF EXHIBITIONISM AND VOYEURISM.

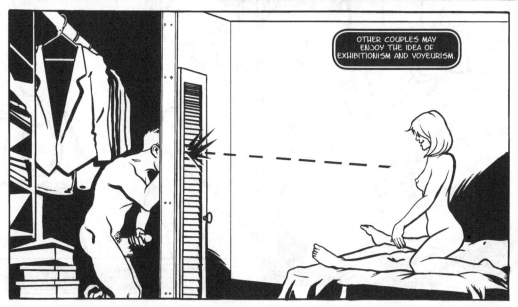

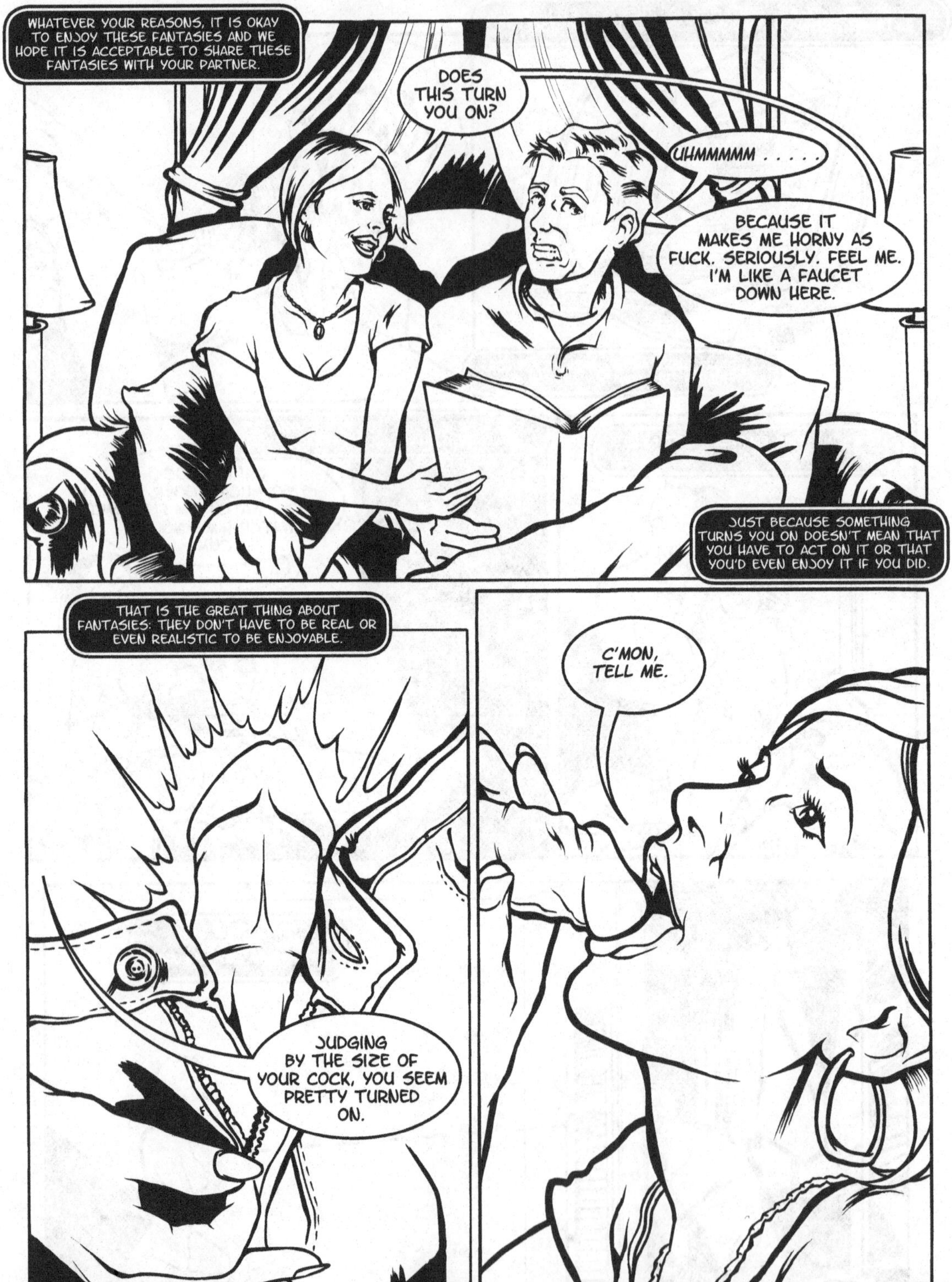
WHATEVER YOUR REASONS, IT IS OKAY TO ENJOY THESE FANTASIES AND WE HOPE IT IS ACCEPTABLE TO SHARE THESE FANTASIES WITH YOUR PARTNER.
DOES THIS TURN YOU ON?
UHMMMMM . . . . .
BECAUSE IT MAKES ME HORNY AS FUCK. SERIOUSLY. FEEL ME. I'M LIKE A FAUCET DOWN HERE.
JUST BECAUSE SOMETHING TURNS YOU ON DOESN'T MEAN THAT YOU HAVE TO ACT ON IT OR THAT YOU'D EVEN ENJOY IT IF YOU DID.
THAT IS THE GREAT THING ABOUT FANTASIES: THEY DON'T HAVE TO BE REAL OR EVEN REALISTIC TO BE ENJOYABLE.
JUDGING BY THE SIZE OF YOUR COCK, YOU SEEM PRETTY TURNED ON.
C'MON, TELL ME.
IN THE FOLLOWING PAGES, WE'LL SHOW YOU HOW TO SIMULATE THE VERY COMMON FANTASY OF CHEATING.

FIRST YOU ARE GOING TO NEED SOME SUPPLIES. GO TO A USED-CLOTHING STORE AND GET A PAIR OF OVERALLS OR OTHER GARMENT THAT A MAN WHO MAY NEED TO VISIT YOUR HOME FOR MAINTENANCE PURPOSES MAY WEAR. THEN GET A BELIEVABLE PROP, LIKE A WRENCH OR OLD-FASHIONED BOTTLE OF MILK IF YOU WANT TO GO FOR THE ULTIMATE ARCHETYPAL MILKMAN FANTASY.

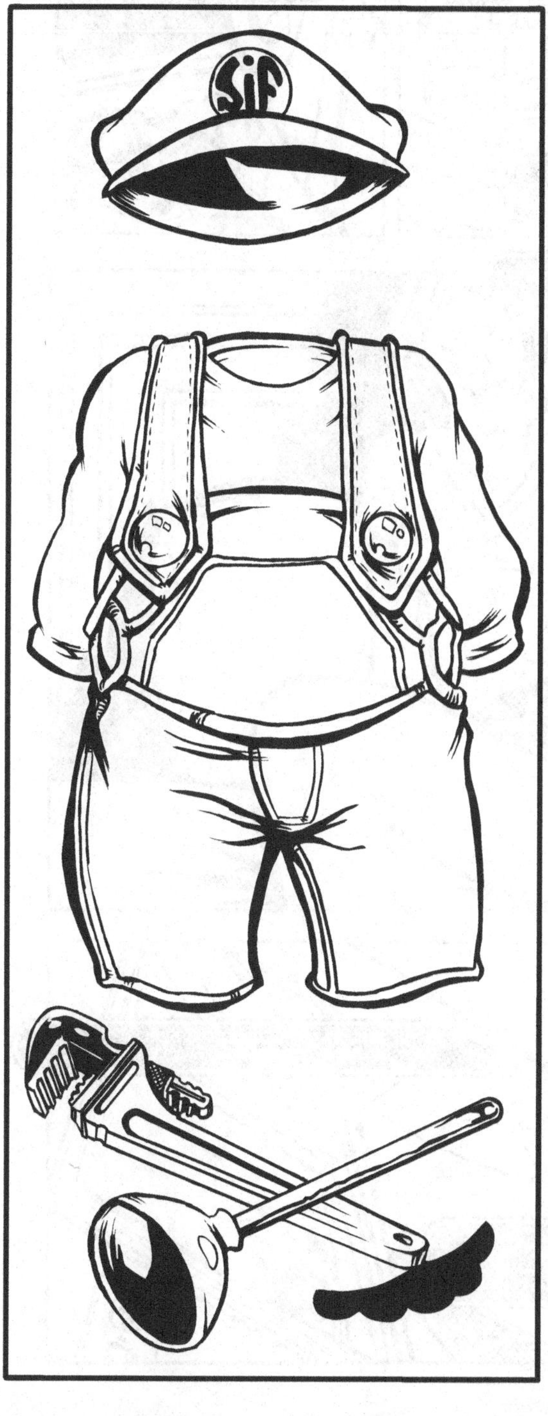
SIF

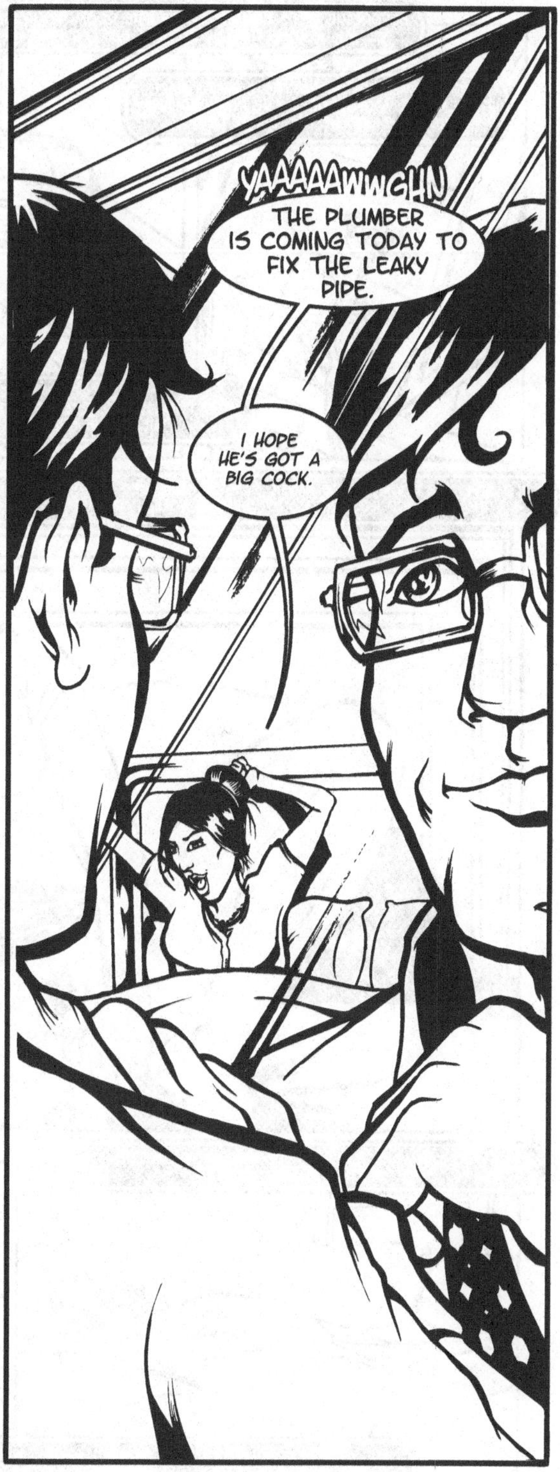
YAAAAAWWGHN
THE PLUMBER IS COMING TODAY TO FIX THE LEAKY PIPE.
I HOPE HE'S GOT A BIG COCK.

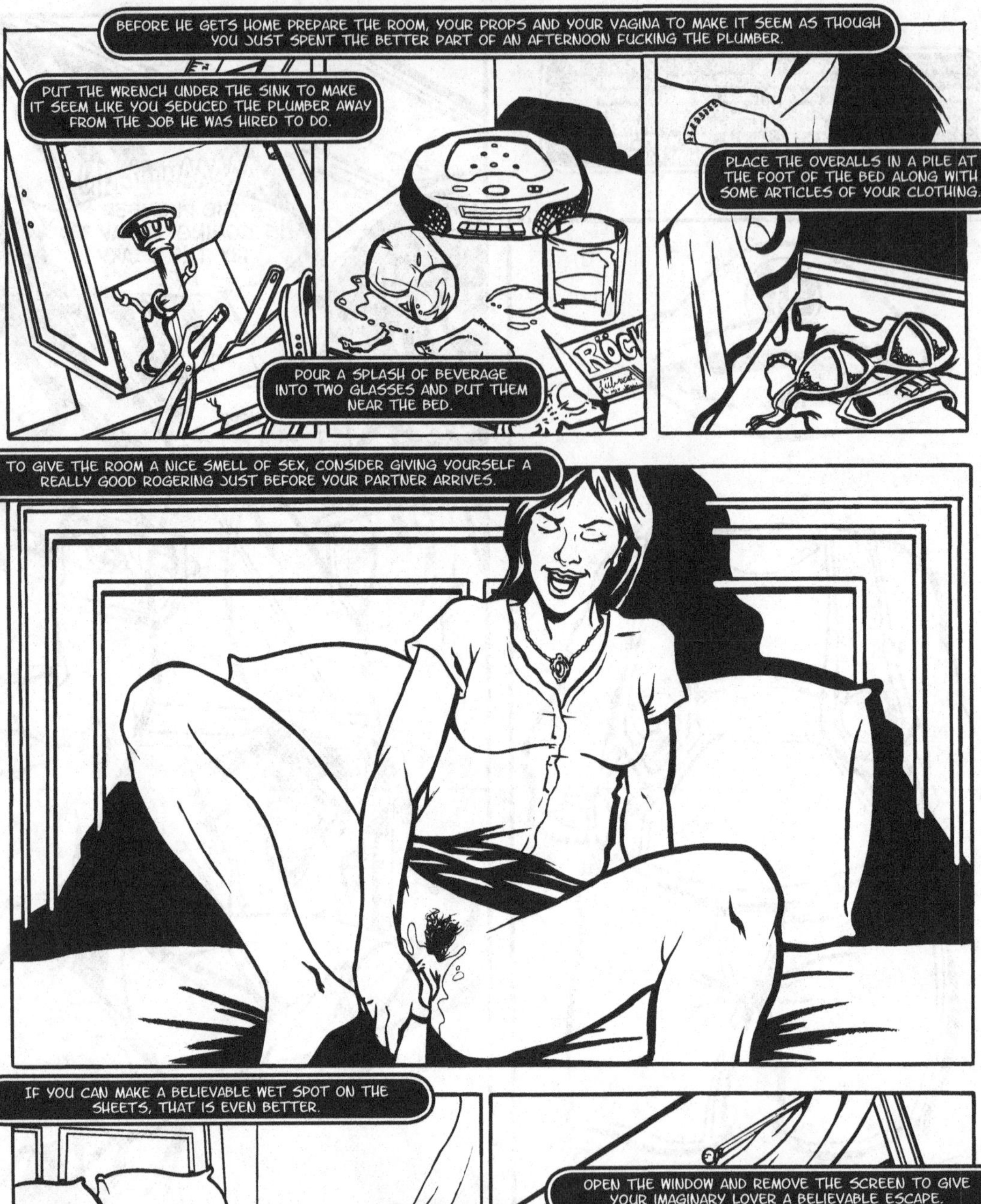
BEFORE HE GETS HOME PREPARE THE ROOM, YOUR PROPS AND YOUR VAGINA TO MAKE IT SEEM AS THOUGH YOU JUST SPENT THE BETTER PART OF AN AFTERNOON FUCKING THE PLUMBER.
PUT THE WRENCH UNDER THE SINK TO MAKE IT SEEM LIKE YOU SEDUCED THE PLUMBER AWAY FROM THE JOB HE WAS HIRED TO DO.
POUR A SPLASH OF BEVERAGE INTO TWO GLASSES AND PUT THEM NEAR THE BED.
PLACE THE OVERALLS IN A PILE AT THE FOOT OF THE BED ALONG WITH SOME ARTICLES OF YOUR CLOTHING.
TO GIVE THE ROOM A NICE SMELL OF SEX, CONSIDER GIVING YOURSELF A REALLY GOOD ROGERING JUST BEFORE YOUR PARTNER ARRIVES.
IF YOU CAN MAKE A BELIEVABLE WET SPOT ON THE SHEETS, THAT IS EVEN BETTER.
IF YOUR BEDROOM IS ON THE SECOND STORY, WHERE JUMPING OUT THE WINDOW IS NOT AS BELIEVABLE, JUST PRETEND THAT YOUR LOVER LEFT JUST BEFORE YOUR PARTNER GOT HOME. REMEMBER! FANTASY IS ALL ABOUT THE SUSPENSION OF DISBELIEF.
OPEN THE WINDOW AND REMOVE THE SCREEN TO GIVE YOUR IMAGINARY LOVER A BELIEVABLE ESCAPE.

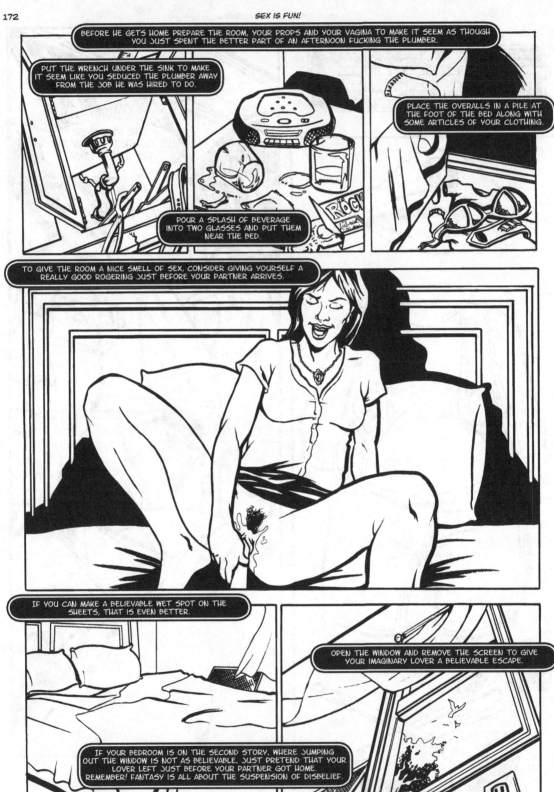

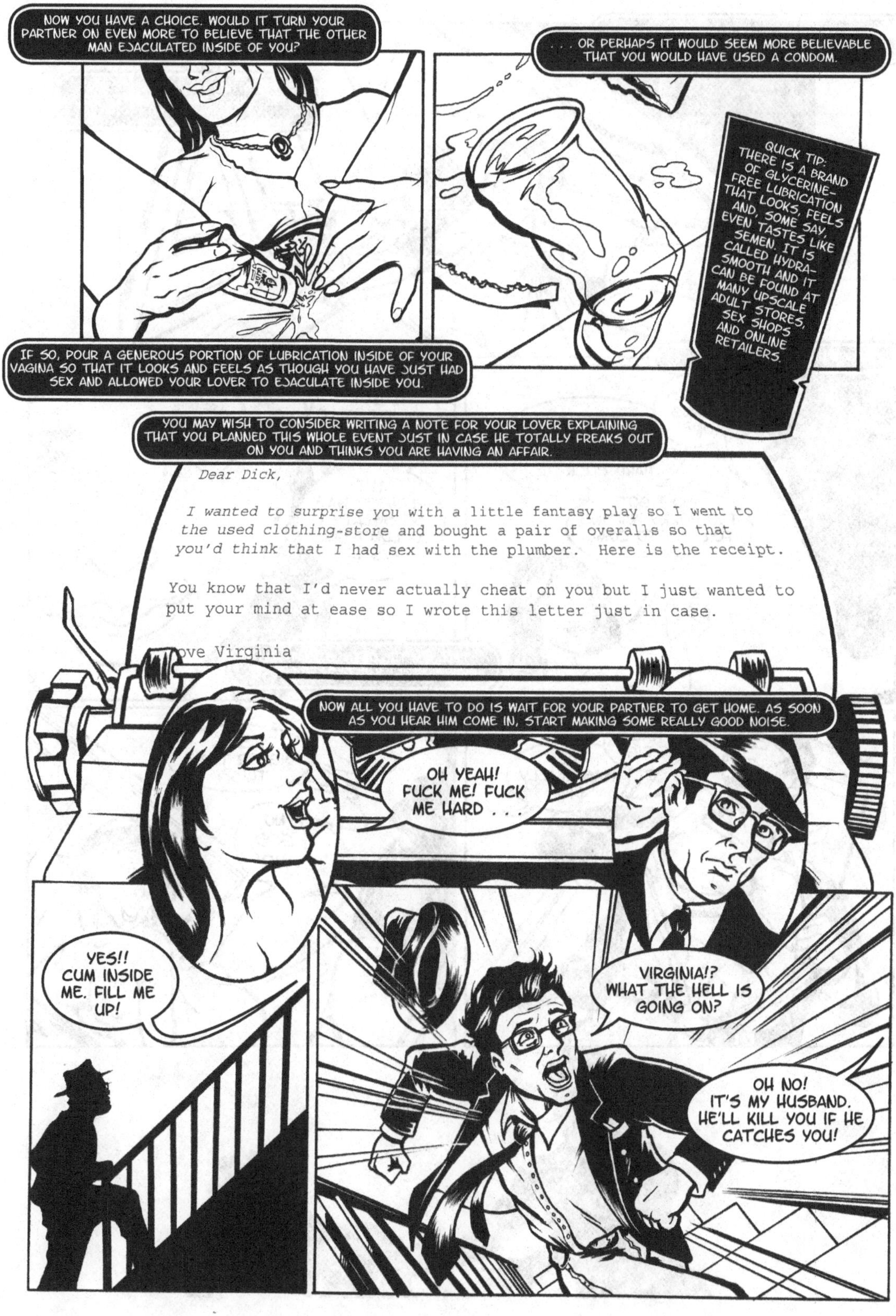

NOW YOU HAVE A CHOICE. WOULD IT TURN YOUR PARTNER ON EVEN MORE TO BELIEVE THAT THE OTHER MAN EJACULATED INSIDE OF YOU?
IF SO, POUR A GENEROUS PORTION OF LUBRICATION INSIDE OF YOUR VAGINA SO THAT IT LOOKS AND FEELS AS THOUGH YOU HAVE JUST HAD SEX AND ALLOWED YOUR LOVER TO EJACULATE INSIDE YOU.
. . . OR PERHAPS IT WOULD SEEM MORE BELIEVABLE THAT YOU WOULD HAVE USED A CONDOM.
QUICK TIP: THERE IS A BRAND OF GLYCERINE-FREE LUBRICATION THAT LOOKS, FEELS AND, SOME SAY, EVEN TASTES LIKE SEMEN. IT IS CALLED HYDRA-SMOOTH AND IT CAN BE FOUND AT MANY UPSCALE ADULT STORES, SEX SHOPS AND ONLINE RETAILERS.
YOU MAY WISH TO CONSIDER WRITING A NOTE FOR YOUR LOVER EXPLAINING THAT YOU PLANNED THIS WHOLE EVENT JUST IN CASE HE TOTALLY FREAKS OUT ON YOU AND THINKS YOU ARE HAVING AN AFFAIR.
Dear Dick,
I wanted to surprise you with a little fantasy play so I went to the used clothing-store and bought a pair of overalls so that you'd think that I had sex with the plumber. Here is the receipt.
You know that I'd never actually cheat on you but I just wanted to put your mind at ease so I wrote this letter just in case.
ove Virginia
NOW ALL YOU HAVE TO DO IS WAIT FOR YOUR PARTNER TO GET HOME. AS SOON AS YOU HEAR HIM COME IN, START MAKING SOME REALLY GOOD NOISE.
OH YEAH! FUCK ME! FUCK ME HARD . . .
YES!! CUM INSIDE ME. FILL ME UP!
VIRGINIA!? WHAT THE HELL IS GOING ON?
OH NO! IT'S MY HUSBAND. HE'LL KILL YOU IF HE CATCHES YOU!

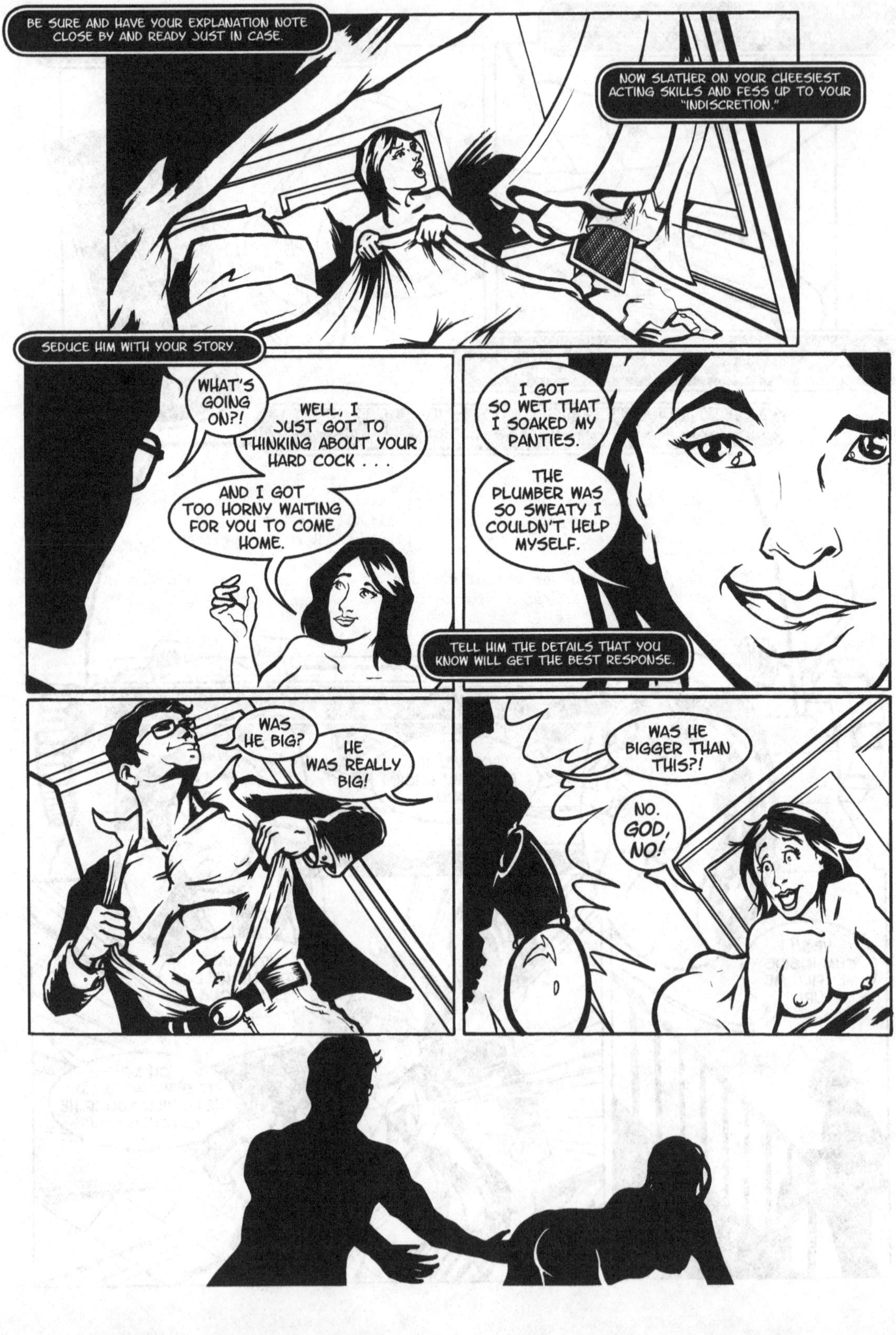
BE SURE AND HAVE YOUR EXPLANATION NOTE CLOSE BY AND READY JUST IN CASE.
NOW SLATHER ON YOUR CHEESIEST ACTING SKILLS AND FESS UP TO YOUR "INDISCRETION."
SEDUCE HIM WITH YOUR STORY.
WHAT'S GOING ON?!
WELL, I JUST GOT TO THINKING ABOUT YOUR HARD COCK . . .
AND I GOT TOO HORNY WAITING FOR YOU TO COME HOME.
I GOT SO WET THAT I SOAKED MY PANTIES.
THE PLUMBER WAS SO SWEATY I COULDN'T HELP MYSELF.
TELL HIM THE DETAILS THAT YOU KNOW WILL GET THE BEST RESPONSE.
WAS HE BIG?
HE WAS REALLY BIG!
WAS HE BIGGER THAN THIS?!
NO. GOD, NO!

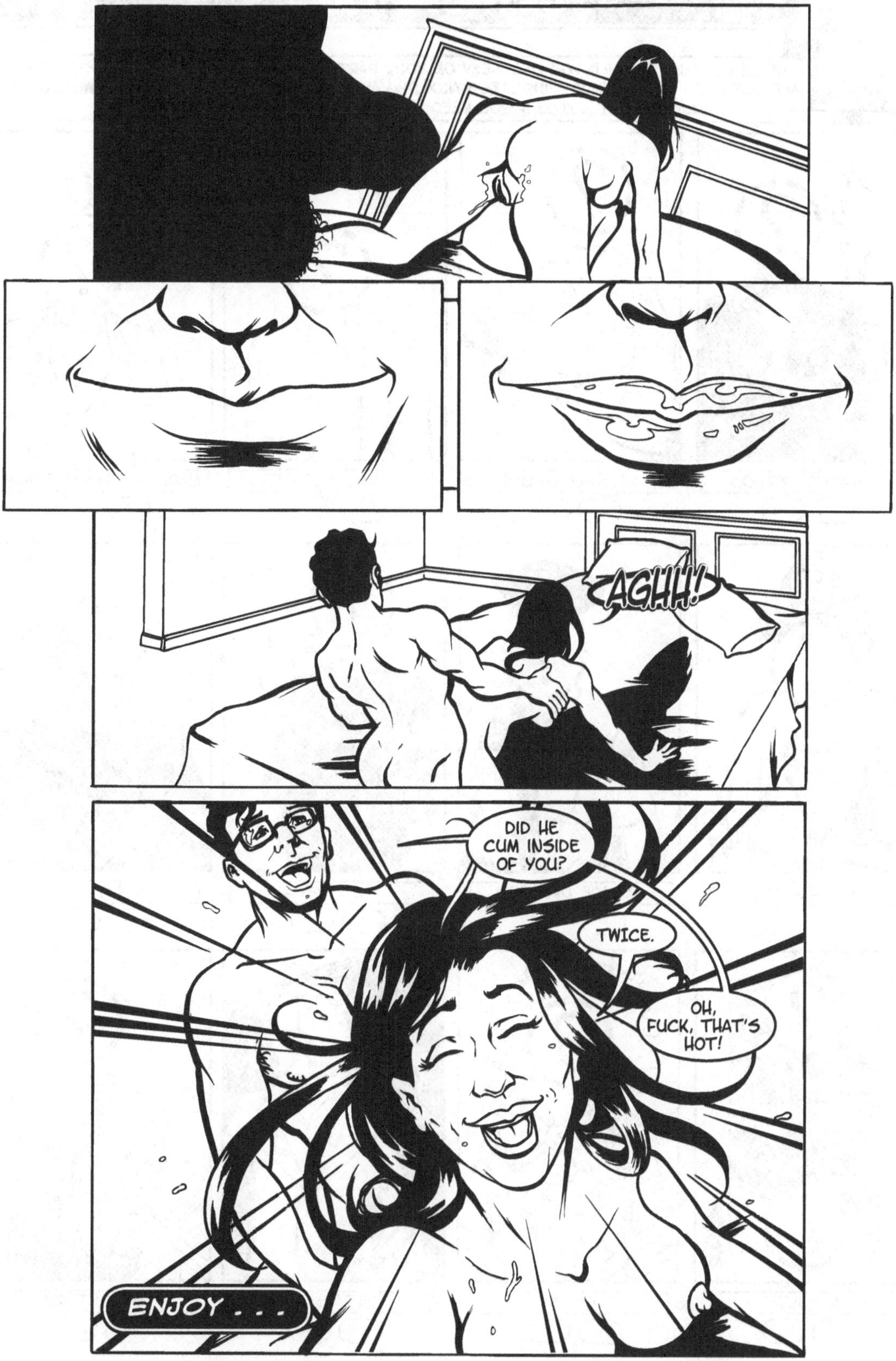
AGHH!
DID HE CUM INSIDE OF YOU?
TWICE.
OH, FUCK, THAT'S HOT!
ENJOY . . .

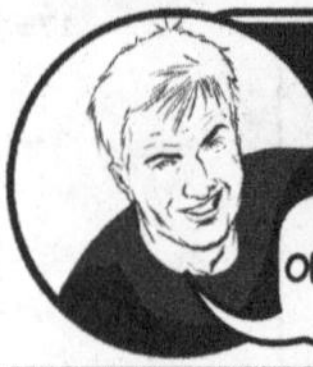

SEXY COSTUMES

WHICH COSTUMES WOULD YOU FIND SEXY ON YOUR PARTNER? RATE THE FOLLOWING COSTUMES ON A SCALE OF 1 TO 10, WITH 10 BEING SUPER-AROUSING AND 1 MEANING THAT YOU COULD LIVE WITHOUT IT. USE POST-IT NOTES IF YOU NEED MORE ROOM FOR YOUR OWN FAVORITES.

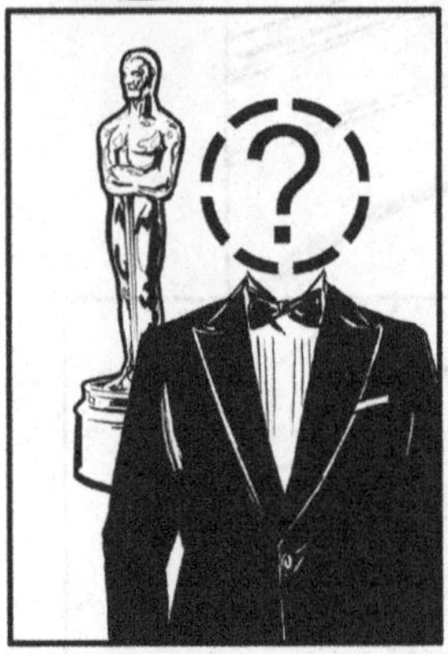

FAMOUS PERSON

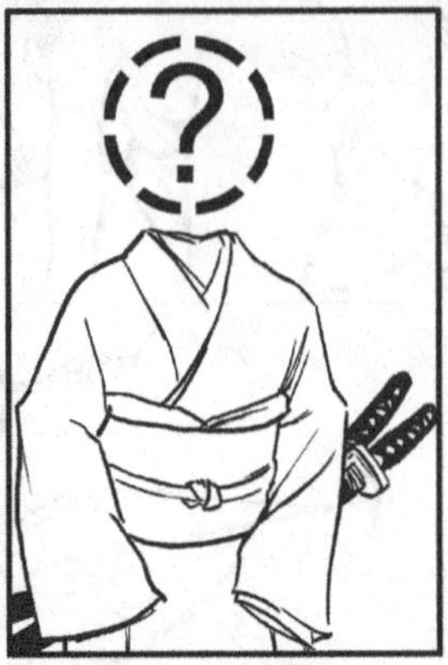

GEISHA/SAMURAI

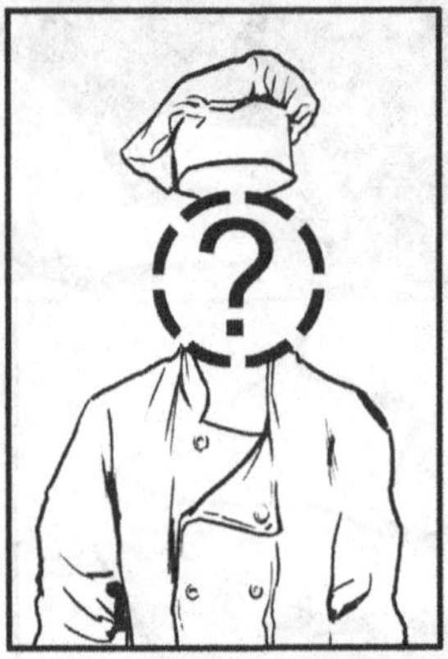

CHEF/SERVER

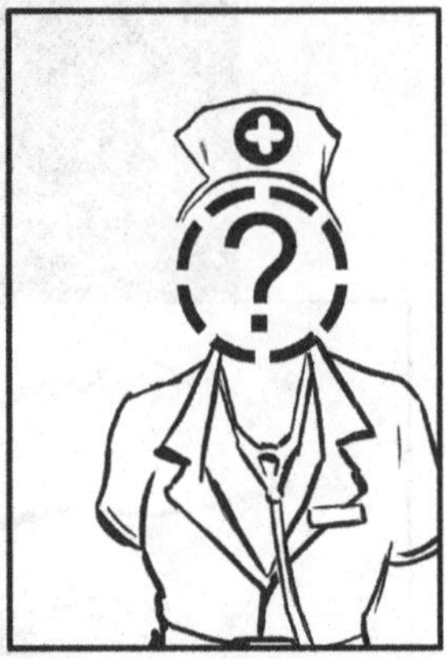

MEDICAL PROFESSIONAL

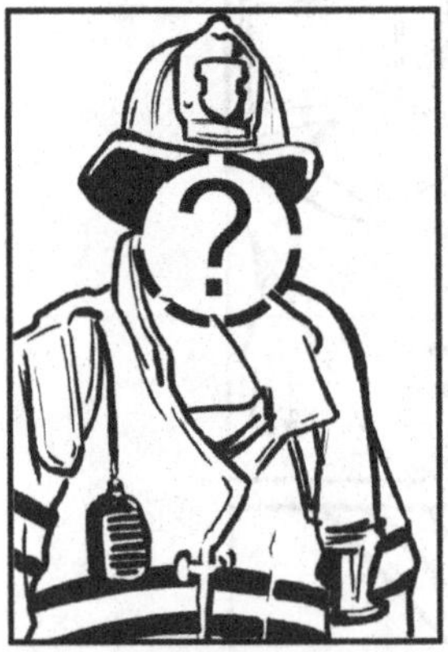

FIREFIGHTER

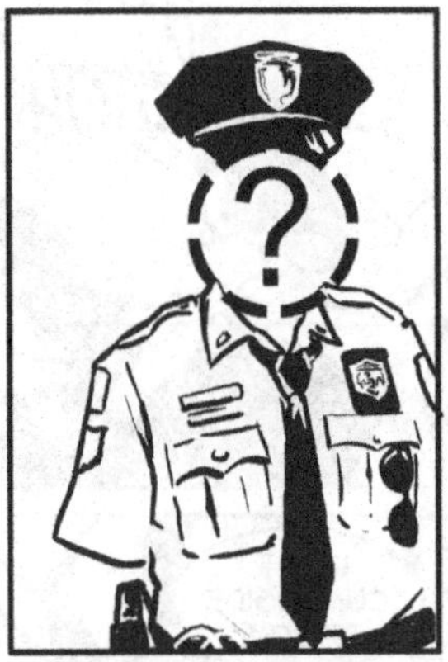

POLICE OFFICER

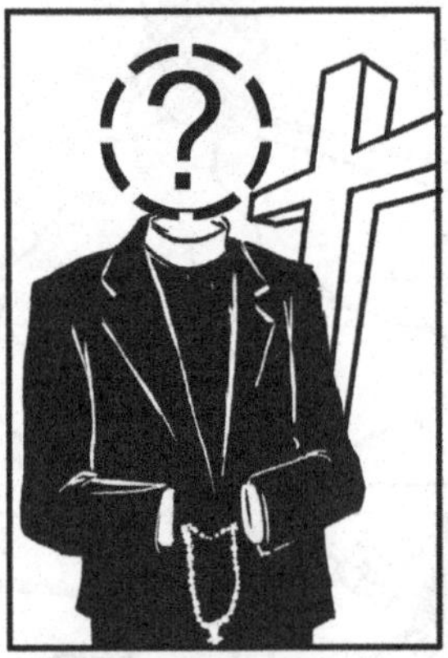

CLERGY

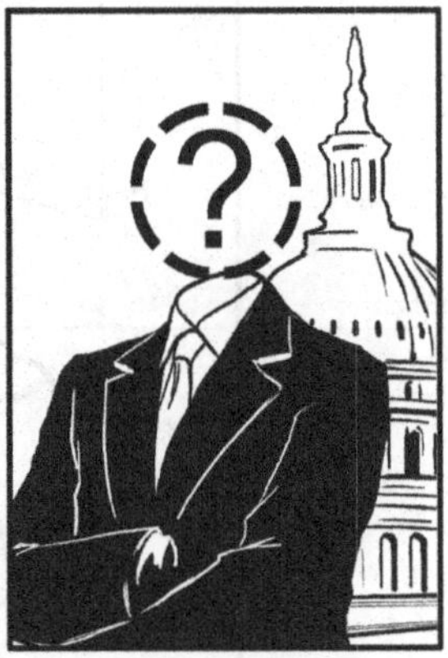

POLITICIAN

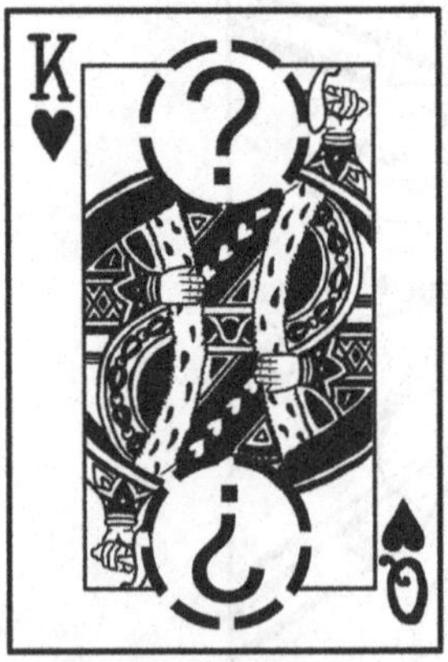

ROYALTY

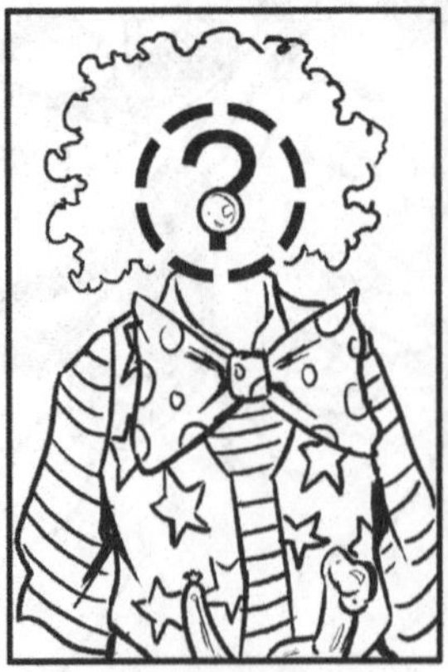

CLOWN

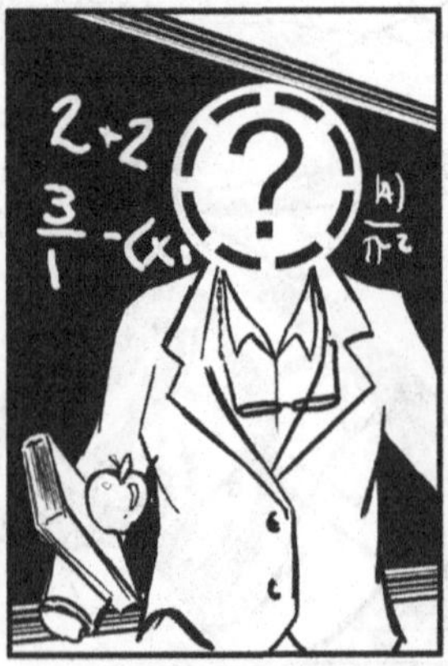
2+2

TEACHER

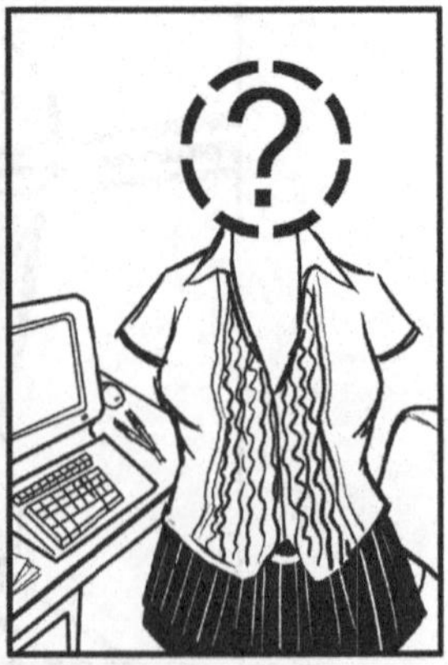

SECRETARY

CHAPTER 34

CAPTURED BY A SUPERVILLAIN

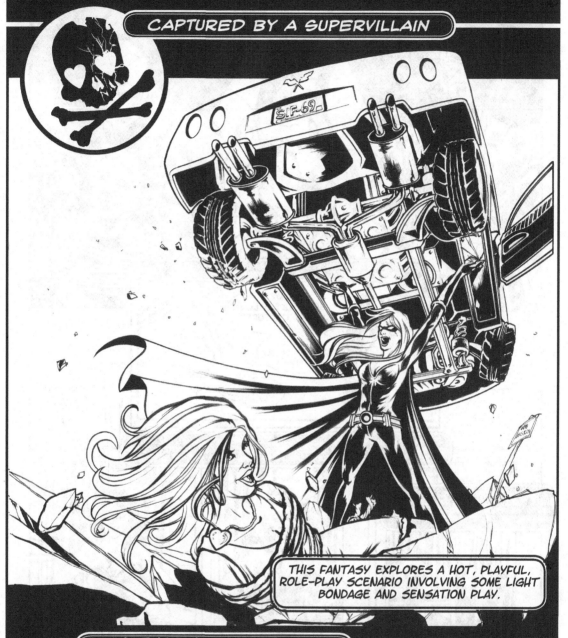

THIS FANTASY EXPLORES A HOT, PLAYFUL, ROLE-PLAY SCENARIO INVOLVING SOME LIGHT BONDAGE AND SENSATION PLAY.

WHAT YOU'LL NEED . . .

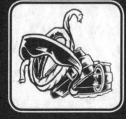

COMFORTABLE RESTRAINTS OR ROPE AND A BLINDFOLD

SUPERVILLAIN COSTUME

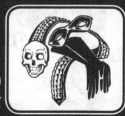

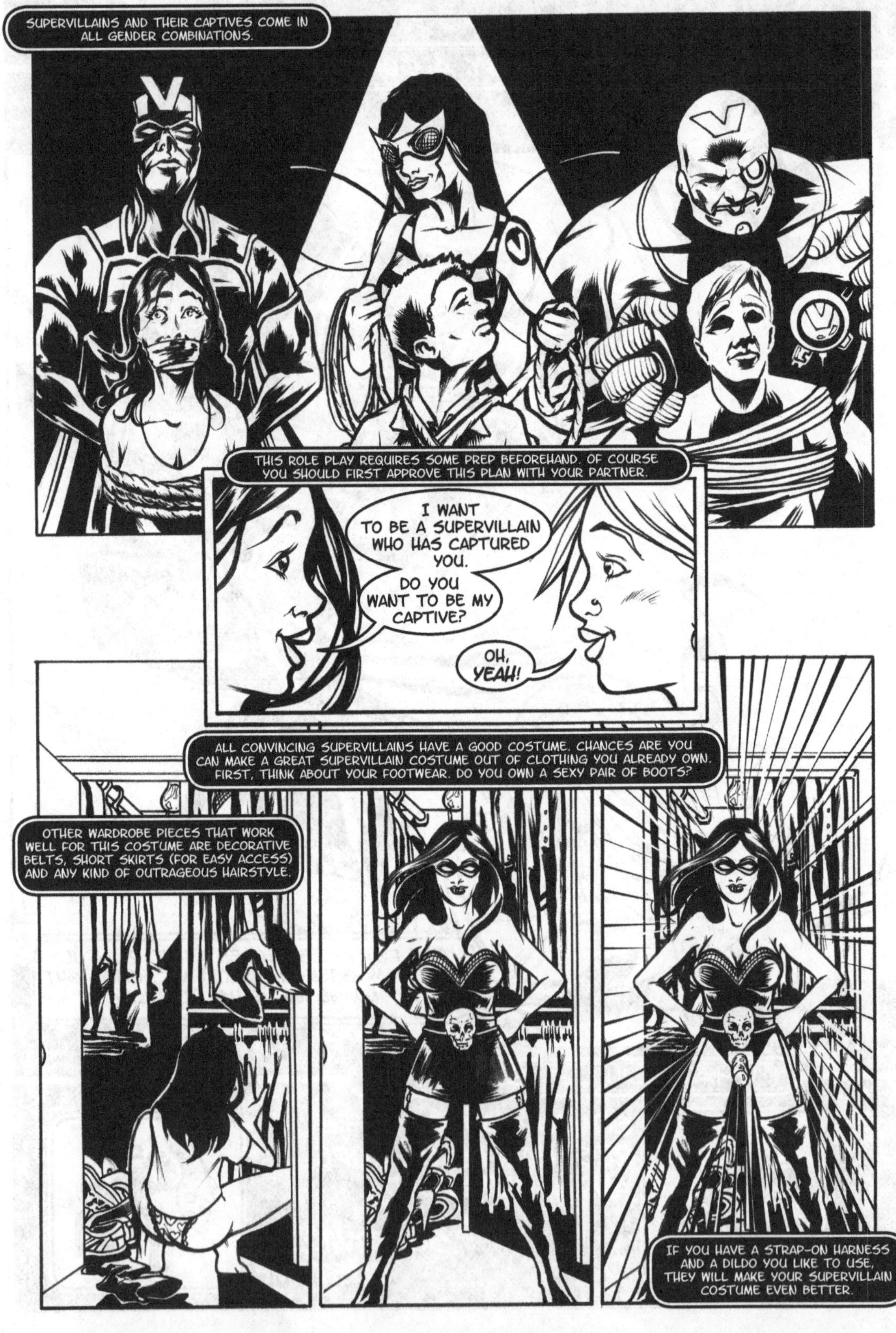
SUPERVILLAINS AND THEIR CAPTIVES COME IN ALL GENDER COMBINATIONS.
THIS ROLE PLAY REQUIRES SOME PREP BEFOREHAND. OF COURSE YOU SHOULD FIRST APPROVE THIS PLAN WITH YOUR PARTNER.
I WANT TO BE A SUPERVILLAIN WHO HAS CAPTURED YOU.
DO YOU WANT TO BE MY CAPTIVE?
OH, YEAH!
ALL CONVINCING SUPERVILLAINS HAVE A GOOD COSTUME. CHANCES ARE YOU CAN MAKE A GREAT SUPERVILLAIN COSTUME OUT OF CLOTHING YOU ALREADY OWN. FIRST, THINK ABOUT YOUR FOOTWEAR. DO YOU OWN A SEXY PAIR OF BOOTS?
OTHER WARDROBE PIECES THAT WORK WELL FOR THIS COSTUME ARE DECORATIVE BELTS, SHORT SKIRTS (FOR EASY ACCESS) AND ANY KIND OF OUTRAGEOUS HAIRSTYLE.
IF YOU HAVE A STRAP-ON HARNESS AND A DILDO YOU LIKE TO USE, THEY WILL MAKE YOUR SUPERVILLAIN COSTUME EVEN BETTER.

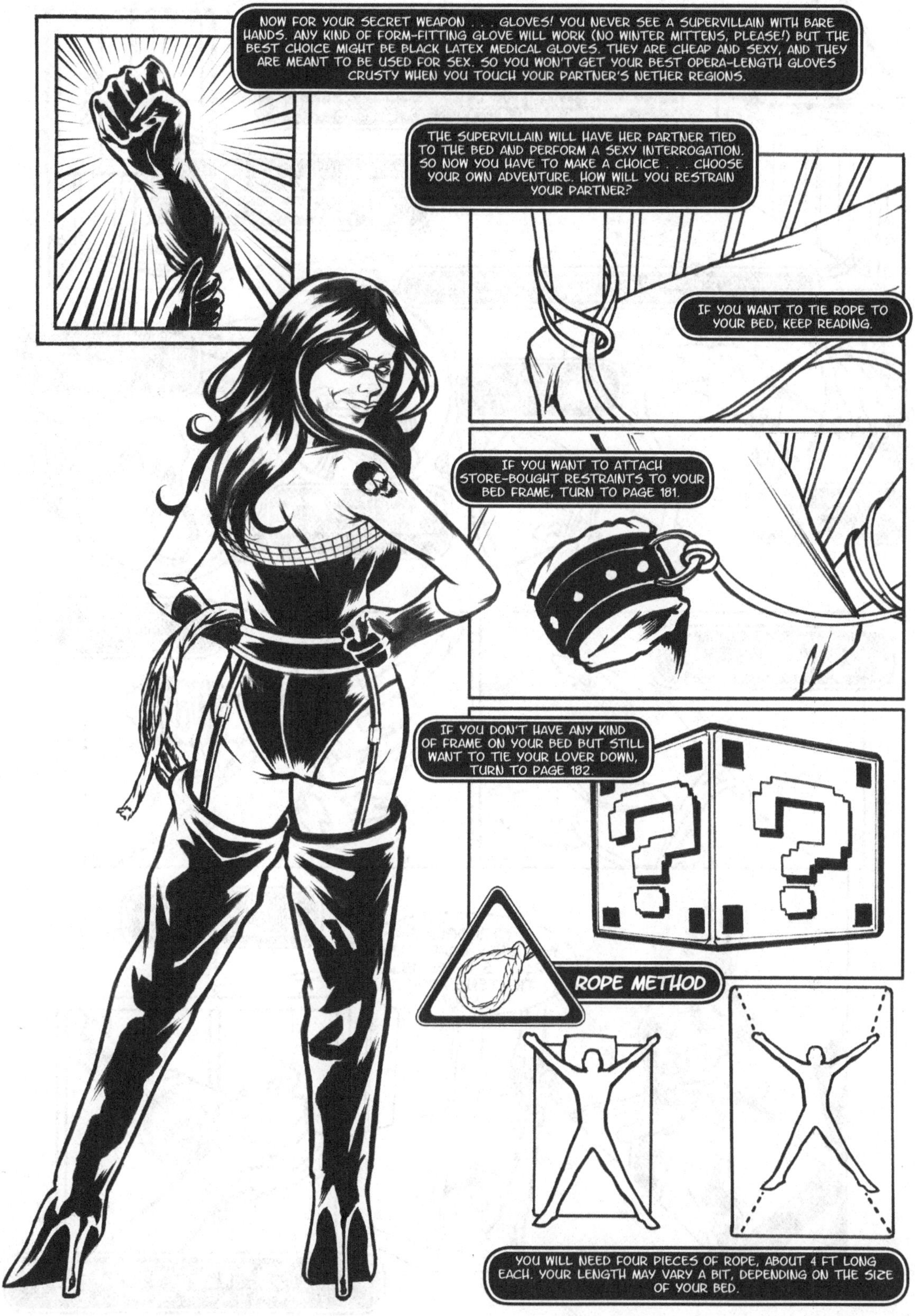
NOW FOR YOUR SECRET WEAPON . . . GLOVES! YOU NEVER SEE A SUPERVILLAIN WITH BARE HANDS. ANY KIND OF FORM-FITTING GLOVE WILL WORK (NO WINTER MITTENS, PLEASE!) BUT THE BEST CHOICE MIGHT BE BLACK LATEX MEDICAL GLOVES. THEY ARE CHEAP AND SEXY, AND THEY ARE MEANT TO BE USED FOR SEX. SO YOU WON'T GET YOUR BEST OPERA-LENGTH GLOVES CRUSTY WHEN YOU TOUCH YOUR PARTNER'S NETHER REGIONS.
THE SUPERVILLAIN WILL HAVE HER PARTNER TIED TO THE BED AND PERFORM A SEXY INTERROGATION. SO NOW YOU HAVE TO MAKE A CHOICE . . . CHOOSE YOUR OWN ADVENTURE. HOW WILL YOU RESTRAIN YOUR PARTNER?
IF YOU WANT TO TIE ROPE TO YOUR BED, KEEP READING.
IF YOU WANT TO ATTACH STORE-BOUGHT RESTRAINTS TO YOUR BED FRAME, TURN TO PAGE 181.
IF YOU DON'T HAVE ANY KIND OF FRAME ON YOUR BED BUT STILL WANT TO TIE YOUR LOVER DOWN, TURN TO PAGE 182.
ROPE METHOD
YOU WILL NEED FOUR PIECES OF ROPE, ABOUT 4 FT LONG EACH. YOUR LENGTH MAY VARY A BIT, DEPENDING ON THE SIZE OF YOUR BED.

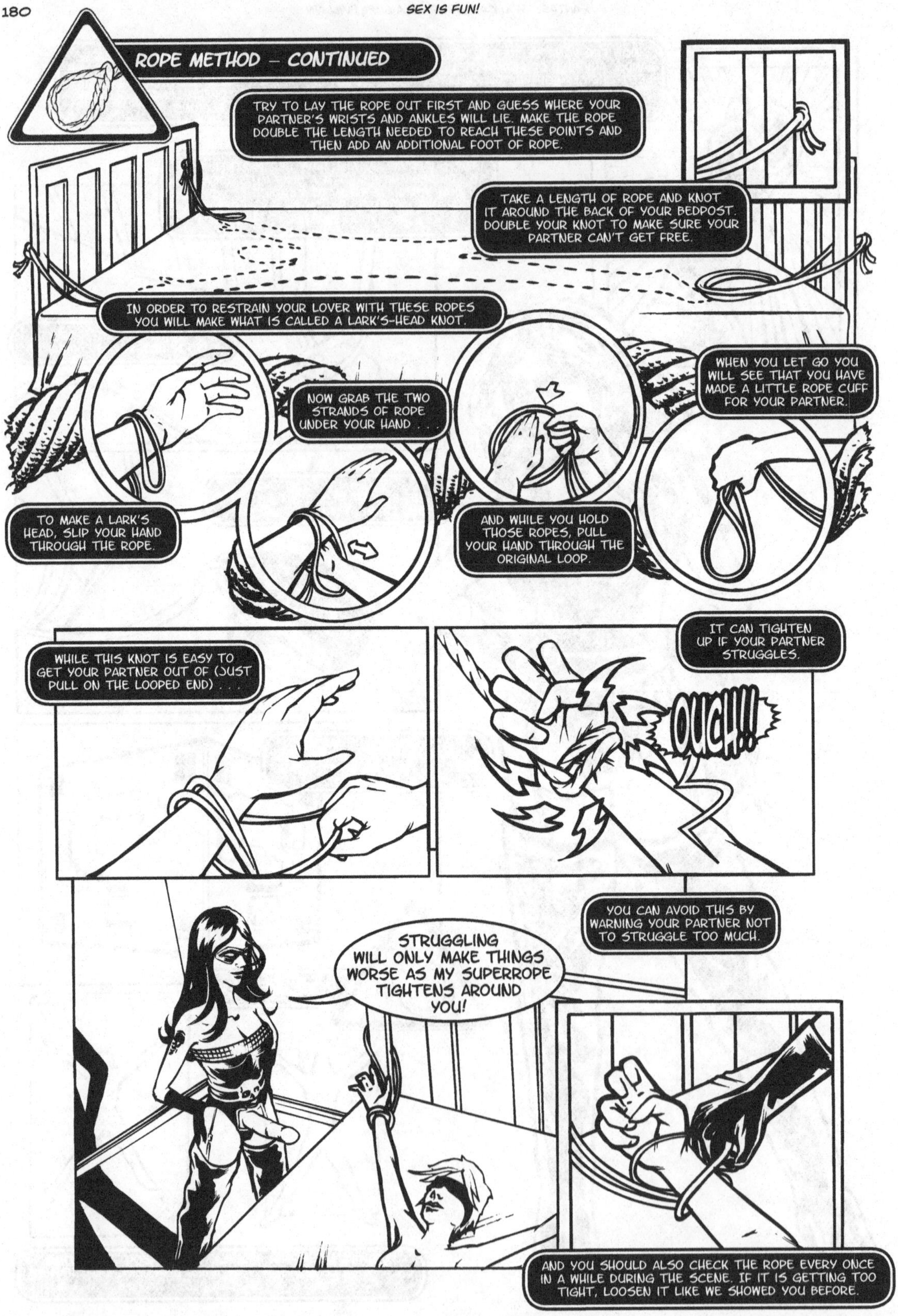
ROPE METHOD – CONTINUED
TRY TO LAY THE ROPE OUT FIRST AND GUESS WHERE YOUR PARTNER'S WRISTS AND ANKLES WILL LIE. MAKE THE ROPE DOUBLE THE LENGTH NEEDED TO REACH THESE POINTS AND THEN ADD AN ADDITIONAL FOOT OF ROPE.
TAKE A LENGTH OF ROPE AND KNOT IT AROUND THE BACK OF YOUR BEDPOST. DOUBLE YOUR KNOT TO MAKE SURE YOUR PARTNER CAN'T GET FREE.
IN ORDER TO RESTRAIN YOUR LOVER WITH THESE ROPES YOU WILL MAKE WHAT IS CALLED A LARK'S-HEAD KNOT.
TO MAKE A LARK'S HEAD, SLIP YOUR HAND THROUGH THE ROPE.
NOW GRAB THE TWO STRANDS OF ROPE UNDER YOUR HAND . . .
AND WHILE YOU HOLD THOSE ROPES, PULL YOUR HAND THROUGH THE ORIGINAL LOOP.
WHEN YOU LET GO YOU WILL SEE THAT YOU HAVE MADE A LITTLE ROPE CUFF FOR YOUR PARTNER.
WHILE THIS KNOT IS EASY TO GET YOUR PARTNER OUT OF (JUST PULL ON THE LOOPED END) . . .
IT CAN TIGHTEN UP IF YOUR PARTNER STRUGGLES.
OUCH!!
YOU CAN AVOID THIS BY WARNING YOUR PARTNER NOT TO STRUGGLE TOO MUCH.
STRUGGLING WILL ONLY MAKE THINGS WORSE AS MY SUPERROPE TIGHTENS AROUND YOU!
AND YOU SHOULD ALSO CHECK THE ROPE EVERY ONCE IN A WHILE DURING THE SCENE. IF IT IS GETTING TOO TIGHT, LOOSEN IT LIKE WE SHOWED YOU BEFORE.

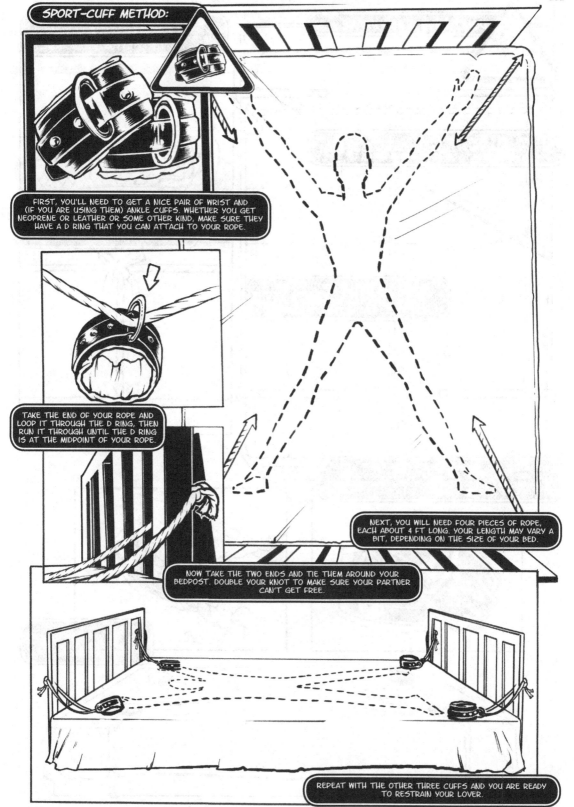

SPORT-CUFF METHOD:

FIRST, YOU'LL NEED TO GET A NICE PAIR OF WRIST AND (IF YOU ARE USING THEM) ANKLE CUFFS. WHETHER YOU GET NEOPRENE OR LEATHER OR SOME OTHER KIND, MAKE SURE THEY HAVE A D RING THAT YOU CAN ATTACH TO YOUR ROPE.

TAKE THE END OF YOUR ROPE AND LOOP IT THROUGH THE D RING, THEN RUN IT THROUGH UNTIL THE D RING IS AT THE MIDPOINT OF YOUR ROPE.

NEXT, YOU WILL NEED FOUR PIECES OF ROPE, EACH ABOUT 4 FT LONG. YOUR LENGTH MAY VARY A BIT, DEPENDING ON THE SIZE OF YOUR BED.

NOW TAKE THE TWO ENDS AND TIE THEM AROUND YOUR BEDPOST. DOUBLE YOUR KNOT TO MAKE SURE YOUR PARTNER CAN'T GET FREE.

REPEAT WITH THE OTHER THREE CUFFS AND YOU ARE READY TO RESTRAIN YOUR LOVER.

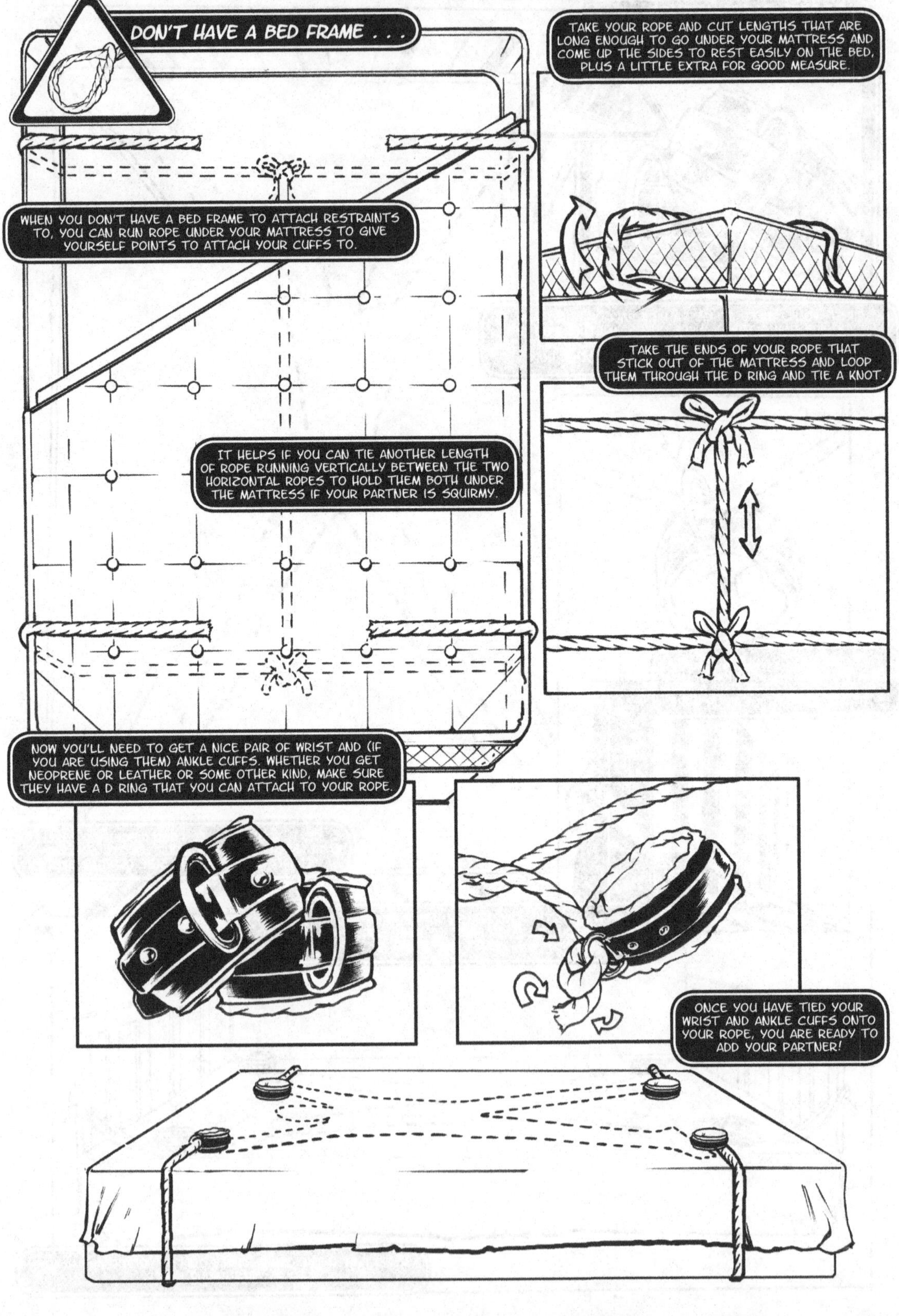
DON'T HAVE A BED FRAME . . .
WHEN YOU DON'T HAVE A BED FRAME TO ATTACH RESTRAINTS TO, YOU CAN RUN ROPE UNDER YOUR MATTRESS TO GIVE YOURSELF POINTS TO ATTACH YOUR CUFFS TO.
IT HELPS IF YOU CAN TIE ANOTHER LENGTH OF ROPE RUNNING VERTICALLY BETWEEN THE TWO HORIZONTAL ROPES TO HOLD THEM BOTH UNDER THE MATTRESS IF YOUR PARTNER IS SQUIRMY.
TAKE YOUR ROPE AND CUT LENGTHS THAT ARE LONG ENOUGH TO GO UNDER YOUR MATTRESS AND COME UP THE SIDES TO REST EASILY ON THE BED, PLUS A LITTLE EXTRA FOR GOOD MEASURE.
TAKE THE ENDS OF YOUR ROPE THAT STICK OUT OF THE MATTRESS AND LOOP THEM THROUGH THE D RING AND TIE A KNOT.
NOW YOU'LL NEED TO GET A NICE PAIR OF WRIST AND (IF YOU ARE USING THEM) ANKLE CUFFS. WHETHER YOU GET NEOPRENE OR LEATHER OR SOME OTHER KIND, MAKE SURE THEY HAVE A D RING THAT YOU CAN ATTACH TO YOUR ROPE.
ONCE YOU HAVE TIED YOUR WRIST AND ANKLE CUFFS ONTO YOUR ROPE, YOU ARE READY TO ADD YOUR PARTNER!

THE PLOT THICKENS . . .

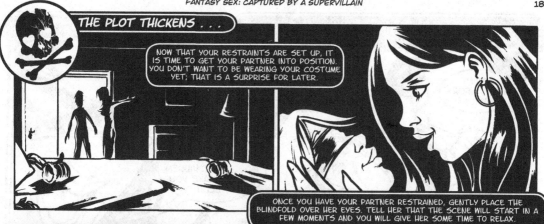

NOW THAT YOUR RESTRAINTS ARE SET UP, IT IS TIME TO GET YOUR PARTNER INTO POSITION. YOU DON'T WANT TO BE WEARING YOUR COSTUME YET; THAT IS A SURPRISE FOR LATER.

ONCE YOU HAVE YOUR PARTNER RESTRAINED, GENTLY PLACE THE BLINDFOLD OVER HER EYES. TELL HER THAT THE SCENE WILL START IN A FEW MOMENTS AND YOU WILL GIVE HER SOME TIME TO RELAX.

TAKE THESE FEW MOMENTS TO CHANGE INTO YOUR SUPERVILLAIN COSTUME. DO THIS IN THE SAME ROOM, SINCE YOU DON'T WANT TO LEAVE YOUR PARTNER TIED UP AND ALONE. BESIDES, SHE IS BLINDFOLDED. SHE CAN'T SEE YOU, ANYWAY.

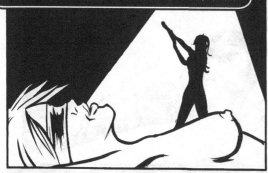

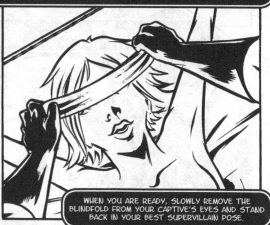

WHEN YOU ARE READY, SLOWLY REMOVE THE BLINDFOLD FROM YOUR CAPTIVE'S EYES AND STAND BACK IN YOUR BEST SUPERVILLAIN POSE.

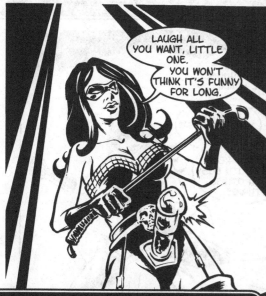

LAUGH ALL YOU WANT, LITTLE ONE. YOU WON'T THINK IT'S FUNNY FOR LONG.

YOUR CAPTIVE MAY LAUGH (BECAUSE IT IS FUNNY, AFTER ALL). IF SHE DOES, YOU CAN USE THIS TO YOUR ADVANTAGE BY MAKING A THREAT AND ESTABLISHING YOUR ROLE RIGHT AWAY.

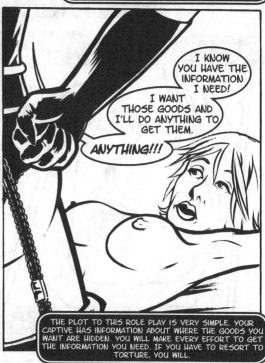

I KNOW YOU HAVE THE INFORMATION I NEED!

I WANT THOSE GOODS AND I'LL DO ANYTHING TO GET THEM.

ANYTHING!!!

THE PLOT TO THIS ROLE PLAY IS VERY SIMPLE. YOUR CAPTIVE HAS INFORMATION ABOUT WHERE THE GOODS YOU WANT ARE HIDDEN. YOU WILL MAKE EVERY EFFORT TO GET THE INFORMATION YOU NEED. IF YOU HAVE TO RESORT TO TORTURE, YOU WILL.

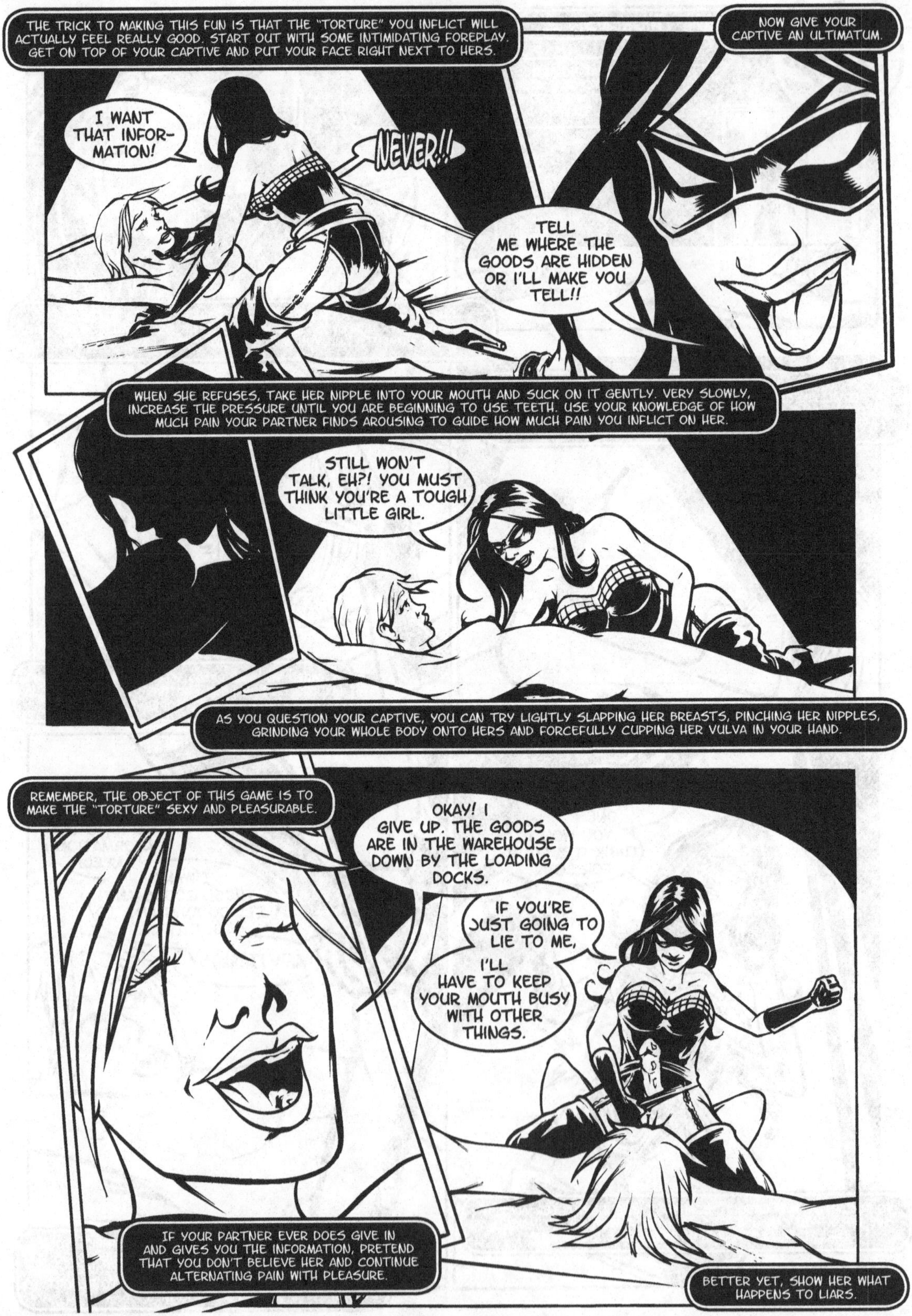
THE TRICK TO MAKING THIS FUN IS THAT THE "TORTURE" YOU INFLICT WILL ACTUALLY FEEL REALLY GOOD. START OUT WITH SOME INTIMIDATING FOREPLAY. GET ON TOP OF YOUR CAPTIVE AND PUT YOUR FACE RIGHT NEXT TO HERS.
I WANT THAT INFORMATION!
NEVER!!
NOW GIVE YOUR CAPTIVE AN ULTIMATUM.
TELL ME WHERE THE GOODS ARE HIDDEN OR I'LL MAKE YOU TELL!!
WHEN SHE REFUSES, TAKE HER NIPPLE INTO YOUR MOUTH AND SUCK ON IT GENTLY. VERY SLOWLY, INCREASE THE PRESSURE UNTIL YOU ARE BEGINNING TO USE TEETH. USE YOUR KNOWLEDGE OF HOW MUCH PAIN YOUR PARTNER FINDS AROUSING TO GUIDE HOW MUCH PAIN YOU INFLICT ON HER.
STILL WON'T TALK, EH?! YOU MUST THINK YOU'RE A TOUGH LITTLE GIRL.
AS YOU QUESTION YOUR CAPTIVE, YOU CAN TRY LIGHTLY SLAPPING HER BREASTS, PINCHING HER NIPPLES, GRINDING YOUR WHOLE BODY ONTO HERS AND FORCEFULLY CUPPING HER VULVA IN YOUR HAND.
REMEMBER, THE OBJECT OF THIS GAME IS TO MAKE THE "TORTURE" SEXY AND PLEASURABLE.
OKAY! I GIVE UP. THE GOODS ARE IN THE WAREHOUSE DOWN BY THE LOADING DOCKS.
IF YOU'RE JUST GOING TO LIE TO ME,
I'LL HAVE TO KEEP YOUR MOUTH BUSY WITH OTHER THINGS.
IF YOUR PARTNER EVER DOES GIVE IN AND GIVES YOU THE INFORMATION, PRETEND THAT YOU DON'T BELIEVE HER AND CONTINUE ALTERNATING PAIN WITH PLEASURE.
BETTER YET, SHOW HER WHAT HAPPENS TO LIARS.

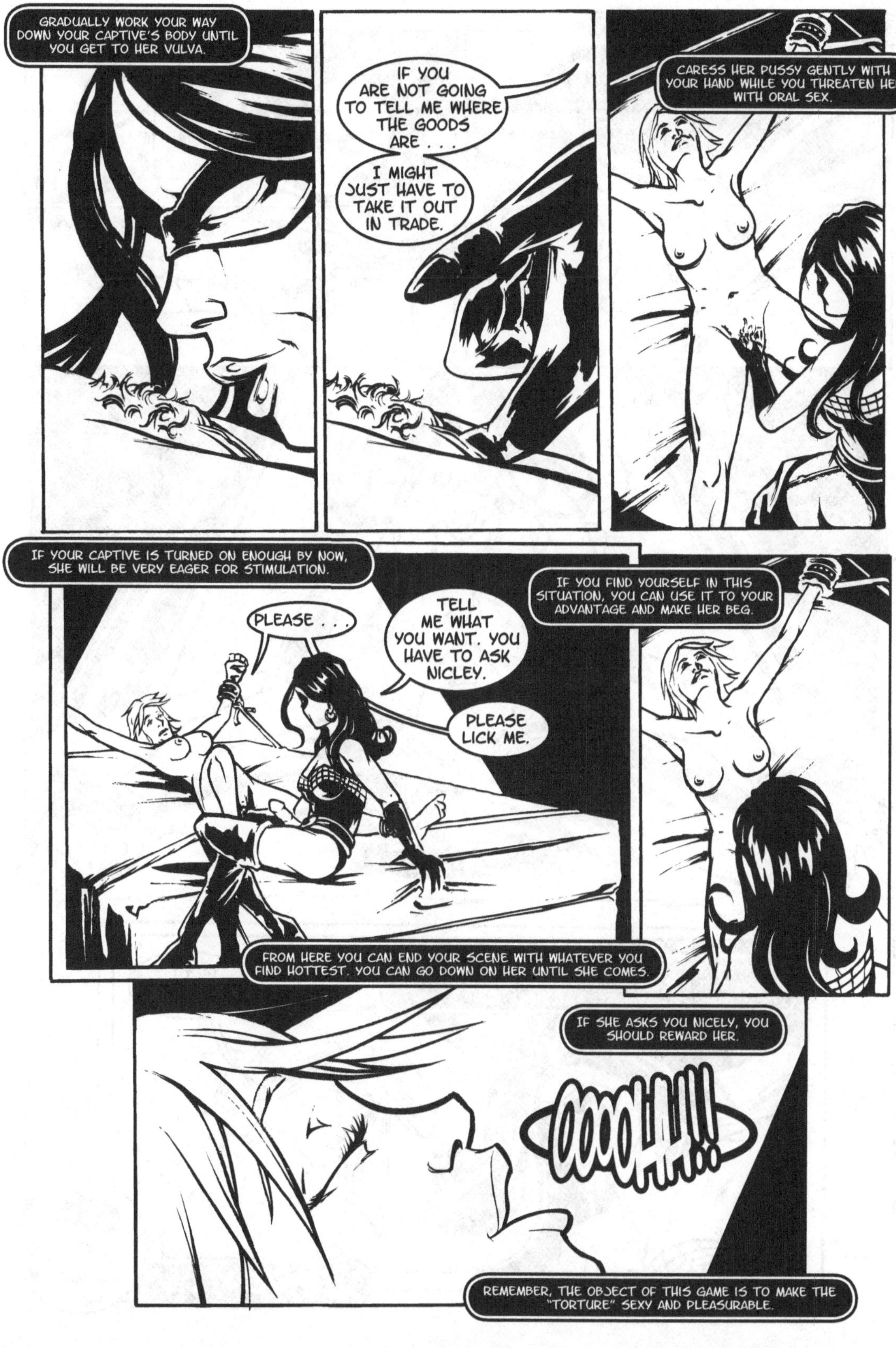
GRADUALLY WORK YOUR WAY DOWN YOUR CAPTIVE'S BODY UNTIL YOU GET TO HER VULVA.
IF YOU ARE NOT GOING TO TELL ME WHERE THE GOODS ARE . . .
I MIGHT JUST HAVE TO TAKE IT OUT IN TRADE.
CARESS HER PUSSY GENTLY WITH YOUR HAND WHILE YOU THREATEN HER WITH ORAL SEX.
IF YOUR CAPTIVE IS TURNED ON ENOUGH BY NOW, SHE WILL BE VERY EAGER FOR STIMULATION.
PLEASE . . .
TELL ME WHAT YOU WANT. YOU HAVE TO ASK NICLEY.
PLEASE LICK ME.
IF YOU FIND YOURSELF IN THIS SITUATION, YOU CAN USE IT TO YOUR ADVANTAGE AND MAKE HER BEG.
FROM HERE YOU CAN END YOUR SCENE WITH WHATEVER YOU FIND HOTTEST. YOU CAN GO DOWN ON HER UNTIL SHE COMES.
IF SHE ASKS YOU NICELY, YOU SHOULD REWARD HER.
OOOHHH!!
REMEMBER, THE OBJECT OF THIS GAME IS TO MAKE THE "TORTURE" SEXY AND PLEASURABLE.

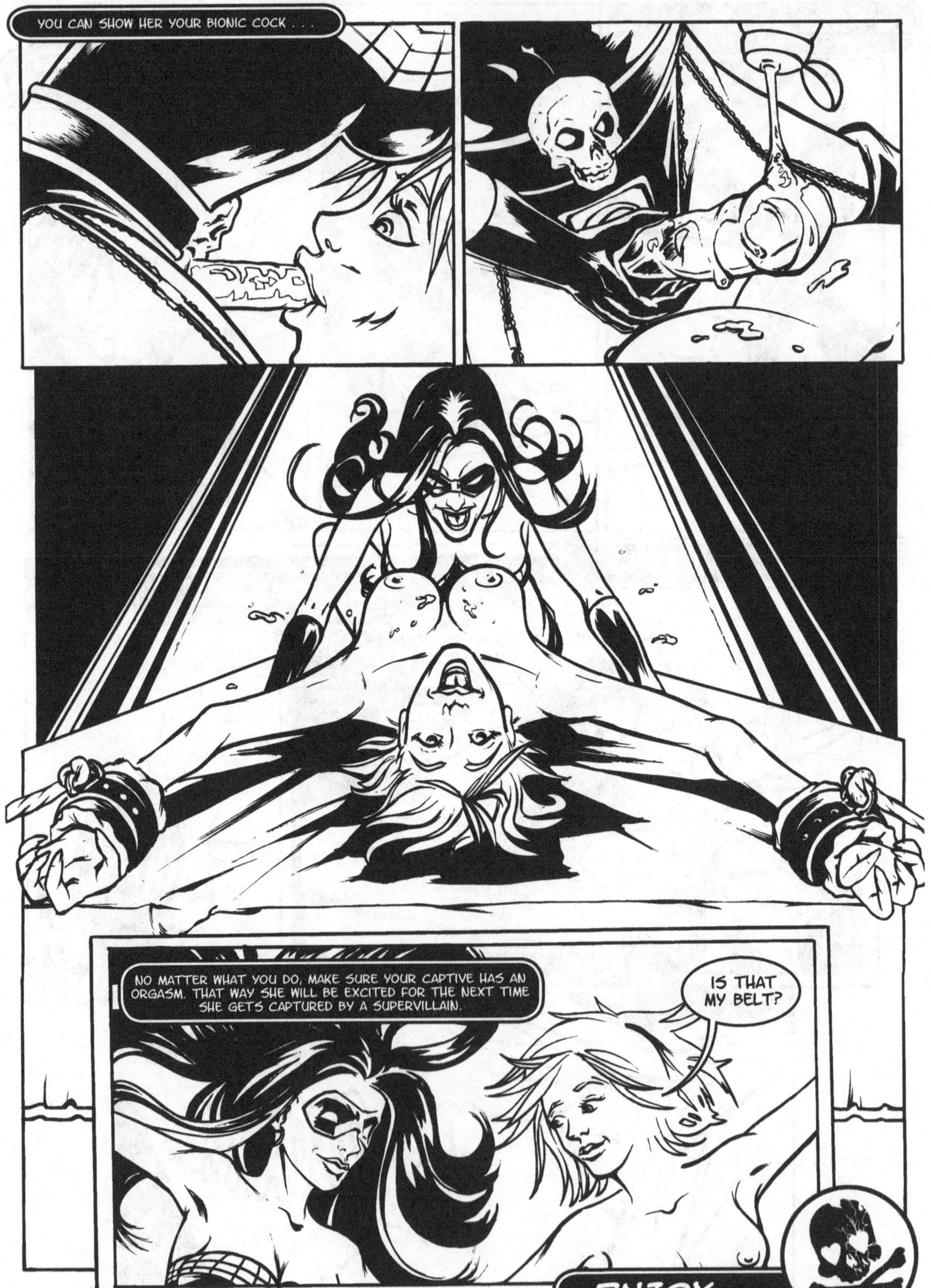
YOU CAN SHOW HER YOUR BIONIC COCK . . .
NO MATTER WHAT YOU DO, MAKE SURE YOUR CAPTIVE HAS AN ORGASM. THAT WAY SHE WILL BE EXCITED FOR THE NEXT TIME SHE GETS CAPTURED BY A SUPERVILLAIN.
IS THAT MY BELT?
ENJOY . . .

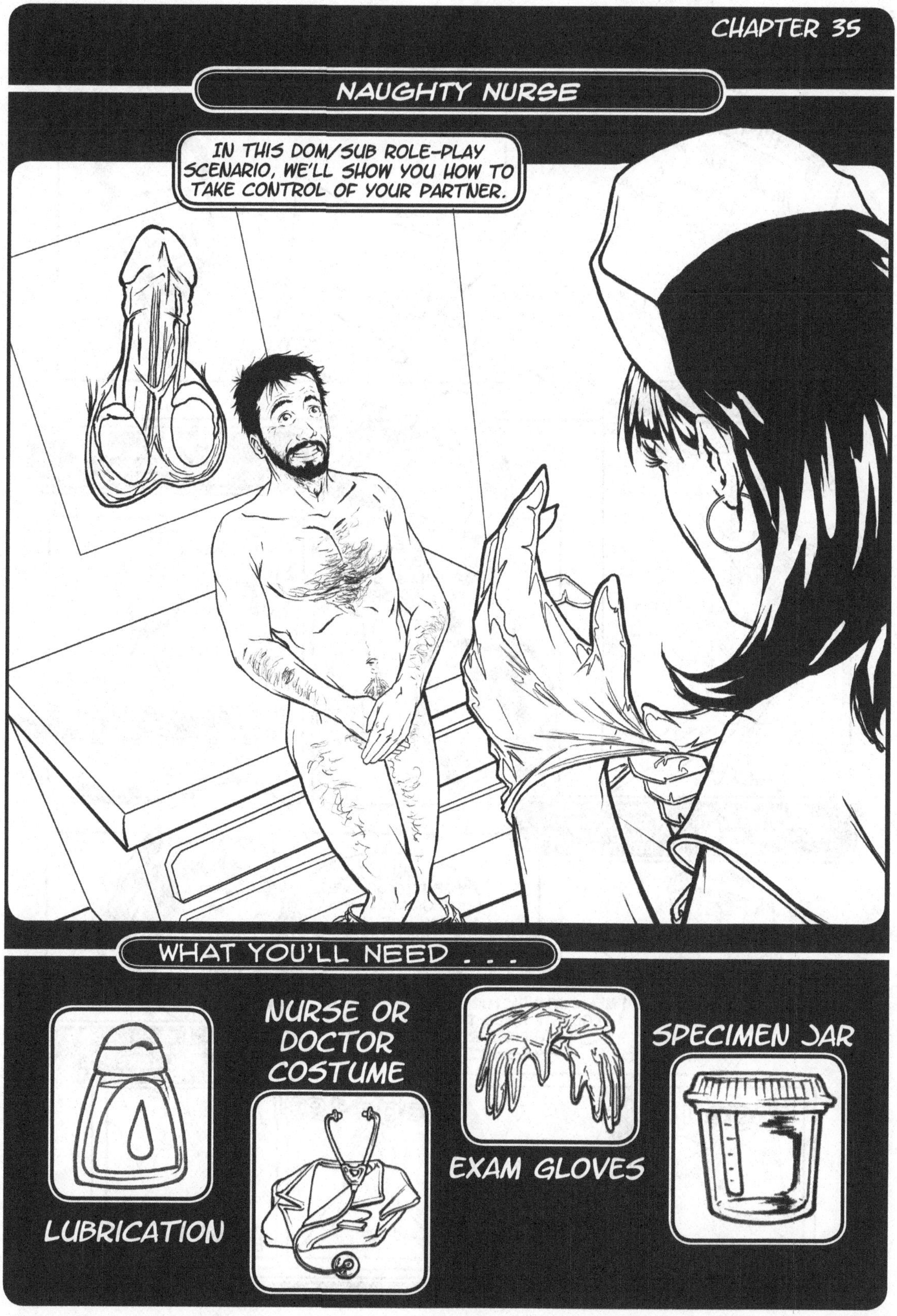
CHAPTER 35
NAUGHTY NURSE
IN THIS DOM/SUB ROLE-PLAY SCENARIO, WE'LL SHOW YOU HOW TO TAKE CONTROL OF YOUR PARTNER.
WHAT YOU'LL NEED . . .
LUBRICATION
NURSE OR DOCTOR COSTUME
EXAM GLOVES
SPECIMEN JAR

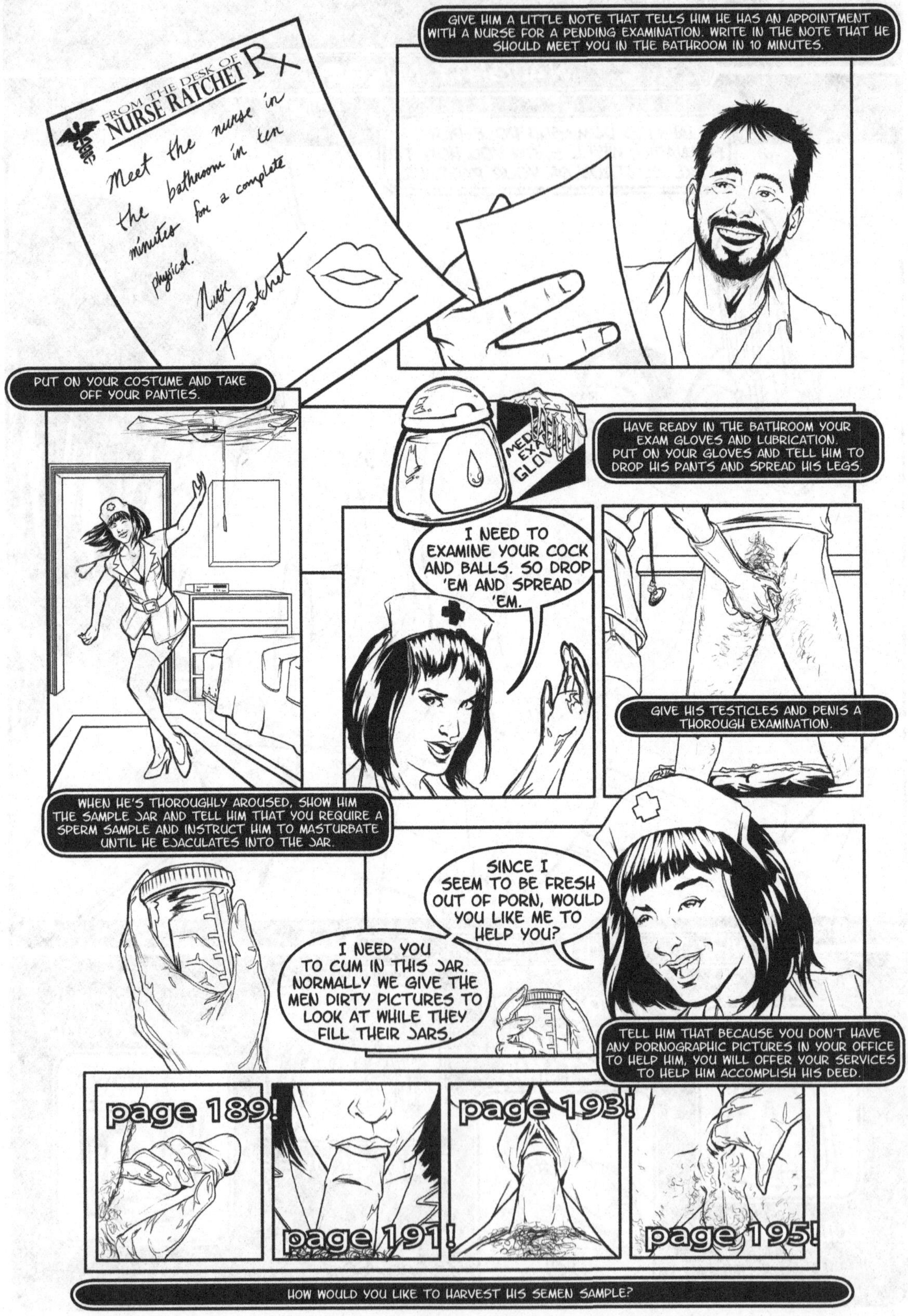
GIVE HIM A LITTLE NOTE THAT TELLS HIM HE HAS AN APPOINTMENT WITH A NURSE FOR A PENDING EXAMINATION. WRITE IN THE NOTE THAT HE SHOULD MEET YOU IN THE BATHROOM IN 10 MINUTES.
FROM THE DESK OF NURSE RATCHET Rx
Meet the nurse in the bathroom in ten minutes for a complete physical.
Nurse Ratchet
PUT ON YOUR COSTUME AND TAKE OFF YOUR PANTIES.
HAVE READY IN THE BATHROOM YOUR EXAM GLOVES AND LUBRICATION. PUT ON YOUR GLOVES AND TELL HIM TO DROP HIS PANTS AND SPREAD HIS LEGS.
I NEED TO EXAMINE YOUR COCK AND BALLS. SO DROP 'EM AND SPREAD 'EM.
GIVE HIS TESTICLES AND PENIS A THOROUGH EXAMINATION.
WHEN HE'S THOROUGHLY AROUSED, SHOW HIM THE SAMPLE JAR AND TELL HIM THAT YOU REQUIRE A SPERM SAMPLE AND INSTRUCT HIM TO MASTURBATE UNTIL HE EJACULATES INTO THE JAR.
I NEED YOU TO CUM IN THIS JAR. NORMALLY WE GIVE THE MEN DIRTY PICTURES TO LOOK AT WHILE THEY FILL THEIR JARS.
SINCE I SEEM TO BE FRESH OUT OF PORN, WOULD YOU LIKE ME TO HELP YOU?
TELL HIM THAT BECAUSE YOU DON'T HAVE ANY PORNOGRAPHIC PICTURES IN YOUR OFFICE TO HELP HIM, YOU WILL OFFER YOUR SERVICES TO HELP HIM ACCOMPLISH HIS DEED.
page 189!
page 191!
page 193!
page 195!
HOW WOULD YOU LIKE TO HARVEST HIS SEMEN SAMPLE?

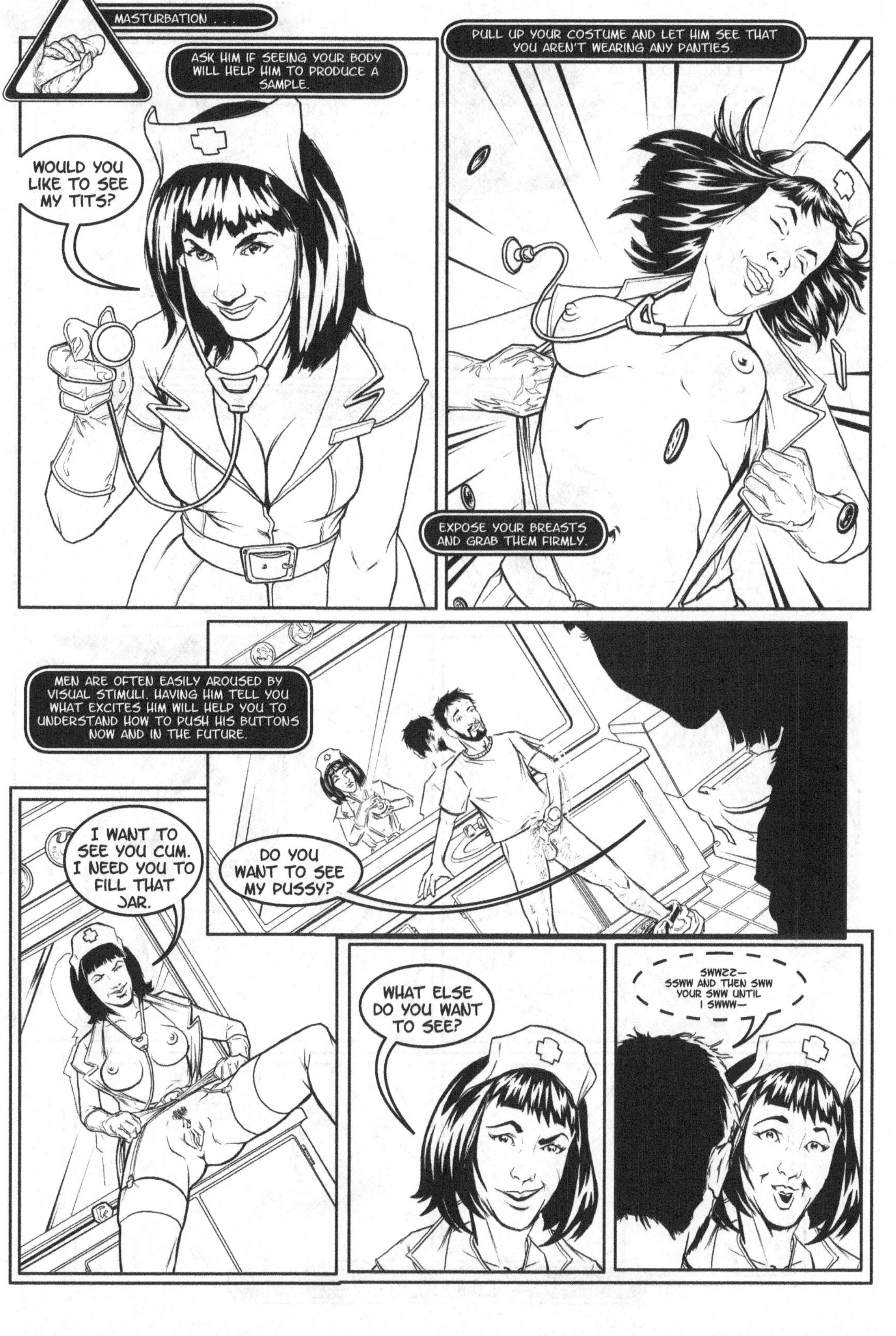
MASTURBATION . . .
ASK HIM IF SEEING YOUR BODY WILL HELP HIM TO PRODUCE A SAMPLE.
WOULD YOU LIKE TO SEE MY TITS?
PULL UP YOUR COSTUME AND LET HIM SEE THAT YOU AREN'T WEARING ANY PANTIES.
EXPOSE YOUR BREASTS AND GRAB THEM FIRMLY.
MEN ARE OFTEN EASILY AROUSED BY VISUAL STIMULI. HAVING HIM TELL YOU WHAT EXCITES HIM WILL HELP YOU TO UNDERSTAND HOW TO PUSH HIS BUTTONS NOW AND IN THE FUTURE.
DO YOU WANT TO SEE MY PUSSY?
I WANT TO SEE YOU CUM. I NEED YOU TO FILL THAT JAR.
WHAT ELSE DO YOU WANT TO SEE?
SWWZZ— SSWW AND THEN SWW YOUR SWW UNTIL I SWWW—

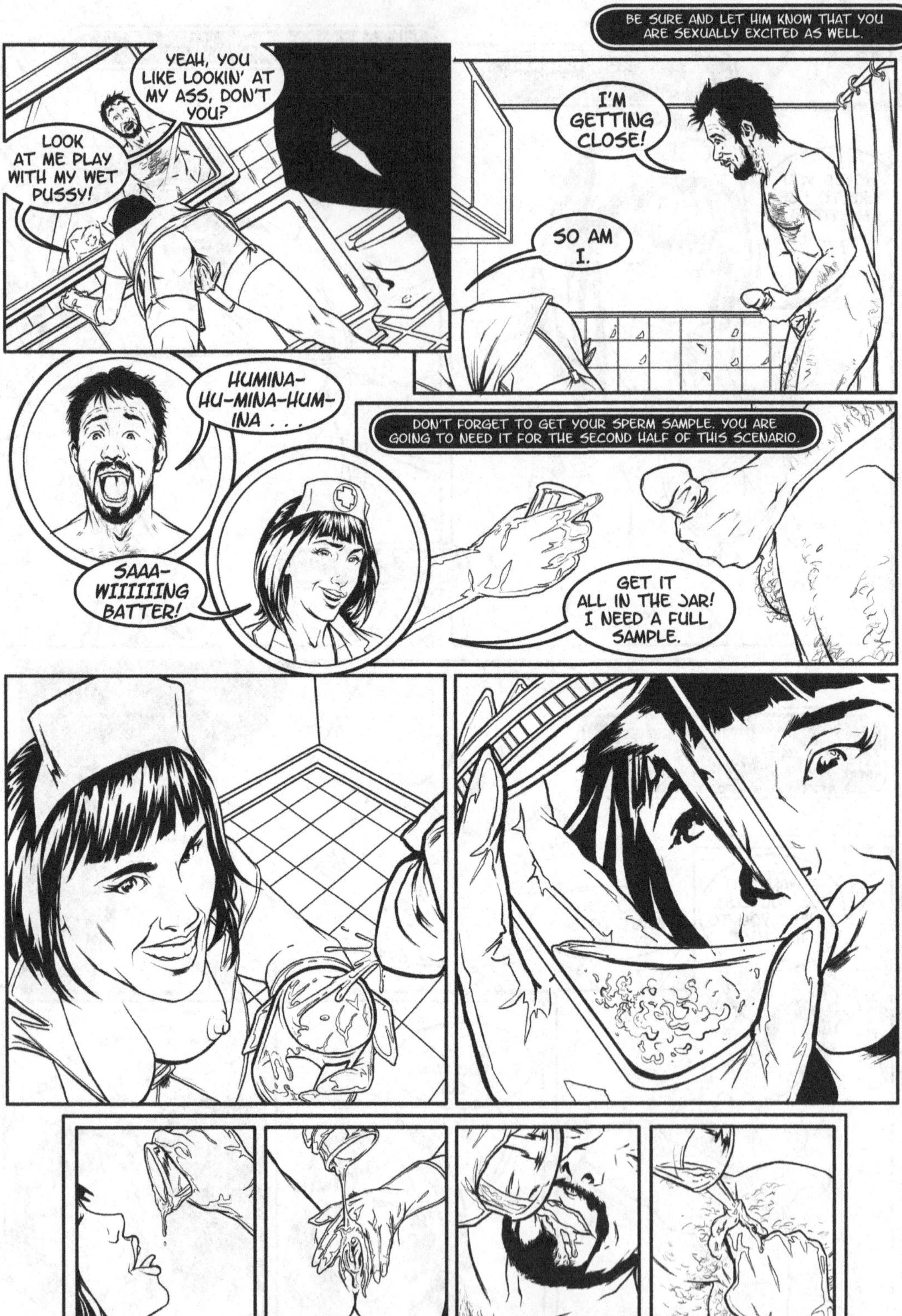
YEAH, YOU LIKE LOOKIN' AT MY ASS, DON'T YOU?
LOOK AT ME PLAY WITH MY WET PUSSY!
BE SURE AND LET HIM KNOW THAT YOU ARE SEXUALLY EXCITED AS WELL.
I'M GETTING CLOSE!
SO AM I.
HUMINA-HU-MINA-HUM-INA . . .
SAAA-WIIIIIING BATTER!
DON'T FORGET TO GET YOUR SPERM SAMPLE. YOU ARE GOING TO NEED IT FOR THE SECOND HALF OF THIS SCENARIO.
GET IT ALL IN THE JAR! I NEED A FULL SAMPLE.
CONTINUE YOUR ADVENTURE ONLINE.
WWW.SEXISFUN.NET/NAUGHTYNURSE

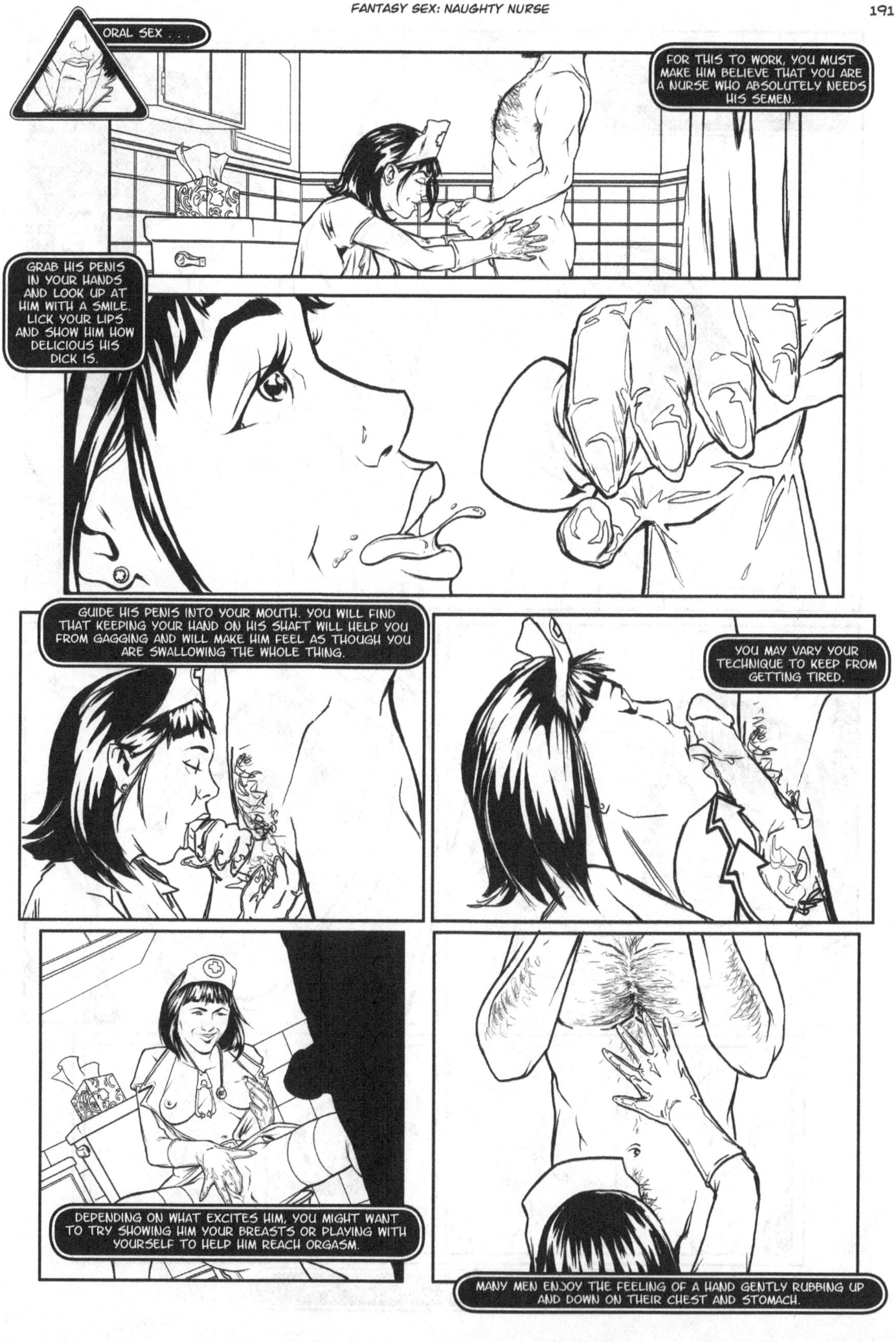
ORAL SEX . . .
FOR THIS TO WORK, YOU MUST MAKE HIM BELIEVE THAT YOU ARE A NURSE WHO ABSOLUTELY NEEDS HIS SEMEN.
GRAB HIS PENIS IN YOUR HANDS AND LOOK UP AT HIM WITH A SMILE. LICK YOUR LIPS AND SHOW HIM HOW DELICIOUS HIS DICK IS.
GUIDE HIS PENIS INTO YOUR MOUTH. YOU WILL FIND THAT KEEPING YOUR HAND ON HIS SHAFT WILL HELP YOU FROM GAGGING AND WILL MAKE HIM FEEL AS THOUGH YOU ARE SWALLOWING THE WHOLE THING.
YOU MAY VARY YOUR TECHNIQUE TO KEEP FROM GETTING TIRED.
DEPENDING ON WHAT EXCITES HIM, YOU MIGHT WANT TO TRY SHOWING HIM YOUR BREASTS OR PLAYING WITH YOURSELF TO HELP HIM REACH ORGASM.
MANY MEN ENJOY THE FEELING OF A HAND GENTLY RUBBING UP AND DOWN ON THEIR CHEST AND STOMACH.

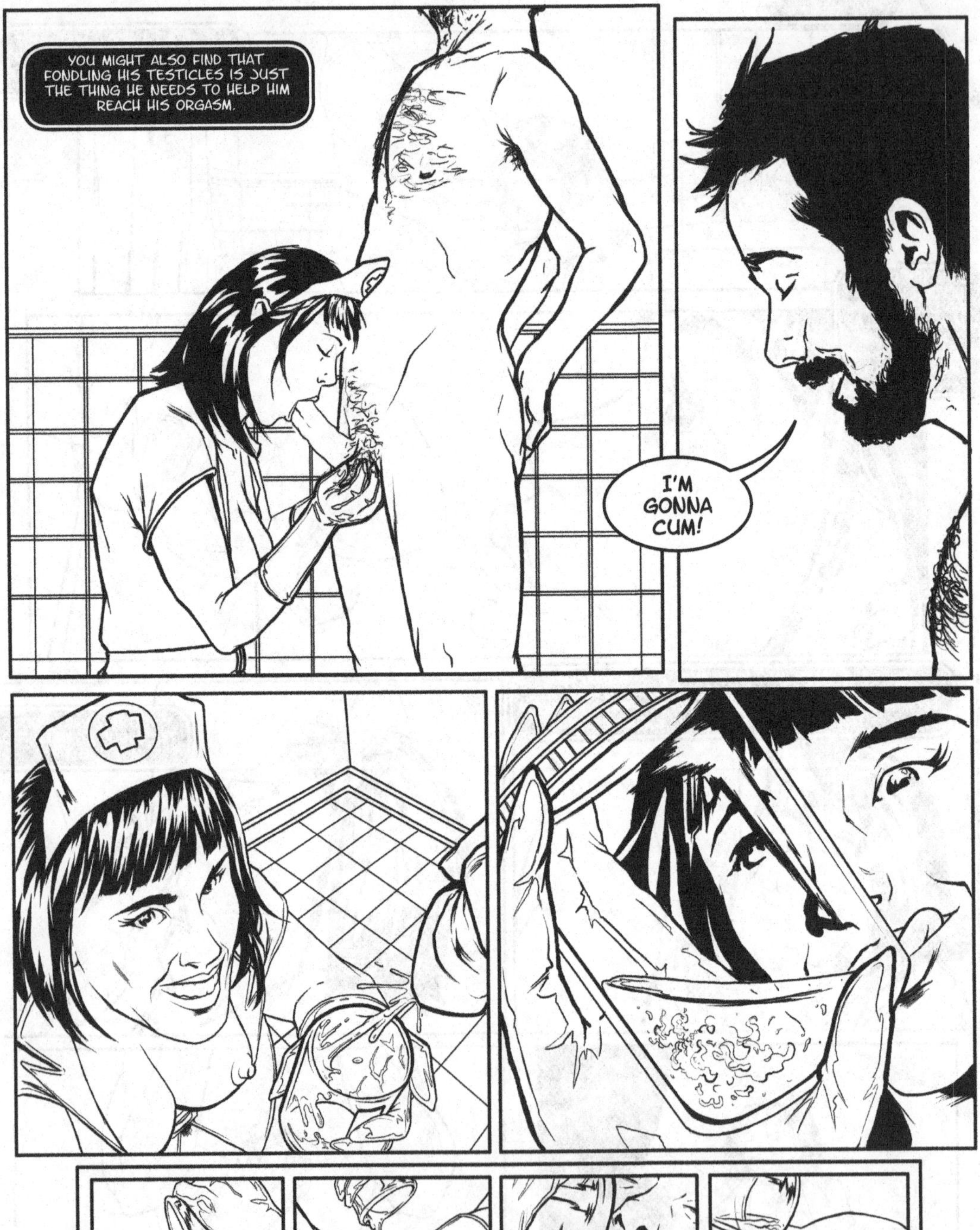
YOU MIGHT ALSO FIND THAT FONDLING HIS TESTICLES IS JUST THE THING HE NEEDS TO HELP HIM REACH HIS ORGASM.
I'M GONNA CUM!

CONTINUE YOUR ADVENTURE ONLINE.
WWW.SEXISFUN.NET/NAUGHTYNURSE

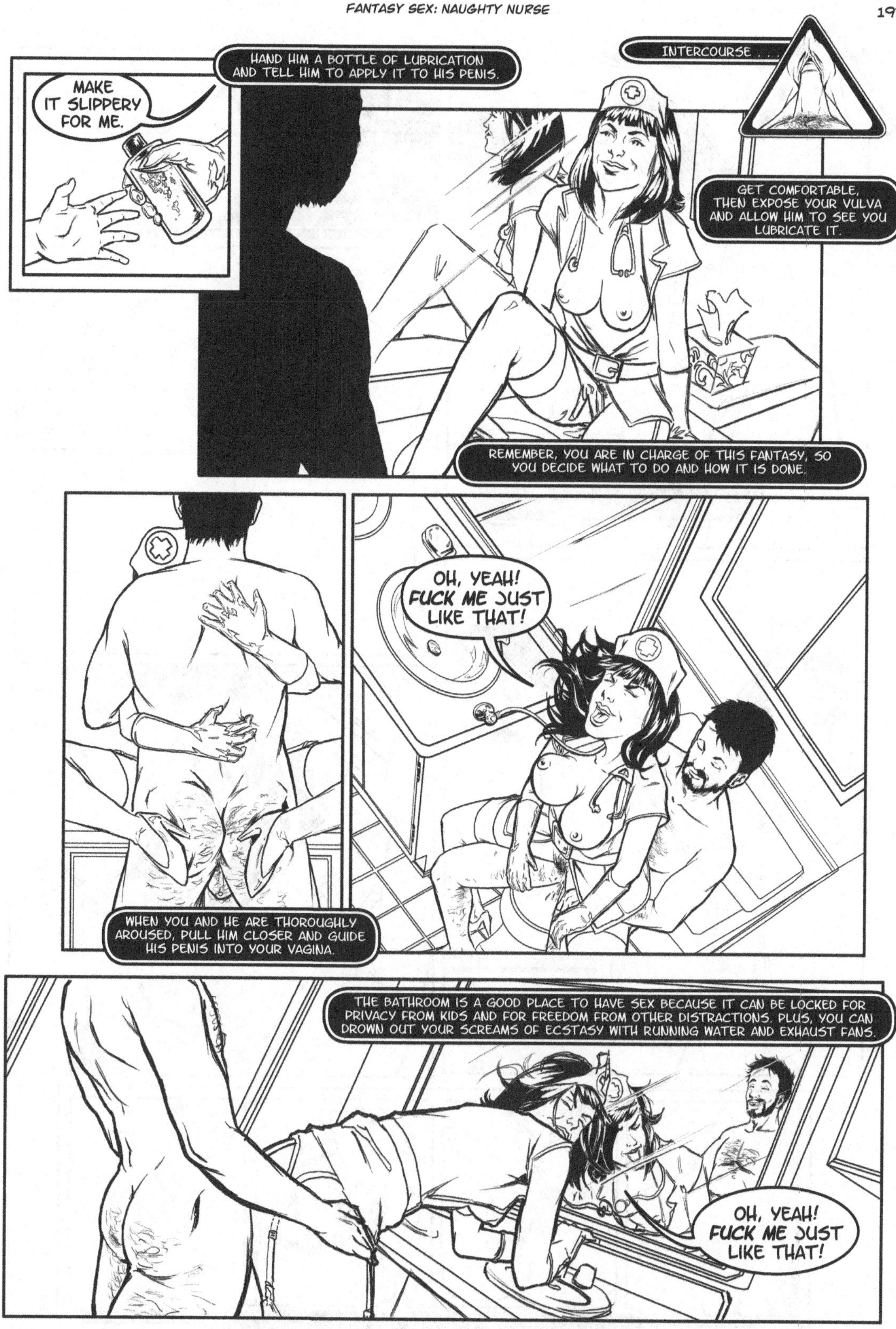
HAND HIM A BOTTLE OF LUBRICATION AND TELL HIM TO APPLY IT TO HIS PENIS.
MAKE IT SLIPPERY FOR ME.
INTERCOURSE . . .
GET COMFORTABLE, THEN EXPOSE YOUR VULVA AND ALLOW HIM TO SEE YOU LUBRICATE IT.
REMEMBER, YOU ARE IN CHARGE OF THIS FANTASY, SO YOU DECIDE WHAT TO DO AND HOW IT IS DONE.
WHEN YOU AND HE ARE THOROUGHLY AROUSED, PULL HIM CLOSER AND GUIDE HIS PENIS INTO YOUR VAGINA.
OH, YEAH! FUCK ME JUST LIKE THAT!
THE BATHROOM IS A GOOD PLACE TO HAVE SEX BECAUSE IT CAN BE LOCKED FOR PRIVACY FROM KIDS AND FOR FREEDOM FROM OTHER DISTRACTIONS. PLUS, YOU CAN DROWN OUT YOUR SCREAMS OF ECSTASY WITH RUNNING WATER AND EXHAUST FANS.
OH, YEAH! FUCK ME JUST LIKE THAT!

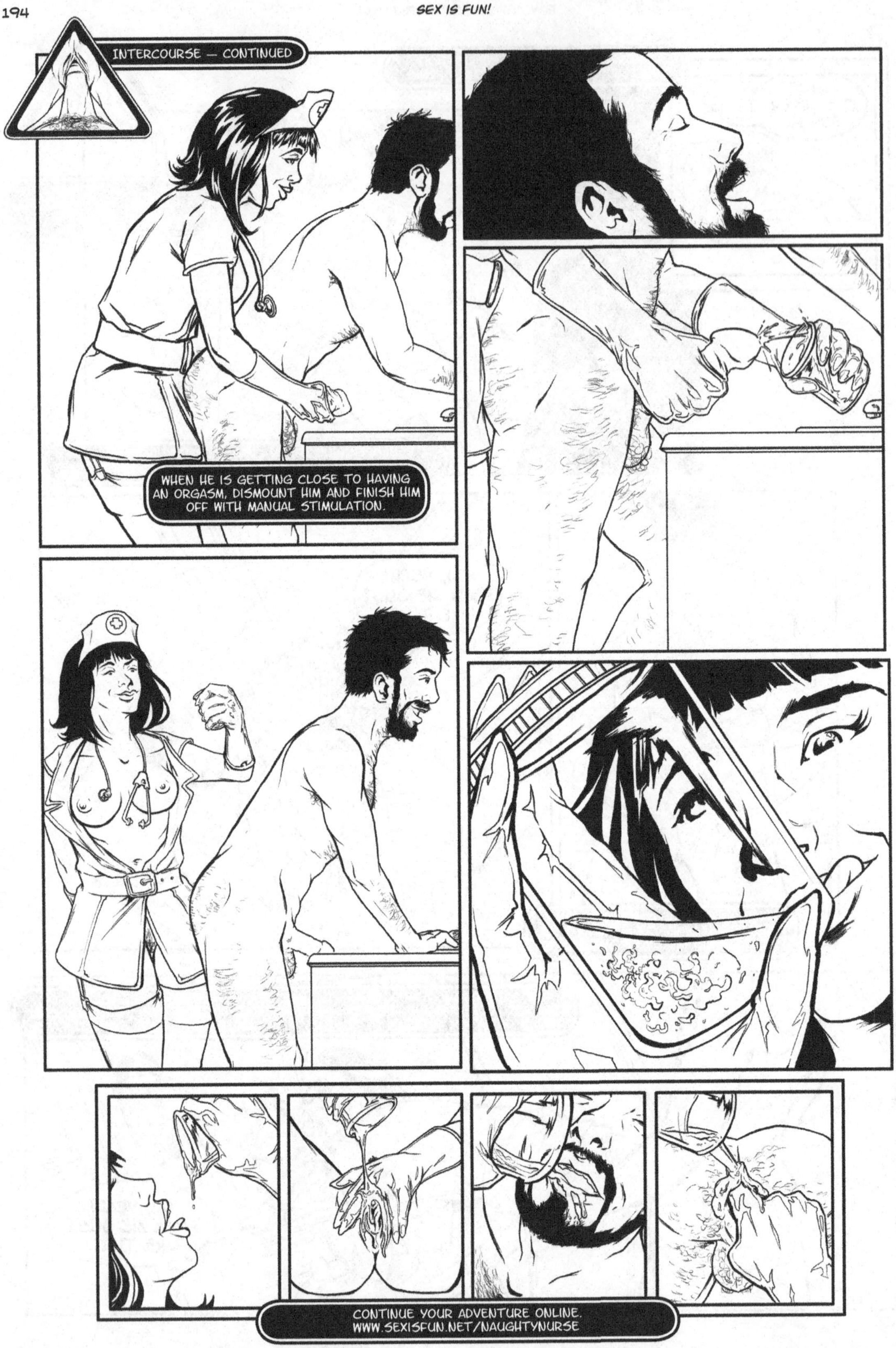
INTERCOURSE — CONTINUED
WHEN HE IS GETTING CLOSE TO HAVING AN ORGASM, DISMOUNT HIM AND FINISH HIM OFF WITH MANUAL STIMULATION.
CONTINUE YOUR ADVENTURE ONLINE. WWW.SEXISFUN.NET/NAUGHTYNURSE

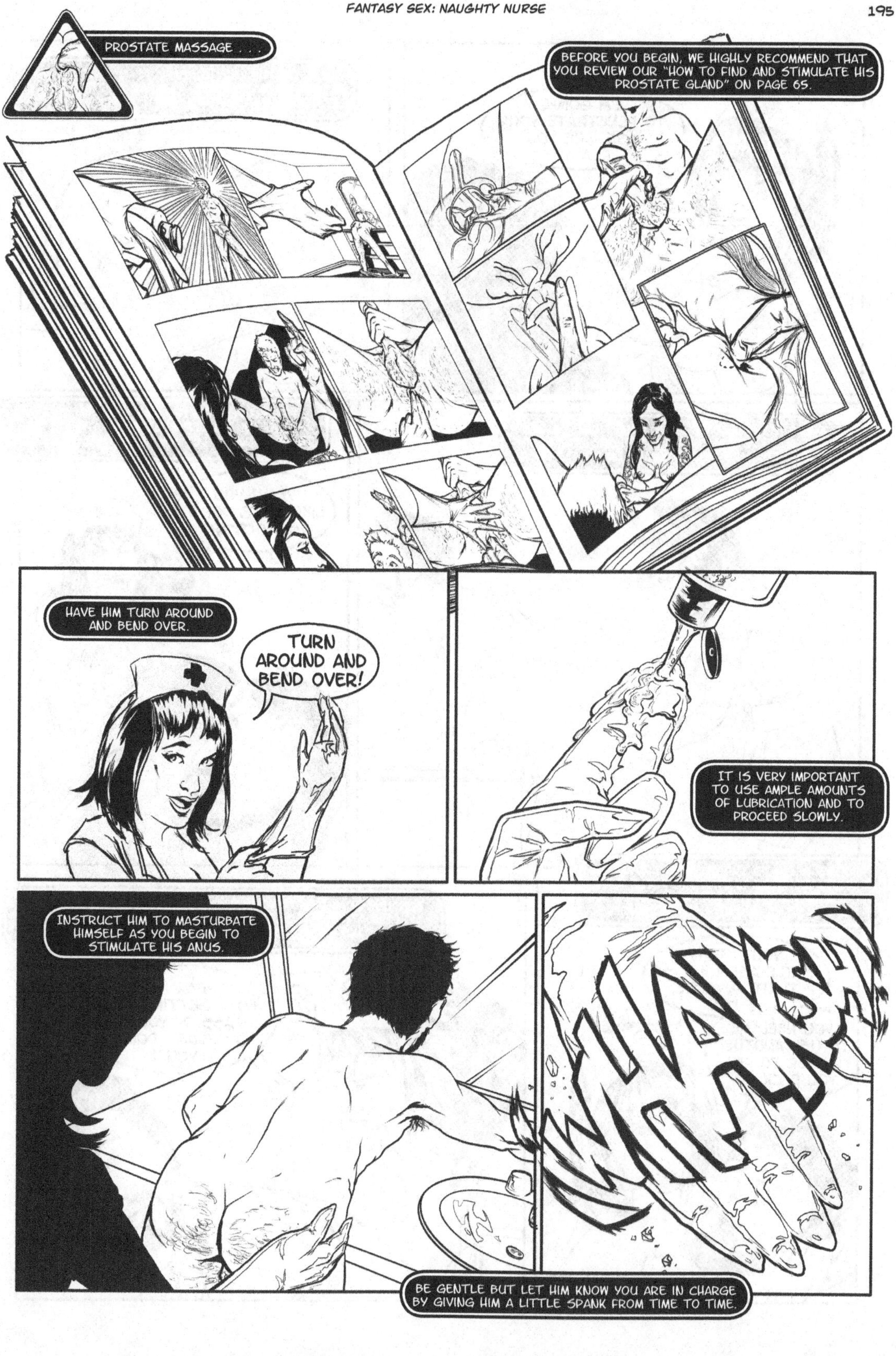
PROSTATE MASSAGE . . .
BEFORE YOU BEGIN, WE HIGHLY RECOMMEND THAT YOU REVIEW OUR "HOW TO FIND AND STIMULATE HIS PROSTATE GLAND" ON PAGE 65.
HAVE HIM TURN AROUND AND BEND OVER.
TURN AROUND AND BEND OVER!
IT IS VERY IMPORTANT TO USE AMPLE AMOUNTS OF LUBRICATION AND TO PROCEED SLOWLY.
INSTRUCT HIM TO MASTURBATE HIMSELF AS YOU BEGIN TO STIMULATE HIS ANUS.
BE GENTLE BUT LET HIM KNOW YOU ARE IN CHARGE BY GIVING HIM A LITTLE SPANK FROM TIME TO TIME.

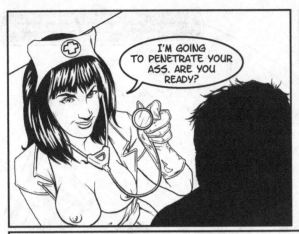

I'M GOING TO PENETRATE YOUR ASS. ARE YOU READY?

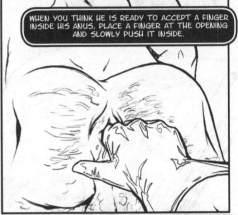

WHEN YOU THINK HE IS READY TO ACCEPT A FINGER INSIDE HIS ANUS, PLACE A FINGER AT THE OPENING AND SLOWLY PUSH IT INSIDE.

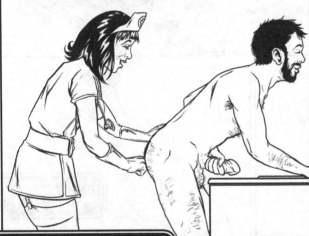

THERE IS NO NEED TO MOVE YOUR FINGER IN AND OUT JUST YET. WHEN HE IS READY HE WILL BEGIN MOVING FORWARD AND BACKWARD ON YOUR FINGER.

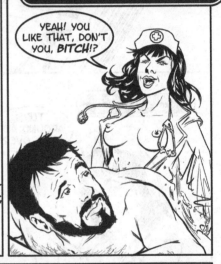

BEING PENETRATED MAY MAKE HIM FEEL AFRAID AND VULNERABLE. BE EMPATHETIC AND REASSURING TO LET HIM KNOW THAT YOU CARE.

YEAH! YOU LIKE THAT, DON'T YOU, *BITCH!*?

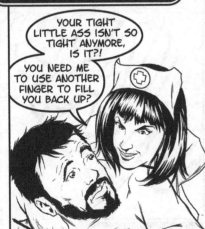

YOU MAY BEGIN TO THRUST INTO HIM AFTER HIS SPEED PICKS UP. WHEN IT FEELS AS THOUGH THERE IS LESS RESISTANCE, ASK HIM IF HE WOULD LIKE YOU TO USE TWO FINGERS.

YOUR TIGHT LITTLE ASS ISN'T SO TIGHT ANYMORE, IS IT?!

YOU NEED ME TO USE ANOTHER FINGER TO FILL YOU BACK UP?

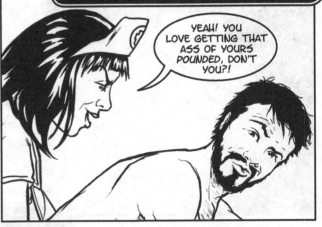

BECAUSE ANAL PENETRATION WRONGFULLY CARRIES WITH IT SO MUCH NEGATIVE STIGMA, IT MIGHT BE A GOOD IDEA TO REASSURE HIM OF HIS MASCULINITY AS YOU PERFORM THIS EXERCISE.

YEAH! YOU LOVE GETTING THAT ASS OF YOURS POUNDED, DON'T YOU?!

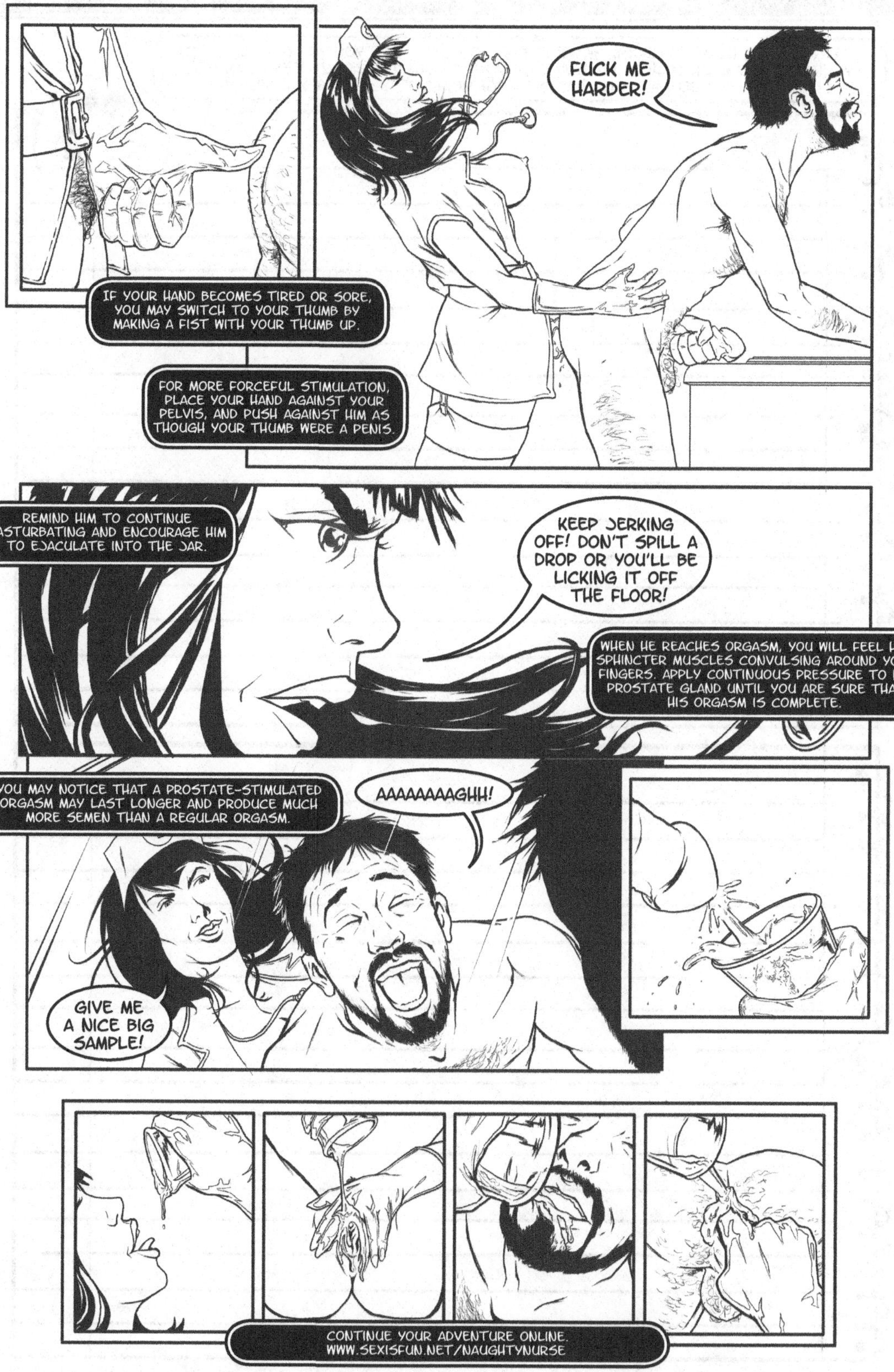
FUCK ME HARDER!
IF YOUR HAND BECOMES TIRED OR SORE, YOU MAY SWITCH TO YOUR THUMB BY MAKING A FIST WITH YOUR THUMB UP.
FOR MORE FORCEFUL STIMULATION, PLACE YOUR HAND AGAINST YOUR PELVIS, AND PUSH AGAINST HIM AS THOUGH YOUR THUMB WERE A PENIS.
REMIND HIM TO CONTINUE MASTURBATING AND ENCOURAGE HIM TO EJACULATE INTO THE JAR.
KEEP JERKING OFF! DON'T SPILL A DROP OR YOU'LL BE LICKING IT OFF THE FLOOR!
WHEN HE REACHES ORGASM, YOU WILL FEEL HIS SPHINCTER MUSCLES CONVULSING AROUND YOUR FINGERS. APPLY CONTINUOUS PRESSURE TO HIS PROSTATE GLAND UNTIL YOU ARE SURE THAT HIS ORGASM IS COMPLETE.
YOU MAY NOTICE THAT A PROSTATE-STIMULATED ORGASM MAY LAST LONGER AND PRODUCE MUCH MORE SEMEN THAN A REGULAR ORGASM.
AAAAAAAAGHH!
GIVE ME A NICE BIG SAMPLE!
CONTINUE YOUR ADVENTURE ONLINE.
WWW.SEXISFUN.NET/NAUGHTYNURSE

WHAT HAVE WE LEARNED???

AS THIS BOOK NEARS A CLOSE, WHAT WOULD YOU SAY THAT YOU'VE LEARNED ABOUT YOURSELF AND EACH OTHER? HAVE ANY OF YOUR THOUGHTS ABOUT SEX CHANGED? HAS THE WAY YOU AND YOUR PARTNER COMMUNICATE ABOUT SEX CHANGED?

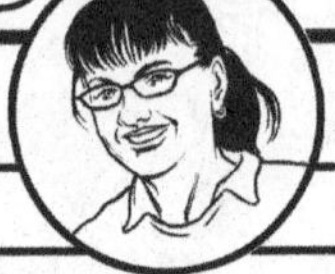

CHAPTER 36

TWO HEADS ARE BETTER THAN ONE

IN THIS SCENARIO, WE'LL SHOW YOU HOW TO USE A FEW SEX TOYS AND SOME INGENUITY TO SIMULATE BEING PENETRATED BY MULTIPLE PARTNERS AT ONE TIME.

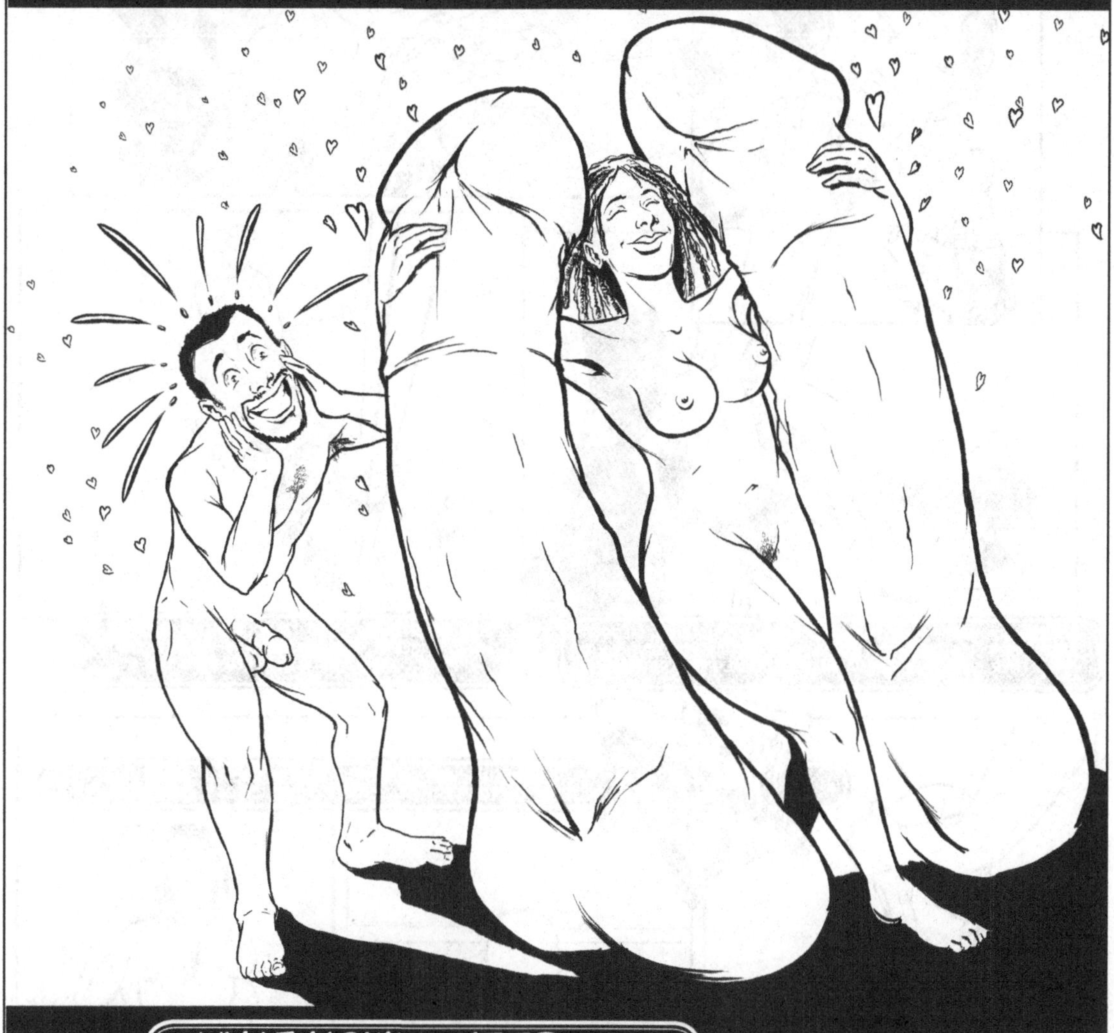

WHAT YOU'LL NEED . . .

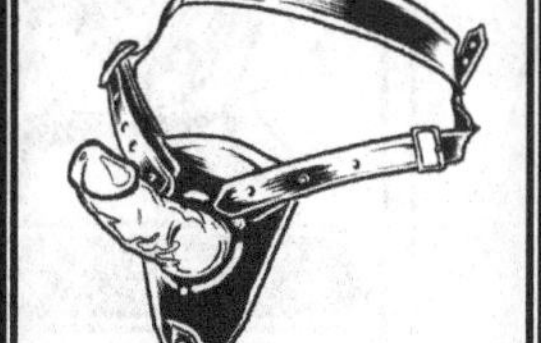

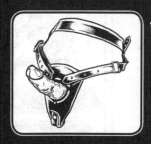

DILDO AND HARNESS

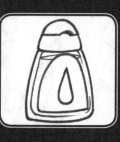

LUBRICATION

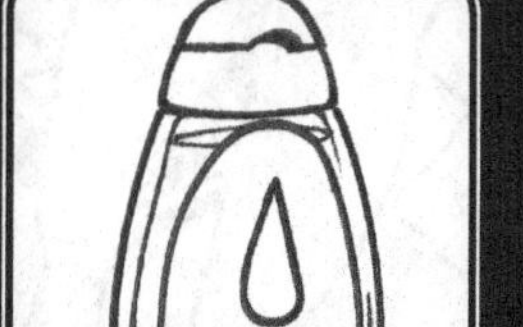

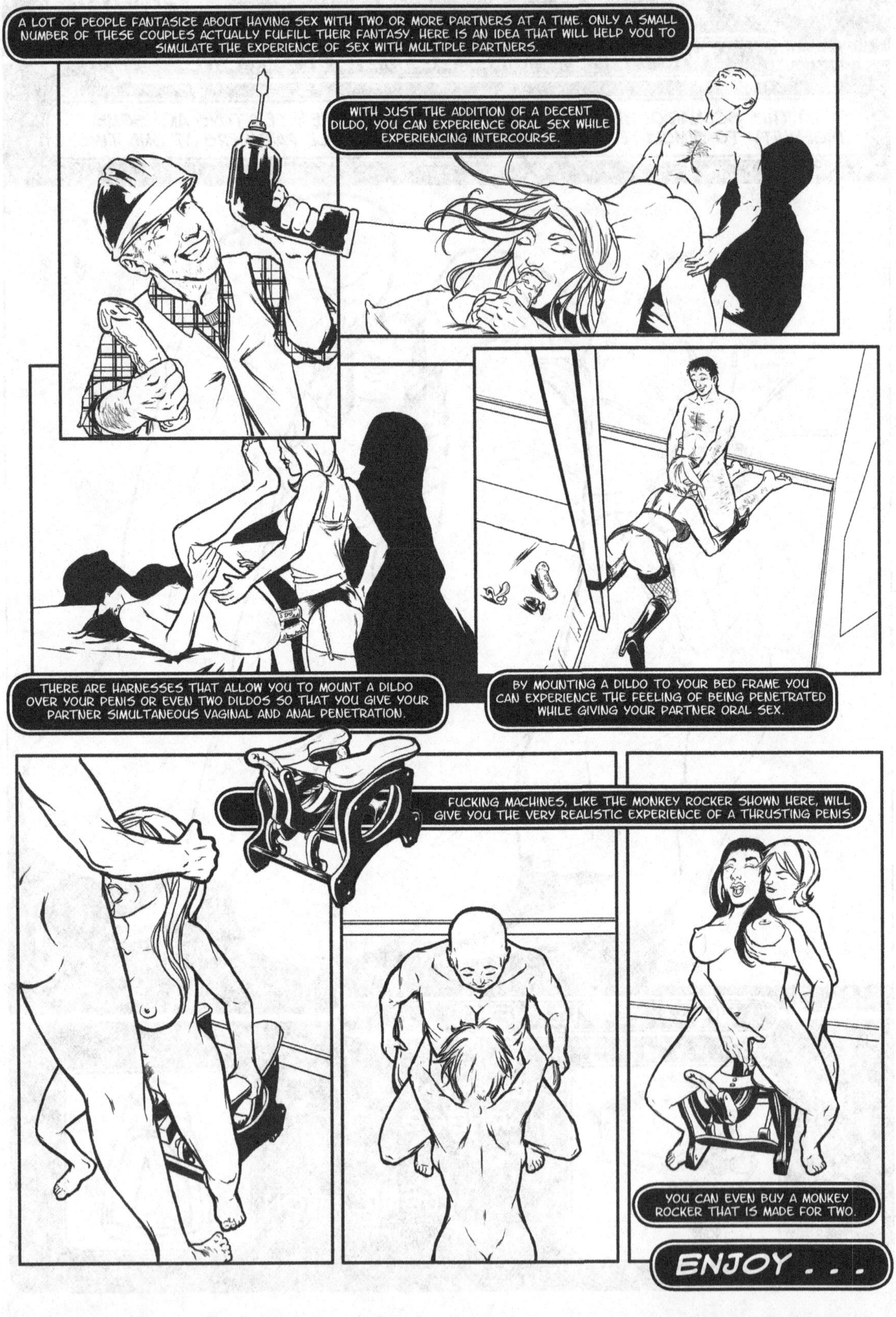
A LOT OF PEOPLE FANTASIZE ABOUT HAVING SEX WITH TWO OR MORE PARTNERS AT A TIME. ONLY A SMALL NUMBER OF THESE COUPLES ACTUALLY FULFILL THEIR FANTASY. HERE IS AN IDEA THAT WILL HELP YOU TO SIMULATE THE EXPERIENCE OF SEX WITH MULTIPLE PARTNERS.
WITH JUST THE ADDITION OF A DECENT DILDO, YOU CAN EXPERIENCE ORAL SEX WHILE EXPERIENCING INTERCOURSE.
THERE ARE HARNESSES THAT ALLOW YOU TO MOUNT A DILDO OVER YOUR PENIS OR EVEN TWO DILDOS SO THAT YOU GIVE YOUR PARTNER SIMULTANEOUS VAGINAL AND ANAL PENETRATION.
BY MOUNTING A DILDO TO YOUR BED FRAME YOU CAN EXPERIENCE THE FEELING OF BEING PENETRATED WHILE GIVING YOUR PARTNER ORAL SEX.
FUCKING MACHINES, LIKE THE MONKEY ROCKER SHOWN HERE, WILL GIVE YOU THE VERY REALISTIC EXPERIENCE OF A THRUSTING PENIS.
YOU CAN EVEN BUY A MONKEY ROCKER THAT IS MADE FOR TWO.
ENJOY . . .

CHAPTER 37

YES, MISTRESS HELGA

FOR SOME, TAKING THE DOMINANT ROLE COMES NATURALLY; FOR OTHERS IT CAN BE AWKWARD AND UNCOMFORTABLE. IN THIS SCENARIO, WE'LL SHOW YOU HOW TO COMPLETELY DOMINATE YOUR PARTNER.

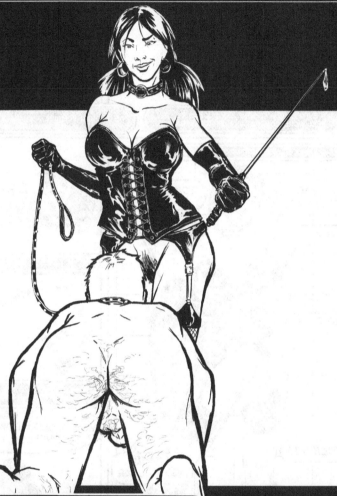

WHAT YOU'LL NEED . . .

 LEASH AND COLLAR

 STRAP-ON HARNESS AND DILDO

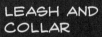 WHIP OR CROP

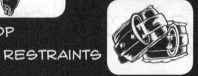 RESTRAINTS

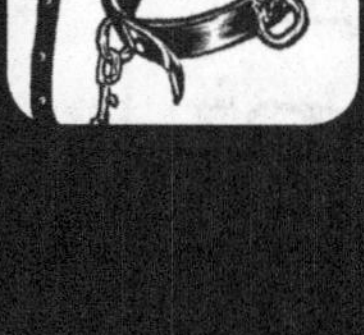

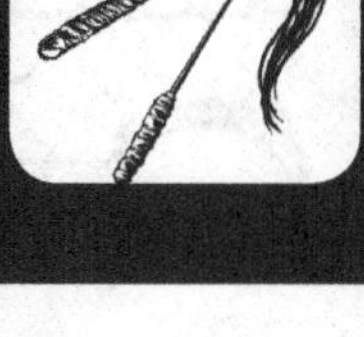

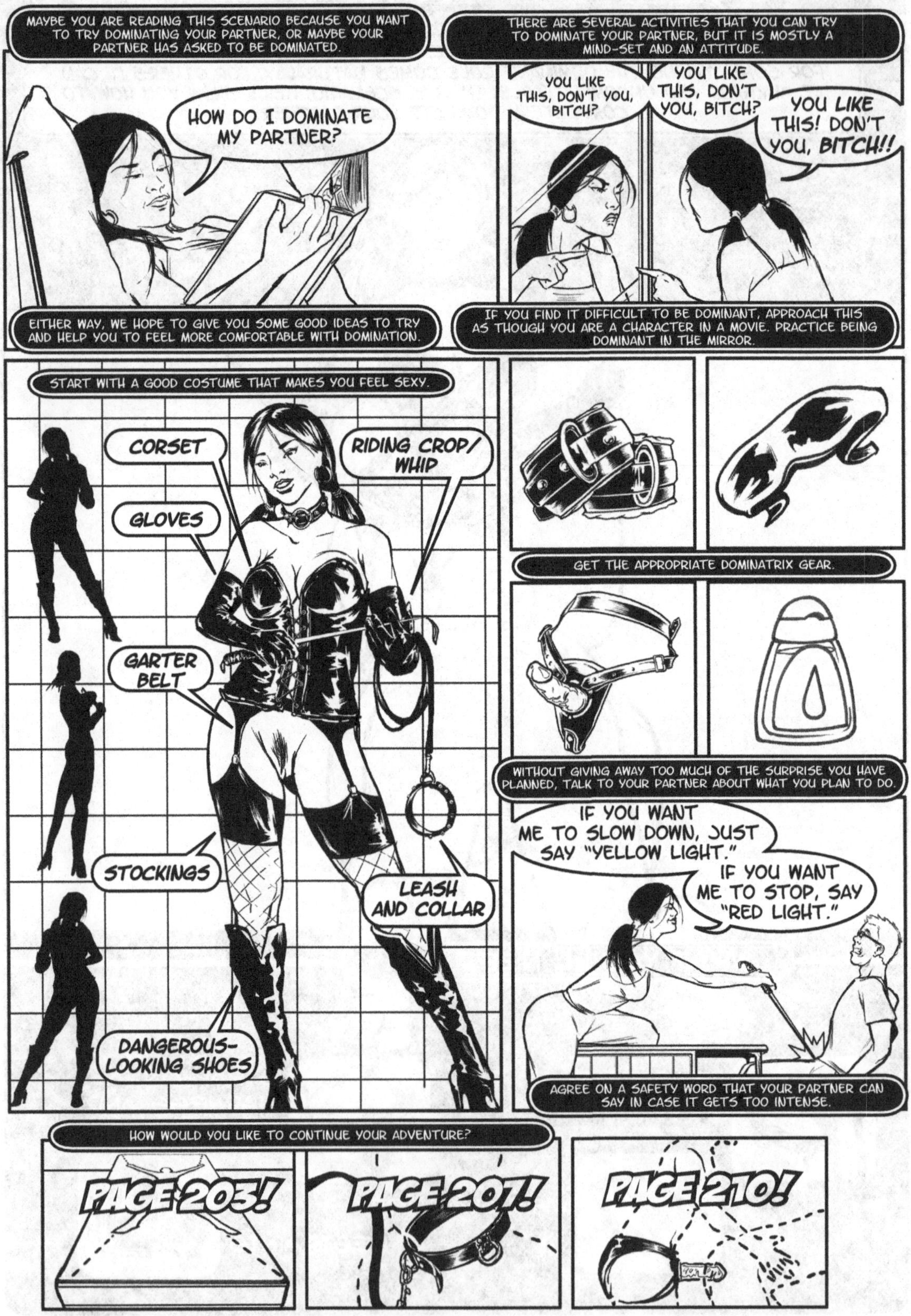
MAYBE YOU ARE READING THIS SCENARIO BECAUSE YOU WANT TO TRY DOMINATING YOUR PARTNER, OR MAYBE YOUR PARTNER HAS ASKED TO BE DOMINATED.
HOW DO I DOMINATE MY PARTNER?
EITHER WAY, WE HOPE TO GIVE YOU SOME GOOD IDEAS TO TRY AND HELP YOU TO FEEL MORE COMFORTABLE WITH DOMINATION.
THERE ARE SEVERAL ACTIVITIES THAT YOU CAN TRY TO DOMINATE YOUR PARTNER, BUT IT IS MOSTLY A MIND-SET AND AN ATTITUDE.
YOU LIKE THIS, DON'T YOU, BITCH?
YOU LIKE THIS, DON'T YOU, BITCH?
YOU LIKE THIS! DON'T YOU, BITCH!!
IF YOU FIND IT DIFFICULT TO BE DOMINANT, APPROACH THIS AS THOUGH YOU ARE A CHARACTER IN A MOVIE. PRACTICE BEING DOMINANT IN THE MIRROR.
START WITH A GOOD COSTUME THAT MAKES YOU FEEL SEXY.
CORSET
RIDING CROP/ WHIP
GLOVES
GARTER BELT
STOCKINGS
LEASH AND COLLAR
DANGEROUS-LOOKING SHOES
GET THE APPROPRIATE DOMINATRIX GEAR.
WITHOUT GIVING AWAY TOO MUCH OF THE SURPRISE YOU HAVE PLANNED, TALK TO YOUR PARTNER ABOUT WHAT YOU PLAN TO DO.
IF YOU WANT ME TO SLOW DOWN, JUST SAY "YELLOW LIGHT."
IF YOU WANT ME TO STOP, SAY "RED LIGHT."
AGREE ON A SAFETY WORD THAT YOUR PARTNER CAN SAY IN CASE IT GETS TOO INTENSE.
HOW WOULD YOU LIKE TO CONTINUE YOUR ADVENTURE?
PAGE 203!
PAGE 207!
PAGE 210!

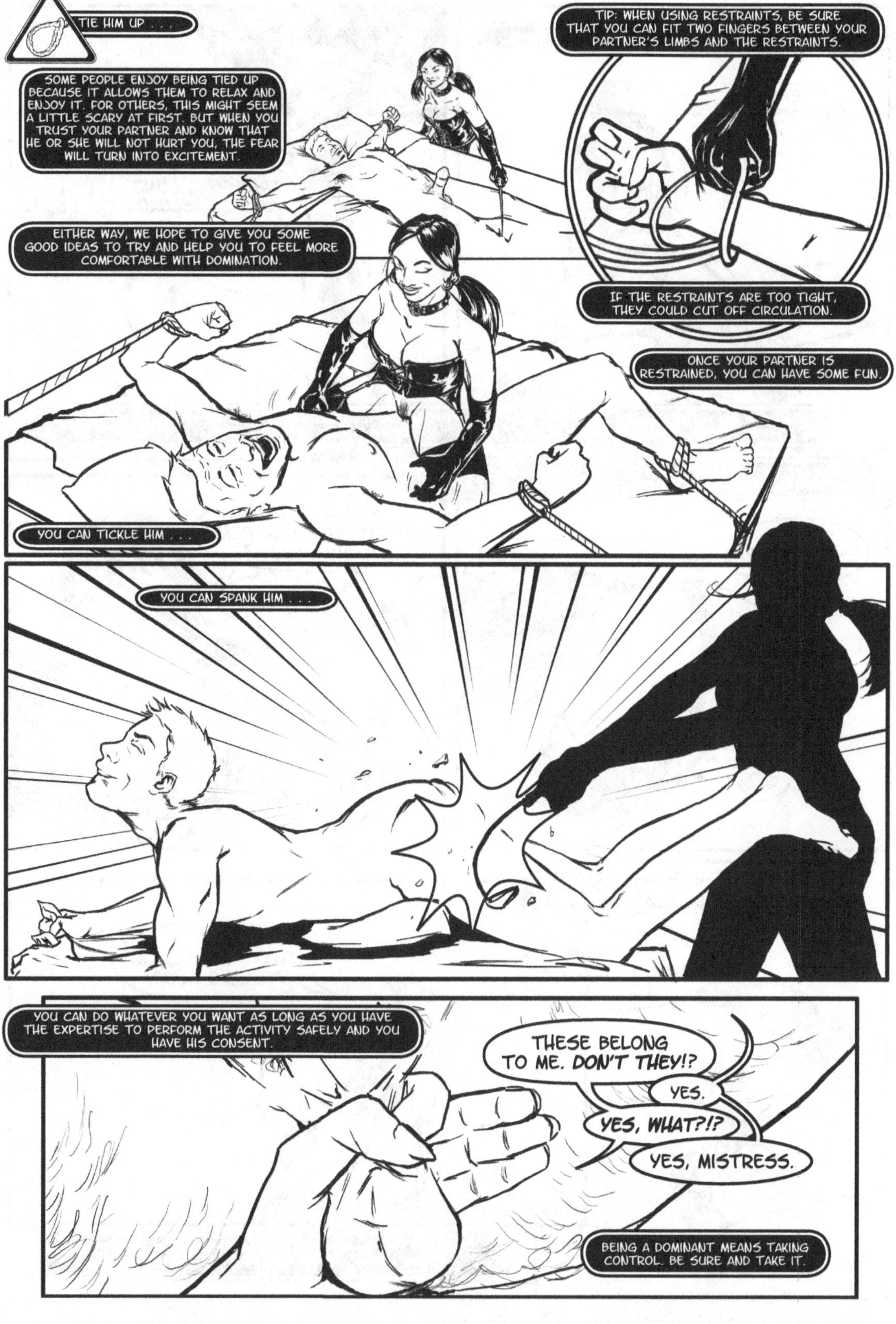
TIE HIM UP . . .
SOME PEOPLE ENJOY BEING TIED UP BECAUSE IT ALLOWS THEM TO RELAX AND ENJOY IT. FOR OTHERS, THIS MIGHT SEEM A LITTLE SCARY AT FIRST. BUT WHEN YOU TRUST YOUR PARTNER AND KNOW THAT HE OR SHE WILL NOT HURT YOU, THE FEAR WILL TURN INTO EXCITEMENT.
TIP: WHEN USING RESTRAINTS, BE SURE THAT YOU CAN FIT TWO FINGERS BETWEEN YOUR PARTNER'S LIMBS AND THE RESTRAINTS.
EITHER WAY, WE HOPE TO GIVE YOU SOME GOOD IDEAS TO TRY AND HELP YOU TO FEEL MORE COMFORTABLE WITH DOMINATION.
IF THE RESTRAINTS ARE TOO TIGHT, THEY COULD CUT OFF CIRCULATION.
ONCE YOUR PARTNER IS RESTRAINED, YOU CAN HAVE SOME FUN.
YOU CAN TICKLE HIM . . .
YOU CAN SPANK HIM . . .
YOU CAN DO WHATEVER YOU WANT AS LONG AS YOU HAVE THE EXPERTISE TO PERFORM THE ACTIVITY SAFELY AND YOU HAVE HIS CONSENT.
THESE BELONG TO ME. DON'T THEY!?
YES.
YES, WHAT?!?
YES, MISTRESS.
BEING A DOMINANT MEANS TAKING CONTROL. BE SURE AND TAKE IT.

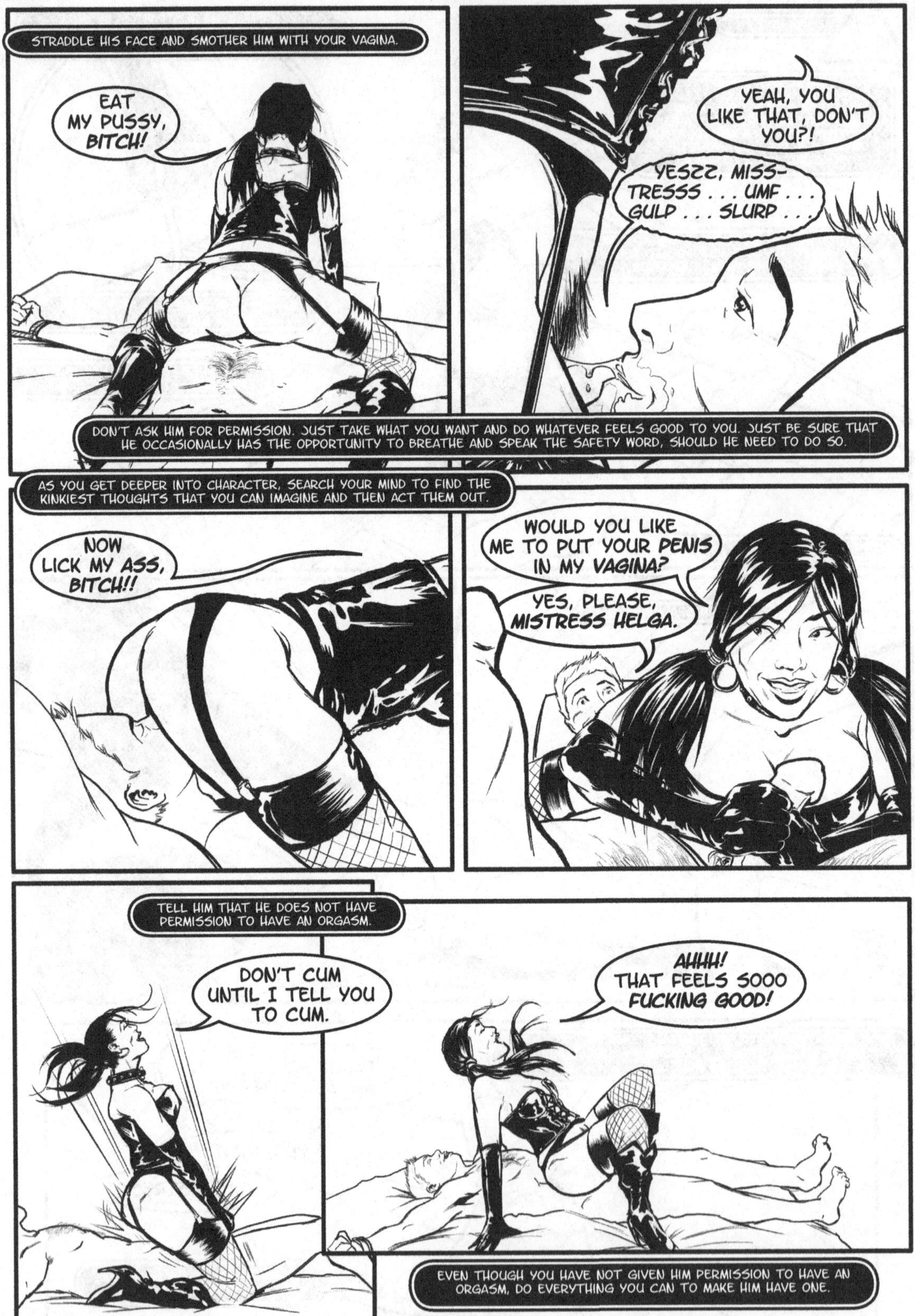
STRADDLE HIS FACE AND SMOTHER HIM WITH YOUR VAGINA.
EAT MY PUSSY, BITCH!
YEAH, YOU LIKE THAT, DON'T YOU?!
YESZZ, MISS-TRESSS . . . UMF . . . GULP . . . SLURP . . .
DON'T ASK HIM FOR PERMISSION. JUST TAKE WHAT YOU WANT AND DO WHATEVER FEELS GOOD TO YOU. JUST BE SURE THAT HE OCCASIONALLY HAS THE OPPORTUNITY TO BREATHE AND SPEAK THE SAFETY WORD, SHOULD HE NEED TO DO SO.
AS YOU GET DEEPER INTO CHARACTER, SEARCH YOUR MIND TO FIND THE KINKIEST THOUGHTS THAT YOU CAN IMAGINE AND THEN ACT THEM OUT.
NOW LICK MY ASS, BITCH!!
WOULD YOU LIKE ME TO PUT YOUR PENIS IN MY VAGINA?
YES, PLEASE, MISTRESS HELGA.
TELL HIM THAT HE DOES NOT HAVE PERMISSION TO HAVE AN ORGASM.
DON'T CUM UNTIL I TELL YOU TO CUM.
AHHH! THAT FEELS SOOO FUCKING GOOD!
EVEN THOUGH YOU HAVE NOT GIVEN HIM PERMISSION TO HAVE AN ORGASM, DO EVERYTHING YOU CAN TO MAKE HIM HAVE ONE.

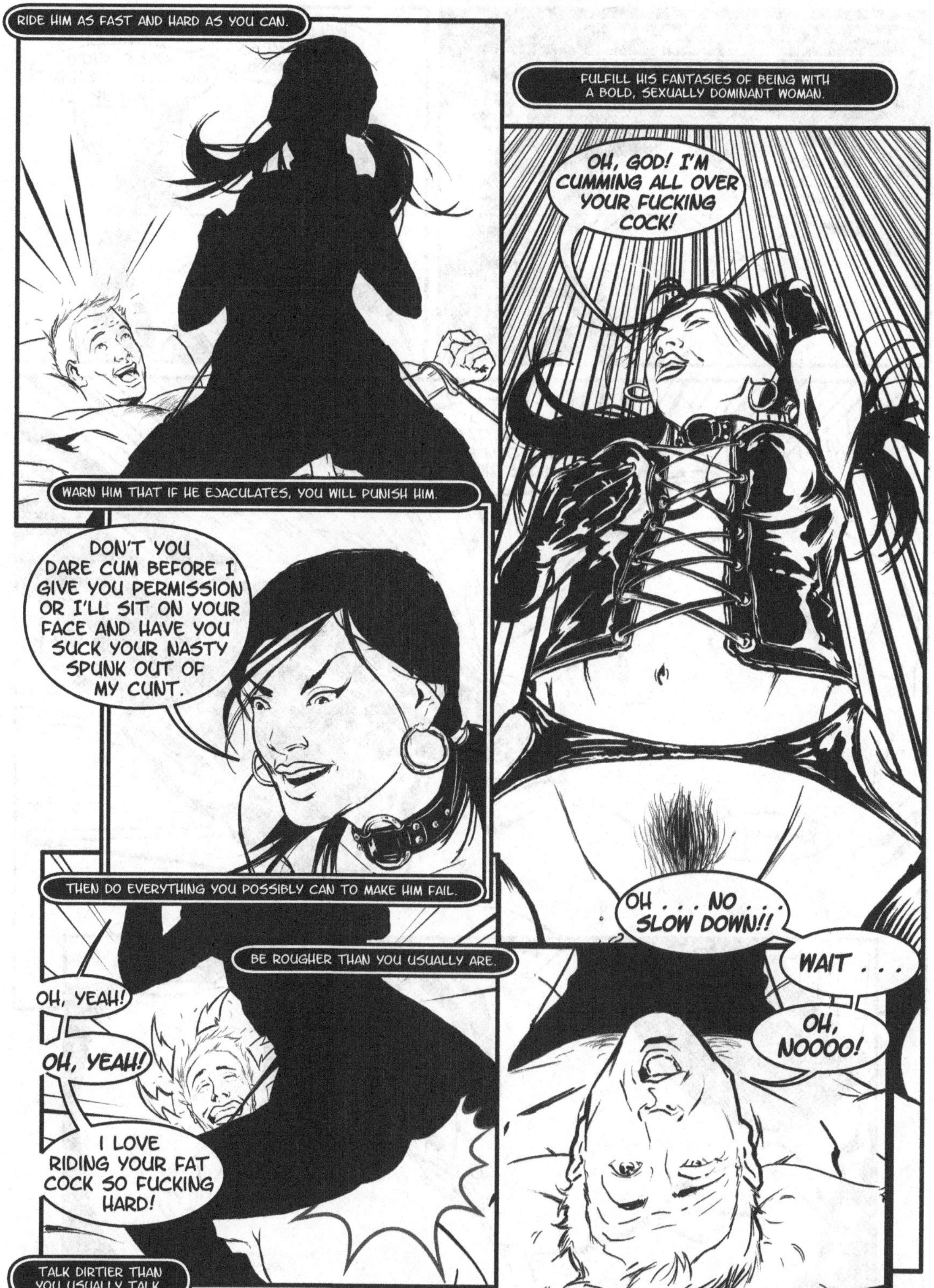
RIDE HIM AS FAST AND HARD AS YOU CAN.
FULFILL HIS FANTASIES OF BEING WITH A BOLD, SEXUALLY DOMINANT WOMAN.
OH, GOD! I'M CUMMING ALL OVER YOUR FUCKING COCK!
WARN HIM THAT IF HE EJACULATES, YOU WILL PUNISH HIM.
DON'T YOU DARE CUM BEFORE I GIVE YOU PERMISSION OR I'LL SIT ON YOUR FACE AND HAVE YOU SUCK YOUR NASTY SPUNK OUT OF MY CUNT.
THEN DO EVERYTHING YOU POSSIBLY CAN TO MAKE HIM FAIL.
OH . . . NO . . . SLOW DOWN!!
WAIT . . .
OH, NOOOO!
BE ROUGHER THAN YOU USUALLY ARE.
OH, YEAH!
OH, YEAH!
I LOVE RIDING YOUR FAT COCK SO FUCKING HARD!
TALK DIRTIER THAN YOU USUALLY TALK.

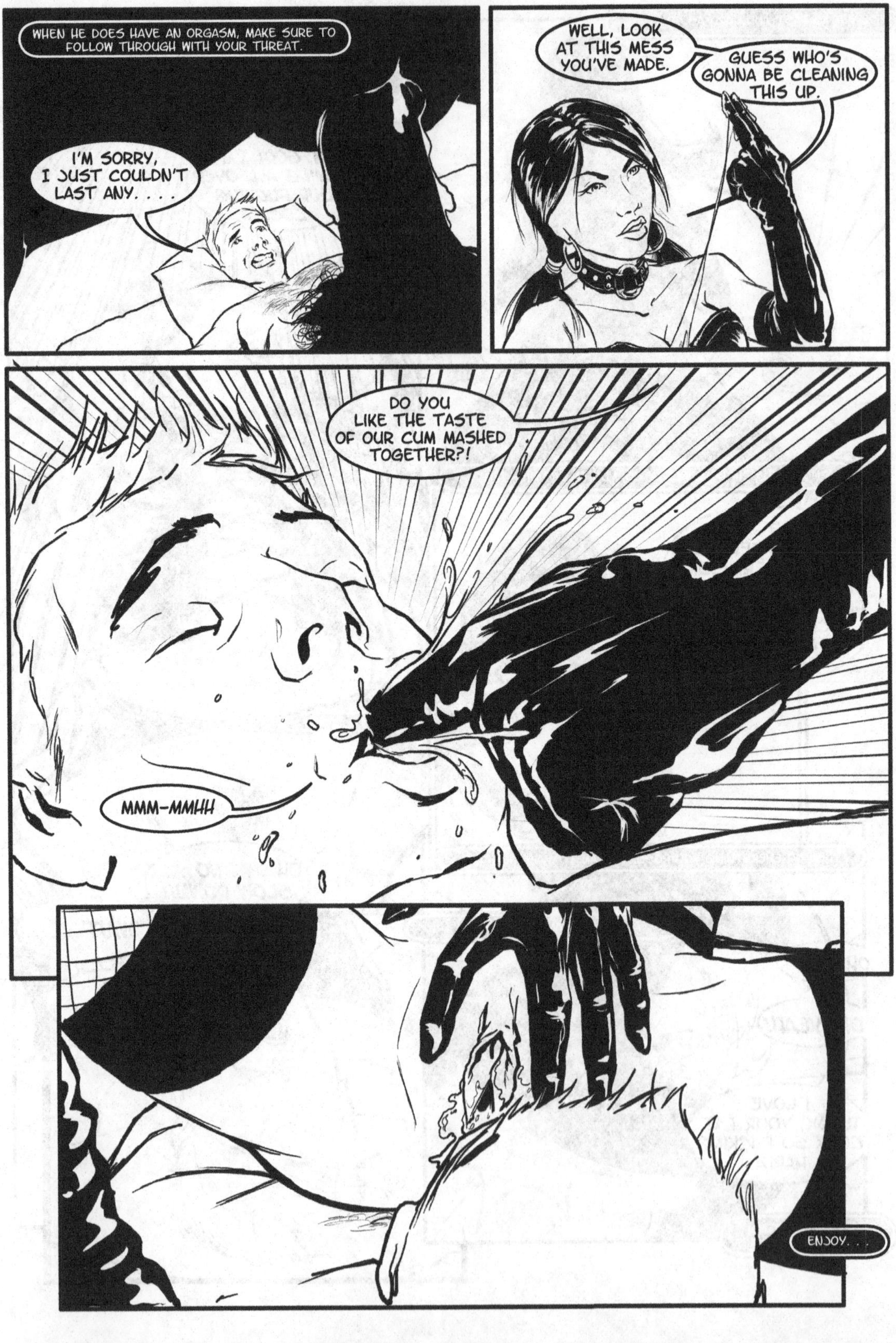
WHEN HE DOES HAVE AN ORGASM, MAKE SURE TO FOLLOW THROUGH WITH YOUR THREAT.
I'M SORRY, I JUST COULDN'T LAST ANY. . . .
WELL, LOOK AT THIS MESS YOU'VE MADE.
GUESS WHO'S GONNA BE CLEANING THIS UP.
DO YOU LIKE THE TASTE OF OUR CUM MASHED TOGETHER?!
MMM-MMHH
ENJOY. . .

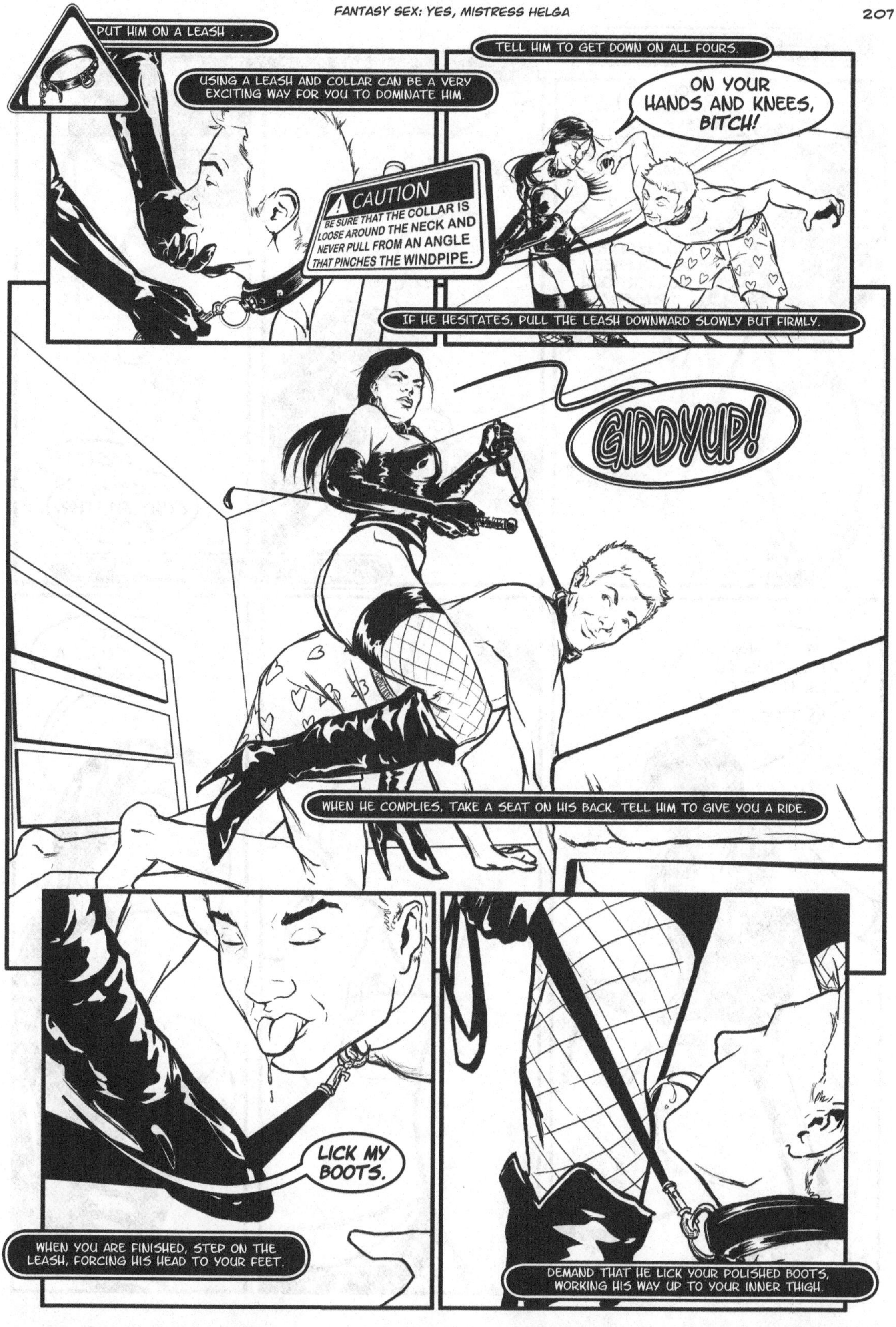
PUT HIM ON A LEASH . . .
USING A LEASH AND COLLAR CAN BE A VERY EXCITING WAY FOR YOU TO DOMINATE HIM.
CAUTION
BE SURE THAT THE COLLAR IS LOOSE AROUND THE NECK AND NEVER PULL FROM AN ANGLE THAT PINCHES THE WINDPIPE.
TELL HIM TO GET DOWN ON ALL FOURS.
ON YOUR HANDS AND KNEES, BITCH!
IF HE HESITATES, PULL THE LEASH DOWNWARD SLOWLY BUT FIRMLY.
GIDDYUP!
WHEN HE COMPLIES, TAKE A SEAT ON HIS BACK. TELL HIM TO GIVE YOU A RIDE.
LICK MY BOOTS.
WHEN YOU ARE FINISHED, STEP ON THE LEASH, FORCING HIS HEAD TO YOUR FEET.
DEMAND THAT HE LICK YOUR POLISHED BOOTS, WORKING HIS WAY UP TO YOUR INNER THIGH.

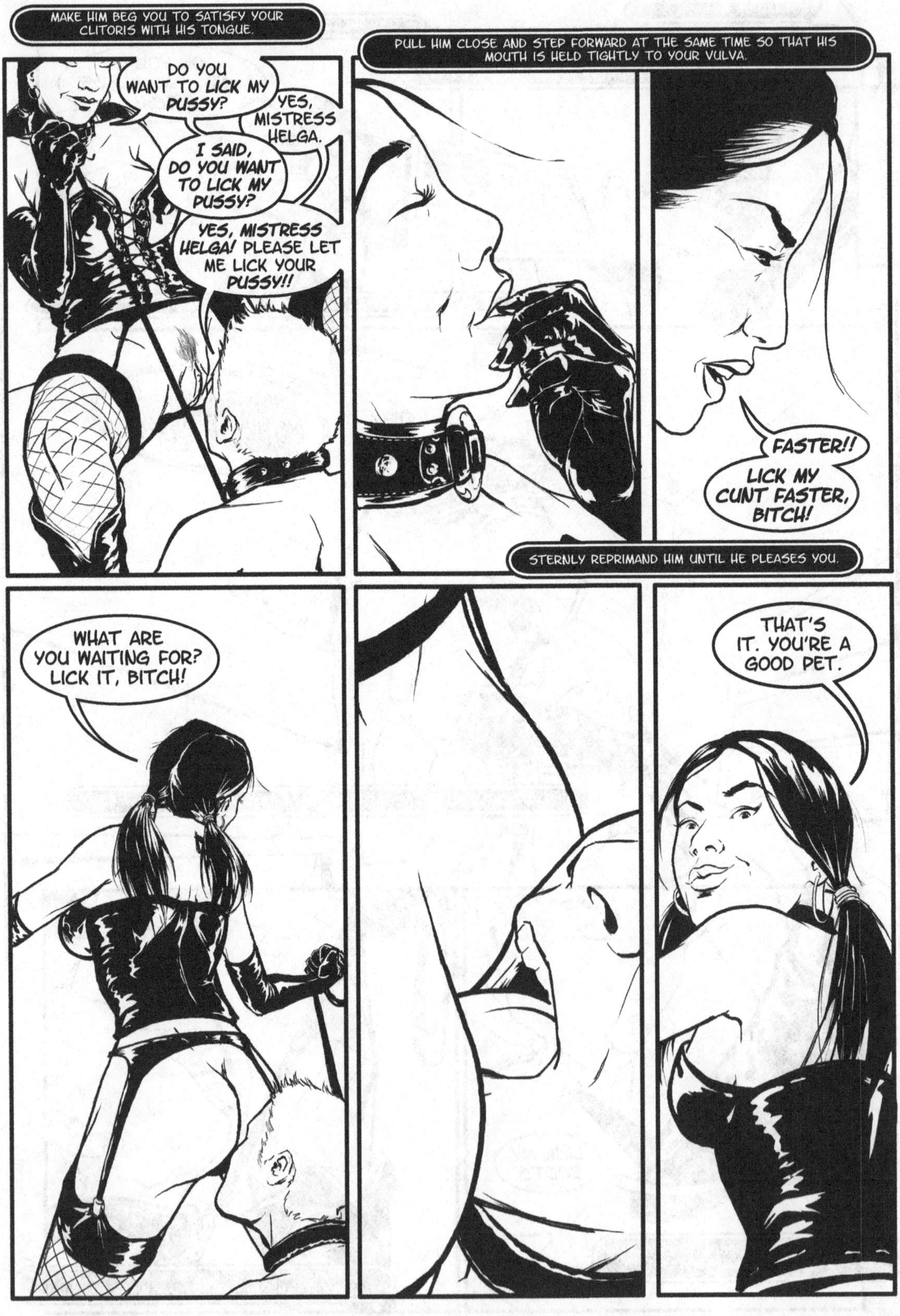
MAKE HIM BEG YOU TO SATISFY YOUR CLITORIS WITH HIS TONGUE.
DO YOU WANT TO LICK MY PUSSY?
YES, MISTRESS HELGA.
I SAID, DO YOU WANT TO LICK MY PUSSY?
YES, MISTRESS HELGA! PLEASE LET ME LICK YOUR PUSSY!!
PULL HIM CLOSE AND STEP FORWARD AT THE SAME TIME SO THAT HIS MOUTH IS HELD TIGHTLY TO YOUR VULVA.
FASTER!!
LICK MY CUNT FASTER, BITCH!
STERNLY REPRIMAND HIM UNTIL HE PLEASES YOU.
WHAT ARE YOU WAITING FOR? LICK IT, BITCH!
THAT'S IT. YOU'RE A GOOD PET.

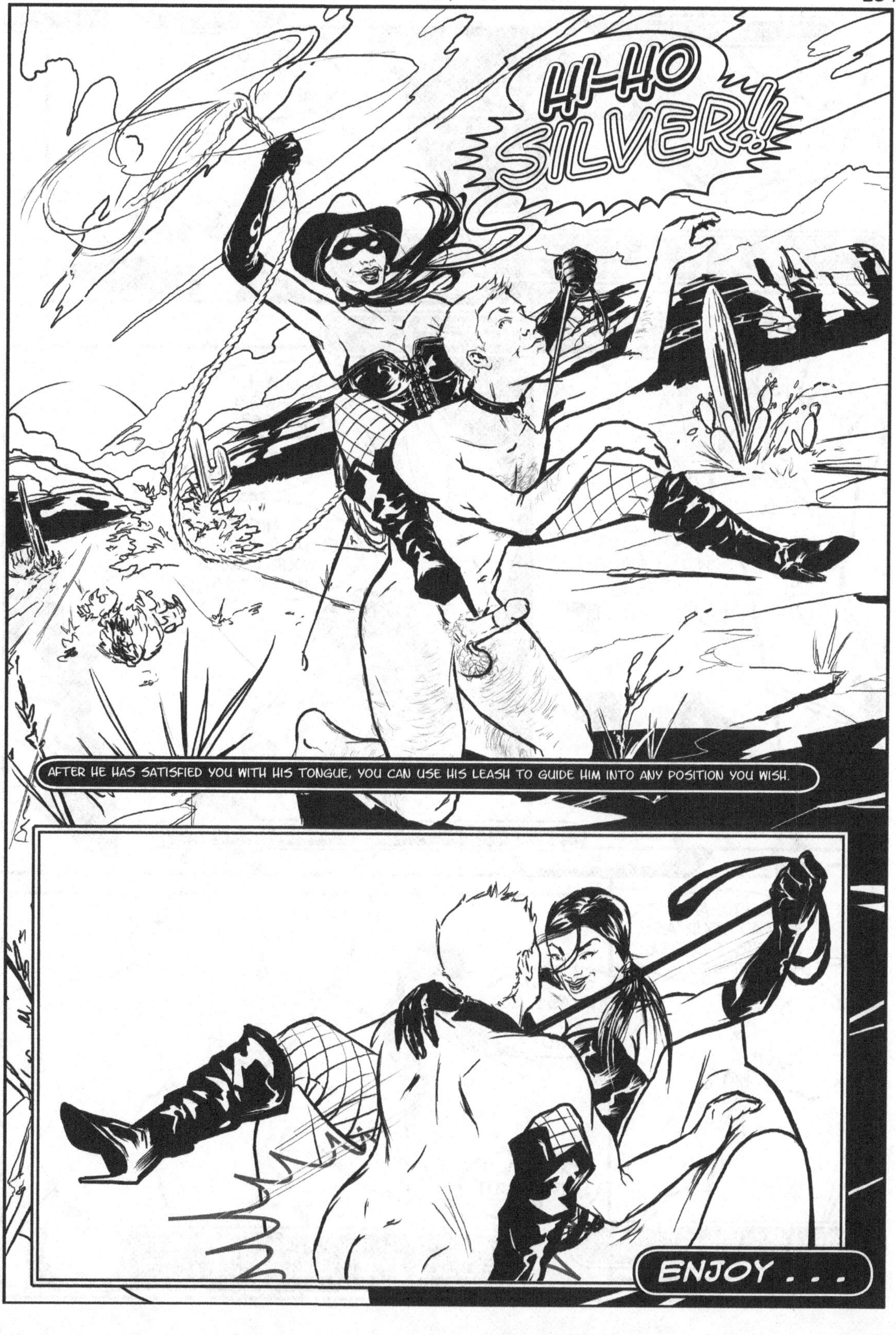
HI-HO SILVER!!
AFTER HE HAS SATISFIED YOU WITH HIS TONGUE, YOU CAN USE HIS LEASH TO GUIDE HIM INTO ANY POSITION YOU WISH.
ENJOY . . .

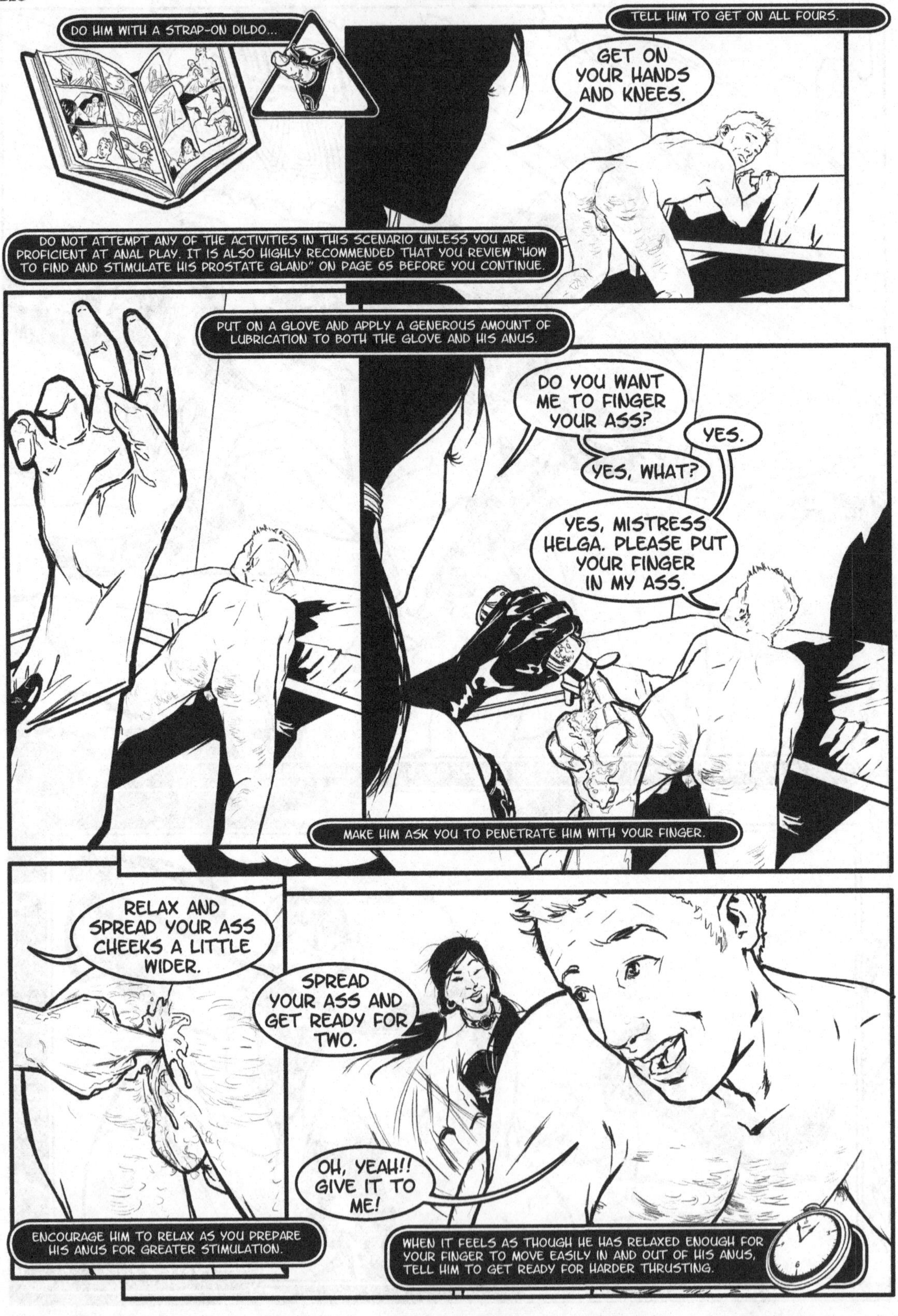
DO HIM WITH A STRAP-ON DILDO...
TELL HIM TO GET ON ALL FOURS.
GET ON YOUR HANDS AND KNEES.
DO NOT ATTEMPT ANY OF THE ACTIVITIES IN THIS SCENARIO UNLESS YOU ARE PROFICIENT AT ANAL PLAY. IT IS ALSO HIGHLY RECOMMENDED THAT YOU REVIEW "HOW TO FIND AND STIMULATE HIS PROSTATE GLAND" ON PAGE 65 BEFORE YOU CONTINUE.
PUT ON A GLOVE AND APPLY A GENEROUS AMOUNT OF LUBRICATION TO BOTH THE GLOVE AND HIS ANUS.
DO YOU WANT ME TO FINGER YOUR ASS?
YES.
YES, WHAT?
YES, MISTRESS HELGA. PLEASE PUT YOUR FINGER IN MY ASS.
MAKE HIM ASK YOU TO PENETRATE HIM WITH YOUR FINGER.
RELAX AND SPREAD YOUR ASS CHEEKS A LITTLE WIDER.
SPREAD YOUR ASS AND GET READY FOR TWO.
OH, YEAH!! GIVE IT TO ME!
ENCOURAGE HIM TO RELAX AS YOU PREPARE HIS ANUS FOR GREATER STIMULATION.
WHEN IT FEELS AS THOUGH HE HAS RELAXED ENOUGH FOR YOUR FINGER TO MOVE EASILY IN AND OUT OF HIS ANUS, TELL HIM TO GET READY FOR HARDER THRUSTING.

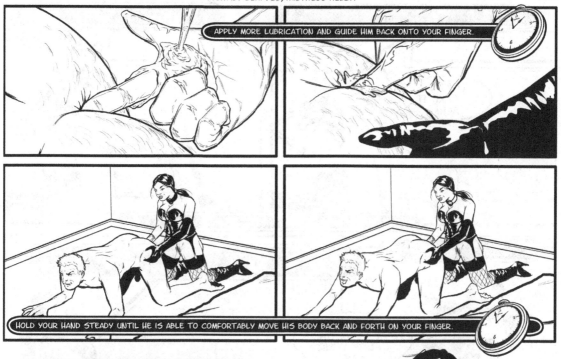

APPLY MORE LUBRICATION AND GUIDE HIM BACK ONTO YOUR FINGER.

HOLD YOUR HAND STEADY UNTIL HE IS ABLE TO COMFORTABLY MOVE HIS BODY BACK AND FORTH ON YOUR FINGER.

WHEN YOU THINK HE'S READY, ASK HIM IF HE WANTS SOMETHING BIGGER.

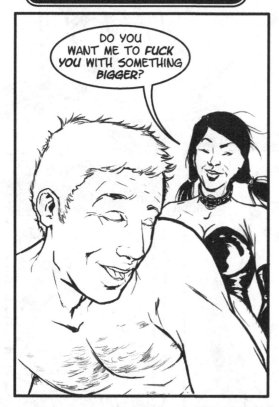

DO YOU WANT ME TO *FUCK* YOU WITH SOMETHING *BIGGER*?

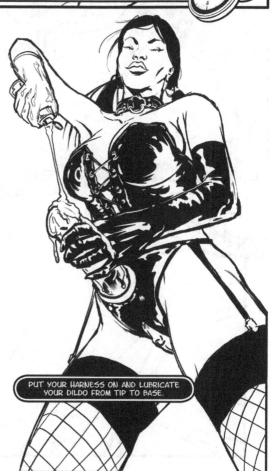

PUT YOUR HARNESS ON AND LUBRICATE YOUR DILDO FROM TIP TO BASE.

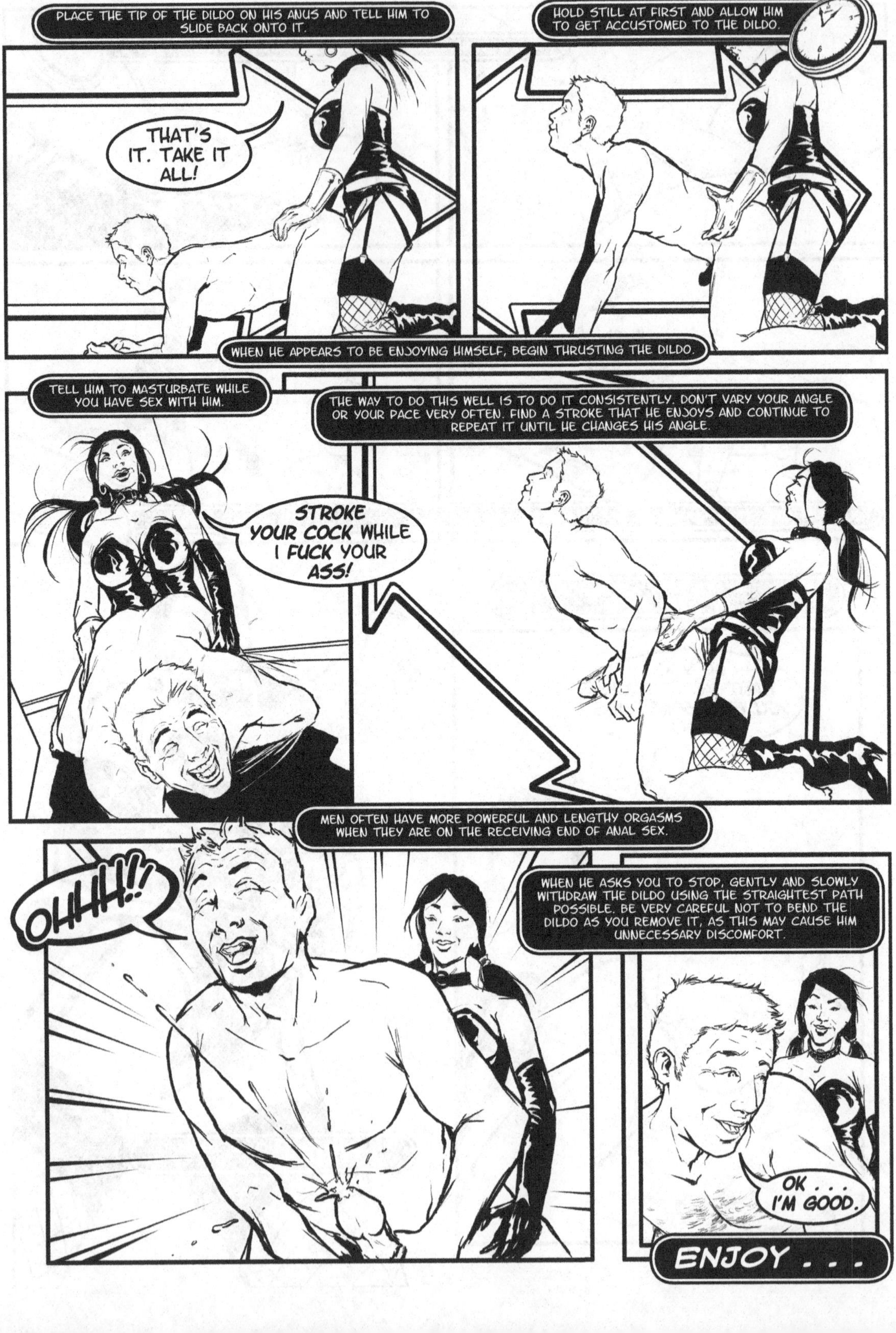
PLACE THE TIP OF THE DILDO ON HIS ANUS AND TELL HIM TO SLIDE BACK ONTO IT.
THAT'S IT. TAKE IT ALL!
HOLD STILL AT FIRST AND ALLOW HIM TO GET ACCUSTOMED TO THE DILDO.
WHEN HE APPEARS TO BE ENJOYING HIMSELF, BEGIN THRUSTING THE DILDO.
TELL HIM TO MASTURBATE WHILE YOU HAVE SEX WITH HIM.
STROKE YOUR COCK WHILE I FUCK YOUR ASS!
THE WAY TO DO THIS WELL IS TO DO IT CONSISTENTLY. DON'T VARY YOUR ANGLE OR YOUR PACE VERY OFTEN. FIND A STROKE THAT HE ENJOYS AND CONTINUE TO REPEAT IT UNTIL HE CHANGES HIS ANGLE.
MEN OFTEN HAVE MORE POWERFUL AND LENGTHY ORGASMS WHEN THEY ARE ON THE RECEIVING END OF ANAL SEX.
OHHH!!
WHEN HE ASKS YOU TO STOP, GENTLY AND SLOWLY WITHDRAW THE DILDO USING THE STRAIGHTEST PATH POSSIBLE. BE VERY CAREFUL NOT TO BEND THE DILDO AS YOU REMOVE IT, AS THIS MAY CAUSE HIM UNNECESSARY DISCOMFORT.
OK . . . I'M GOOD.
ENJOY . . .

THE CLOSING DOWN

All good things must come to an end, and all great things usually end with a climax. We hope that this book has given you and your partner lots of fun ways to play with each other and that it will continue to encourage you to explore new and exciting sexual adventures together. To hear from us each week, log on to sexisfun.net to get our free "Sex Is Fun" podcast.

SEX is FUN
PODCAST

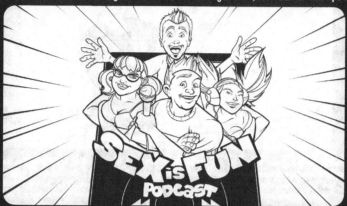

If you enjoyed this book, you may wish to get your hands on a copy of one of the author's sex games that are sold through GreatSexGames.com.

Intense Games DVD
www.GreatSexGames.com
Sex Play
Will you buy this game and have the night of your life?
Sex is Fun
a game of intimate sexual discovery

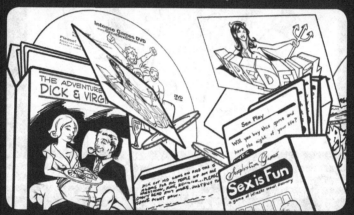

You can also read our online magazine and join our community of sex-positive people just like you at sexisfun.net.

SEX is FUN
Podcast
PacBook

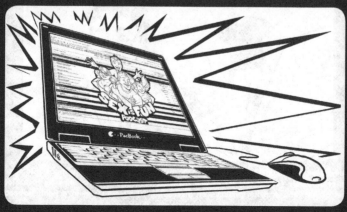

ABOUT THE AUTHORS

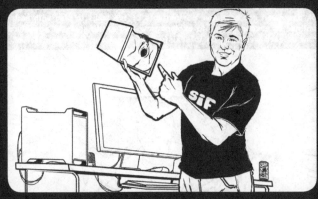

Human sexuality guru Kidder Kaper is the creative genius and head writer for GreatSexGames.com, for which he has written and developed nine sex games. He is also the host of the insanely popular podcast, "Sex Is Fun." Kidder has been theorizing and writing about human sexuality since 1993, when he began work on this book while he was an undergraduate at the University of Minnesota. This book represents Kidder's first collected anthology of his primary goal: "teaching the world to be unafraid to enjoy sex."

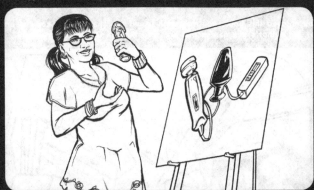

Laura Rad, cohost of the "Sex Is Fun" podcast, has been a sex educator for nearly a decade, presenting classes on topics from birth control to bondage. She has been a proud presenter for the University of Minnesota, BFLAG Minnesota, the Alphabet Soup Conference and Stockholm, Sweden's Pride Festival. She lives in Minneapolis, Minnesota, and spends most of her time singing along to the radio and demonstrating '80s dance moves for her dog.

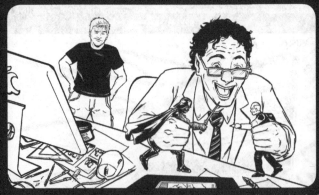

Comic illustrator Josh Lynch was the man who brought the ideas of this book into the visual realm. He is responsible for all the art in this book along with additional inks by Rich Flood. Lynch spends most of his time drawing pictures or discussing who would win in a fight, Robocop or the Terminator? Well, who do you think would win?